S A R S

How a global epidemic
was stopped

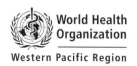

**World Health
Organization**

Western Pacific Region

WHO Library Cataloguing in Publication Data

SARS: how a global epidemic was stopped

1. Severe acute respiratory syndrome -- prevention and control. 2. Disease outbreaks -- prevention and control.

ISBN 92 9061 213 4   (NLM Classification:WC 505)

CONTENTS

OVERVIEW

SARS shook the world. By some standards, the first emerging and readily transmissible disease of the 21st century was not a big killer, but it caused more fear and social disruption than any other outbreak of our time. As I write these words some two years later, memories of how Member States, our partner agencies, and we at the World Health Organization responded to this new threat to global health are still fresh in my mind.

Severe acute respiratory syndrome (SARS) was unique. It showed explosive power, setting off multiple outbreaks around the world, often zeroing in on hospitals, attacking doctors and nurses and bringing some public-health systems to their knees. It buckled economies, crippled international trade and travel, and sent stock markets into a slide.

More than 95% of the SARS cases took place in WHO's Western Pacific Region, where 12 countries or areas were hit, some with devastating force. All of them responded with courage and determination, from the leaders of government through public-health managers to health-care workers and laboratory experts. Many people pushed themselves to the limit, taking sleep only when going on without it would have been impossible. Family life was put on hold. Meals were scrambled affairs and often missed altogether.

I proposed this book because I believe that by identifying the successes and failures of the fight against SARS, our Member States, partners, and WHO will leave an enduring legacy for those who face similar challenges in the future. Already, since SARS, avian influenza has spread across South-East Asia and beyond to pose a new threat to mankind. What will come next? There is, of course, no way of knowing, but one thing is certain: We must all be better prepared than we were when SARS was unleashed.

One way we can do that is to better understand why the SARS coronavirus and the avian influenza H5N1 virus crossed the species barrier from animals to attack humans. What caused this strange migration? The explanation, in my view, lies in part in the way animals are raised for food in Asia, where increasing prosperity has led to a greater demand for meat, and, in some cultures, a taste for the flesh of exotic animals.

In markets where wild animals are sold for the table, creatures that would never meet in their natural habitat are kept in proximity to one another, setting the conditions for the emergence of new viruses. A similar threat lies in the way that chickens, ducks, and pigs are raised together, often in unhygienic conditions and usually with no barriers between them and humans. Such husbandry practices must change, or more viruses are likely to emerge from the animal world.

I don't know if one can decently say that SARS had a silver lining, but if it did, it was that it awakened the global public-health community from a kind of slumber. Before SARS, communicable diseases had been given insufficient attention, with doctors more interested in high-tech fields such as neurosurgery and molecular biology. Awareness levels were low and infection-control procedures had become slack. In sum, public-health systems were simply not ready for what happened.

The silver lining is that since those days many countries and cities have invested extensively in public health. New hospitals have been built. Health-care workers have been drilled in infection-control measures. Better surveillance systems are in place. And research has been intensified. SARS, for all the fear and suffering it caused, has left public-health systems greatly improved.

SARS was the first emerging disease of the age of globalization. I believe that, had it occurred in a time before mass international travel, it would probably have remained a localized problem, with few consequences for global health. But the virus travelled around the world on passenger jets [see the account in Chapter 15 of the consequences of one single flight between Hong Kong and Beijing], making it a true disease of the 21st century. To fight this 21st-century disease, Member States applied 19th-century measures such as contact tracing, quarantine, and isolation. As old fashioned and labour intensive as they were, these measures slowed the virus's spread, and, in the end, contributed to its containment.

But we also had a very modern ally: the Internet. Thousands of email messages flashed around the globe each day. Web pages not only kept the world informed daily, but also offered advice on scores of technical issues. At the same time, international laboratory experts set aside their traditional rivalries and grouped their expertise in a virtual network to decode the virus's secrets. So successful was this unprecedented scientific cooperation that the causative agent, the coronavirus, was identified within weeks, whereas it might have taken months or possibly even years in the days before the Internet.

For WHO, SARS was much more than just a medical challenge. There was also the political, social and economic dimension of disease to deal with, particularly in the area where our mission of safeguarding public health had to be balanced against the genuine interests of Member States. At all levels, WHO worked with Member States to share information and to find common ground in a situation that was new to all of us. On a number of occasions, this required liaising with senior officials, including ministers of health.

In the Philippines, for example, WHO had discussions with authorities after they expressed disappointment at being included in a list of areas with "medium" levels of local transmission when the outbreak there had been limited to hospitals and family contacts. WHO was accused of overstating the problem, and, in retrospect, I suspect we probably did. Like everyone else, we were learning—and we didn't always get things right first time.

On 22 March 2003, I held a frank one-on-one meeting in a hotel in Hong Kong (China) with the Minister of Health of the People's Republic of China. I asked for much more information and better cooperation concerning developments in Guangdong Province, in the south of the country. We didn't get what we needed straight away, but as the number of cases continued to grow, heightening concern both in China and in the international community, things began to change. China went on to make a major contribution to the global fight against SARS through its aggressive control measures and prompt reporting on the situation in the country.

My colleagues and I had occasion to talk on the telephone with the Minister of Health of Singapore as we tried to ascertain how serious a threat the situation there was to global public health and whether there was justification for issuing a travel advisory against Singapore. In the end, we chose not to issue an advisory. It was the right decision.

The possible impact of travel advisories on the economies of affected areas and on the morale of people living there was one of the most difficult issues of the SARS experience. I recall a number of difficult discussions on the subject with WHO's Director-General at the time, Dr Gro Brundtland. In the end, we agreed we would not be fulfilling WHO's mandate if we did not take action when and where we thought it necessary.

So it was that on 1 April 2003 WHO's office in Beijing informed the Chinese authorities that we would be issuing an advisory that day, urging members of the public against unnecessary travel to Guangdong Province. China replied that it accepted the decision. At the same time, our Regional Office in Manila informed the Hong Kong authorities that a similar announcement would be made concerning the Special Administrative Region. The Hong Kong authorities asked if we would wait overnight while they drew up the most comprehensive assessment possible of the situation.

The next day we received the updated information. We concluded that it was not sufficiently persuasive and that the data available on the newly reported cases suggested that travel to the area could contribute to the international spread of SARS. The advisory went out on 2 April, in order to limit further international spread of SARS by restricting travel to areas where there was substantatial risk to travellers. It was a very difficult decision, but WHO's duty to protect global health had to take precedence.

There is no doubt that SARS was a historic challenge. And it produced an unprecedented response from Member States. Viet Nam showed the way, becoming the first country to be declared free of SARS, thanks to prompt recognition of the seriousness of the problem, backed by strong political commitment. In many other Asian countries too, including Malaysia, Mongolia and Thailand, health authorities reacted with commendable vigour. They were supported unstintingly by public-health managers and workers, laboratory technicians and many others. I thank them for their contribution.

Finally, I would like to pay tribute to those who lost their lives in the struggle against SARS. Before transmission of the virus was finally declared over on 5 July 2004, severe acute respiratory syndrome had killed nearly 800 people. Among them were many brave health-care workers, including our own Dr Carlo Urbani, who, while working in Viet Nam in the early days of the outbreak, was the first to raise the alarm about the new disease. These people selflessly gave their lives to protect others. We are all in their debt.

Looking back, I believe that one of the lessons that SARS taught us is that public health around the world has entered an era where it will need to be on constant guard against threats from emerging diseases. It is my hope that this book will help guide generations to come as they take on those challenges.

Shigeru Omi, M.D., Ph.D.
Regional Director

PART I:

OVERALL PERSPECTIVES

1 SARS
CHRONOLOGY

In early February 2003, an apparent outbreak of pneumonia in southern China broke into the news. While WHO was seeking to learn more about the new disease, the virus left China's mainland and started its global spread. Reports of similar outbreaks in Hanoi, Viet Nam, and Hong Kong (China) led WHO to issue a global alert on 12 March. On 15 March, WHO issued a second alert and travel advisory, and named the disease severe acute respiratory syndrome (SARS). Over the next several months, the virus would kill hundreds of people and infect thousands more.

The following is a comprehensive chronology of SARS-related events, starting with the emergence of the new virus in November 2002. It recounts the spread of the virus and its impact on people, describes the control measures taken, and highlights the WHO mobilization—in individual countries, in the Region, and around the world—to stop the epidemic.

16 NOVEMBER 2002

China
: A 45-year-old man in Foshan City, Guangdong, becomes ill with fever and respiratory symptoms, and passes on the infection to four relatives. He is retrospectively identified as the first SARS case.[1]

10 DECEMBER 2002

China
: A 34-year-old restaurant chef working in Shenzhen becomes ill when admitted to Heyuan City People's Hospital. Eight health-care workers who have close contact with him will develop the same illness.

2 JANUARY 2003

China
: The Guangdong Health Bureau receives reports from Heyuan City People's Hospital, saying that it had admitted two pneumonia cases. Because the cases are not getting better in Heyuan, they are transferred for treatment to Guangzhou

General Army Hospital and Guangzhou Medical University Respiratory Diseases Institute. In the afternoon, epidemiologists and clinical experts from Guangdong Health Bureau go to Heyuan to investigate the situation and provide guidance on treatment.

China

A 49-year-old office worker in Guangzhou City, Guangdong becomes ill.[1] By the end of January the number of new cases in Guangzhou will start to increase exponentially.

8 JANUARY

China

A 26-year-old driver for an animal dealer in Guangxi Province (next to Guangdong) becomes ill and infects several family members.[1]

18 JANUARY

China

In the early evening, the Guangdong Health Bureau receives reports from Zhongshan, similar to those from Heyuan. Two hours later, Health Department experts arrive in Zhongshan to start an investigation.

20 JANUARY

China

At the recommendation of the Guangdong Health Bureau, the Guangdong Center for Disease Control and Prevention (CDC) sends a letter to China CDC inviting its experts to provide guidance in Guangdong.

21 JANUARY

China

In the morning, the Guangdong Health Bureau meets with experts to analyse the prevention and control work of the outbreak. A decision is made to send provincial treatment and prevention teams to Zhongshan. The teams are dispatched at 11:30 a.m. To support the work of the provincial teams, Foshan and Heyuan health bureaus are asked to send doctors who have treated cases together with the medical records. In the afternoon, a team of four experts from China CDC arrives in Guangdong to help with the investigation and provide guidance on prevention and control.

23 JANUARY

China   The Guangdong Health Bureau releases an official document on atypical pneumonia, giving a case definition and recommending control actions. The document, *Investigation Reports of Pneumonia Cases of Unknown Cause in Zhongshan,* is sent to health bureaus and medical institutions in the province, prefecture level and above.

30 JANUARY

China   **First known super-spreading event takes place**
Mr ZZF, a 44-year-old seafood seller, is hospitalized in Guangzhou. He will pass on the virus to at least 50 hospital staff members and 19 relatives [see Chapter 13].[2]

9 FEBRUARY

China   The Vice-Minister of Health and the Deputy Director-General of Health (Disease Control Division) lead a team of experts from the Ministry of Health and China CDC to Guangdong to provide guidance on the prevention and control work.

10 FEBRUARY

China   The WHO country office in Beijing receives an email message describing a "strange contagious disease" that "already left more than 100 people dead in Guangdong Province in the space of one week". The Global Public Health Intelligence Network (GPHIN) also picks up media reports of an unusual epidemic of fatal pneumonia-like illness in Guangdong.

11 FEBRUARY

China   **Guangdong health authorities report on an outbreak of atypical pneumonia that has sickened 305 people**
At a morning press conference, the Guangzhou Vice-Mayor announces that the city is coping with an epidemic of atypical pneumonia and that no extraordinary measures are needed. Later that day, the Guangdong Health Bureau holds a press conference to report 305 cases (including five deaths) of atypical pneumonia of unknown cause in the province, between 16 November 2002 and 9 February 2003. A third of the cases are health workers who contracted the disease while caring for patients.

Hong Kong	The Department of Health closely monitors the local situation and finds no unusual pattern of influenza-like illness or respiratory tract infection including pneumonia through the established surveillance system. A working group is formed to step up surveillance and advise on pneumonia cases.

12 FEBRUARY

China	The WHO Representative informs the Ministry of Health that WHO Headquarters and the Regional Office have learned of the outbreak in Guangdong, requests the Ministry in writing for epidemiological information, and offers WHO's assistance.
Hong Kong	Hospitals begin to report suspected or confirmed cases of severe community-acquired pneumonia (requiring assisted ventilation or treatment in intensive care units) to the Department of Health for investigation.

14 FEBRUARY

China	The Ministry of Health officially informs WHO that the Guangdong outbreak is coming under control. The letter from the Ministry states that the cause of the outbreak is still not known but is probably viral. Pulmonary anthrax, pneumonic plague, leptospirosis, and haemorrhagic fever [which implies Hantavirus infection in China] have been ruled out. The letter also states that six municipalities in Guangdong Province (Foshan, Heyuan, Zhongshan, Jiangmen, Guangzhou, Shenzhen) have reported cases, but no new ones in the first three localities. The information from the Ministry of Health is posted on the WHO website,[3] and reported in WHO's *Weekly Epidemiological Record*.[4]

17 FEBRUARY

China	The WHO Representative writes a follow-up letter to the Ministry of Health, requesting more detailed epidemiological information and again offering WHO's assistance.

19 FEBRUARY

China	The Ministry of Health replies to WHO's earlier letters: "It is almost ascertained that the causal agent for the atypical pneumonia outbreak in Guangdong is *Chlamydia*... [The]

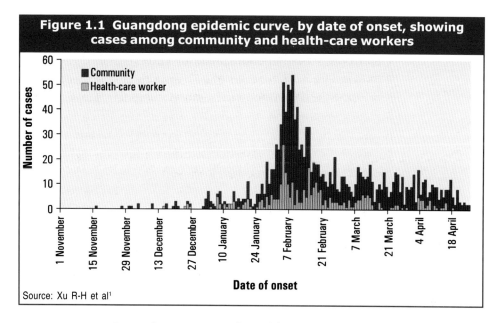

Figure 1.1 Guangdong epidemic curve, by date of onset, showing cases among community and health-care workers

Number of cases

- ■ Community
- ▨ Health-care worker

Date of onset

Source: Xu R-H et al[1]

Guangdong Provincial Health Bureau is collecting, sorting out, and analysing the [epidemiological data]. We will keep you informed of the further developments in due course ... [and] take this opportunity to express our appreciation to WHO for providing the relevant information to the international community."

Hong Kong A possible cause for the outbreak emerges in Hong Kong when the avian influenza A(H5N1) virus is detected in a nine-year-old boy. The boy's family had been visiting Fujian Province, China when he fell ill. His father died on 17 February from an infection with the same virus.[5] His sister died in Fujian on 4 February, presumably also from H5N1 infection, but was not tested for the virus. The case was immediately reported to WHO.

20 FEBRUARY

China WHO's Regional Director of the Western Pacific Regional Office calls the Ministry of Health to request permission for a WHO team to investigate the Guangdong outbreak. The Ministry asks WHO in writing to develop terms of reference for the investigating team, specifying its members, the timing of the visit, and the places to be visited [see 24 February].

21 FEBRUARY

Hong Kong

Index case of the Metropole Hotel outbreak arrives from Guangdong; international spread of virus begins
Professor LJL, a 64-year-old physician from Guangzhou, arrives (infected with the SARS virus) to attend a wedding. He developed flu-like symptoms on 15 February, having been infected in the hospital where he worked [see 30 January]. At least 16 other guests and one visitor are infected during his one-night stay in room 911 of the Metropole Hotel.

22 FEBRUARY

Hong Kong

Professor LJL is admitted to the intensive care unit of the Kwong Wah Hospital for respiratory failure. Besides the hotel guests, three members of his family (wife, daughter, brother-in-law) and one nurse at the hospital are infected. Professor LJL will die on 4 March.

Hong Kong

A 49-year-old woman is transferred to the intensive care unit of Prince of Wales Hospital when her respiratory symptoms worsen; she was admitted to Union Hospital on 17 February on her return from Guangzhou. After being notified, the Hong Kong Department of Health investigated her contacts and followed them up. Blood tests will confirm that she has SARS and has passed it on to one of four family contacts and one nurse at Union Hospital.

23 FEBRUARY

China

WHO team arrives in Beijing to assist WHO country office.

24 FEBRUARY

China

The WHO Regional Office faxes proposed terms of reference for the investigating team for the H5N1 and Guangdong outbreaks to the Ministry of Health. WHO proposes sending three WHO experts to carry out the investigation, first in Beijing and then in Fujian and Guangdong provinces. On 27 February, China will agree to only the Beijing phase of the investigation.

26 FEBRUARY

Viet Nam

Hanoi index case is hospitalized
Mr JC, a 48-year-old merchandise manager from New York, is admitted to the Hanoi-French Hospital. He arrived in Viet Nam on 23 February after travelling to China and Hong Kong. Since

his arrival, he has had fever and respiratory symptoms. The WHO office in Viet Nam will be notified of the case the next morning, and its advice sought.

China
A team in Beijing's Academy of Military Medical Sciences identifies the coronavirus from samples taken from Guangdong patients with atypical pneumonia.[6] As *Chlamydia* is generally believed in China to be the cause, this finding is not publicized and WHO is not informed.

1 MARCH

Singapore
Singapore index case is hospitalized
Ms EM is admitted to Tan Tock Seng Hospital with pneumonia. She has been unwell since returning from a shopping trip to Hong Kong on 25 February. The 22-year-old, who stayed in room 938 at the Metropole Hotel [see 21 February], will pass on the virus to 22 close contacts.

2 MARCH

China
First Beijing index case is hospitalized
A 27-year-old businesswoman from Shanxi Province is admitted to a military hospital in Beijing, and later transferred to an infectious-disease hospital. She is believed to be the first imported case in Beijing [see Chapter 6].[7] She developed symptoms on 22 February in Guangdong and sought medical attention in Shanxi, passing on the virus to two doctors and a nurse there, as well as to 10 health workers at the two Beijing hospitals, and to eight friends and members of her family, including her parents, both of whom will die from SARS.

Hong Kong
A 72-year-old Canadian tourist is admitted to St Paul's Hospital. He was infected during his stay at the Metropole Hotel. He will pass on the virus to three health workers, five visitors, and one patient at St Paul's. Two family contacts of these cases will also be infected. On 8 March, he will be transferred to the intensive care unit of Queen Mary Hospital, where no further transmissions will be recorded.

3 MARCH

Viet Nam
Dr Urbani examines Hanoi index case
In Hanoi, WHO's communicable disease expert in Viet Nam, Dr Carlo Urbani, examines Mr JC, the American businessman

who was admitted to the Hanoi-French Hospital on 26 February with a severe form of pneumonia. Dr Urbani sends a report to WHO's Regional Office, emphasizes the need for strict infection controls, and arranges for Mr JC's serum and throat swabs to be sent to laboratories in Tokyo, Atlanta, and Hanoi.

China

The WHO team, one week after its arrival, starts discussing the H5N1 and Guangdong outbreaks with China's Ministry of Health [see 24 February].

4 March

Hong Kong

Index case of outbreak at Prince of Wales Hospital is hospitalized
A 26-year-old airport worker, Mr CT, is admitted to ward 8A of Prince of Wales Hospital with pneumonia. He has had fever, chills, and rigours since 24 February. His fever and chest condition gradually improves after admission and his case is never categorized as a severe community-acquired pneumonia. Hence, the case is not reported and infection-control measures are not applied. Mr CT was infected when visiting the Metropole Hotel. He will pass on the virus to 143 Hong Kong residents: 50 health workers, 17 medical students, 30 patients in ward 8A, 42 visitors to ward 8A, and four members of his family.

5 March

Viet Nam

Hanoi outbreak begins
In Hanoi, four health-care workers are hospitalized and two more are ill. Their symptoms are similar to those of Mr JC, with whom they were in close contact. By the end of the day, seven hospital staff have been hospitalized. The WHO Representative calls the manager of the Hanoi-French Hospital, who is currently in France, and asks him to return to deal with a situation that is rapidly becoming alarming.

Canada

Toronto index case dies
Ms KSC, 78 years old, dies in her Toronto, Ontario, home. The death certificate attributes her death to heart attack. In fact, she died from SARS acquired at the Metropole Hotel in Hong Kong. Before dying, she has passed the virus on to four members of her extended family, who will then spark the Toronto outbreak.

6 MARCH

Hong Kong   Mr JC, the Hanoi index case who has been medically evacuated, arrives at the Princess Margaret Hospital, where he will die on 13 March. The WHO Regional Office informs Hong Kong and Singapore officials about his transfer. Singapore is informed because the medical evacuation team is from Singapore. Because of strict infection controls, no health worker in the Princess Margaret Hospital is infected by Mr JC.

China   The WHO team meets at the China CDC (6–7 March) and receives clinical, epidemiological, and laboratory information from the investigations on H5N1 in Fujian and the Guangdong outbreak. All agree that the Guangdong outbreak is unlikely to be caused by influenza A(H5N1). The Ministry of Health and China CDC again mention *Chlamydia* as the possible cause.

Singapore   **Three Singapore cases are identified and isolated**
The Ministry of Health receives reports that three travellers from Hong Kong have developed atypical pneumonia. The Ministry advises hospitals to isolate these three patients and to take infection-control measures for any new cases of atypical pneumonia.

7 MARCH

Viet Nam   **Alarming situation evolves in Hanoi**
The situation is rapidly escalating, with 12 Hanoi-French Hospital staff now hospitalized and more falling ill. Three of six employees at Mr JC's office also have high fever. The WHO Representative writes to the Ministry of Health and Hanoi-French Hospital, urging them to control the outbreak by creating a task force, strengthening infection controls, and closing the hospital to other patients. WHO sends out an alert about the Hanoi outbreak to the Global Outbreak Alert and Response Network (GOARN) and requests assistance.

WHO   **Regional Office mobilizes**
The WHO Western Pacific Regional Office forms an ad hoc team to deal with the developing emergency. The team is composed at first of staff members recruited from other parts of the Combating Communicable Disease Division. The team will continue to grow to respond to the outbreaks [see Chapter 3].

The country offices will also start to mobilize, and daily teleconferences will be held between the country offices in outbreak sites, the Regional Office, and Headquarters.

Canada | Mr TCK, the 44-year-old son of Ms KSC [see 5 March], arrives at the emergency department of Scarborough Hospital, Grace division, in Toronto. He complains of high fever, severe cough, and breathing difficulties. While waiting 18 to 20 hours to be admitted, he passes on the virus to three other people in the emergency department. Mr TCK is isolated after a respirologist suspects tuberculosis.

Canada | Mr CKL, a 55-year-old former guest at the Metropole Hotel in Hong Kong, is admitted to Vancouver General Hospital. Because of his travel history, infection-control procedures are implemented. The virus does not spread in Vancouver.

9 MARCH

Viet Nam | WHO convinces the Vice-Minister of Health that urgent action is needed. The Ministry of Health agrees to the visit of WHO's Regional Adviser for Communicable Disease and an influenza expert from the Centers for Disease Control and Prevention (CDC) in the United States of America to help investigate the outbreak. They will arrive on 10 and 11 March, respectively.

10 MARCH

Hong Kong | **Outbreak at Prince of Wales Hospital begins**
Seven doctors and four nurses from ward 8A in the Prince of Wales Hospital report sick. Management immediately closes the ward to patients and visitors.

China | The WHO team, in a debriefing at the Ministry of Health, recommends further investigation in Guangdong and Fujian. WHO informs the Ministry about the Hanoi outbreak, which appears similar to the ongoing Guangdong outbreak, and about the trips of the index case (Mr JC) to Shanghai and Hong Kong.

Viet Nam | At least 22 staff members of the Hanoi-French Hospital are ill; 20 have pneumonia, and one of these is in critical condition.

11 MARCH

Hong Kong

Department of Health investigates Prince of Wales outbreak; WHO is notified
The Department of Health interviews 26 of 36 staff members on sick leave. By the end of the day, 50 are on sick leave. All are recalled for medical examination, and 23 are hospitalized and isolated. The Department continues active case finding and disease surveillance in collaboration with the Prince of Wales Hospital. WHO is officially notified of the outbreak, and alarm bells ring: outbreaks in Guangdong, Hong Kong, and Viet Nam all have similar features.

China

The WHO Director-General contacts the WHO Representative to express the Member States' concern about the lack of information from China about the Guangdong outbreak. She asks the WHO Representative to express these concerns to the Minister of Health.

Viet Nam

Dr Urbani leaves for Bangkok, where he is to give a presentation at a meeting on tropical diseases the next day. He has a fever and is immediately isolated and hospitalized on arrival. He infects no other passengers on his flight or health workers.

12 MARCH

WHO

WHO issues first global alert
Increasingly concerned about the evolving outbreak in Hanoi, and prompted by the Prince of Wales outbreak reported by Hong Kong, WHO issues a rare global alert about atypical pneumonia.[8] WHO informs national health authorities about cases of acute respiratory syndrome with unknown aetiology in Viet Nam, Hong Kong, and Guangdong, which appear to place health workers at high risk. [See Appendix 1 for the full text of the press release.]

At the WHO Regional Office in Manila, the first of many people who will come to help combat SARS throughout the Region arrives.

China

The WHO Representative requests a meeting with the Health Minister to convey the concerns of the Director-General and Member States and to request more information about the Guangdong outbreak.

Viet Nam	The WHO team holds an emergency meeting with the Vice-Minister of Health and Ministry of Health officials to recommend ways of controlling the outbreak. The influenza expert explains that Dr Urbani's summaries of the epidemiology and clinical features of early cases at the Hanoi-French Hospital indicate that the outbreak is not due to human influenza or avian influenza H5N1, but is a new disease most likely caused by a new respiratory virus. The Vice-Minister of Health agrees to invite a larger WHO team and acts immediately on WHO's recommendations to control the outbreak. Meanwhile, the Hanoi-French Hospital discharges all other patients and limits new admissions to staff members suspected of having the infection. Now, 26 staff members are ill, five in critical condition.
Hong Kong	A preliminary investigation of the Prince of Wales outbreak by the Department of Health suggests that the disease has an incubation period of one to seven days and is spread through droplets and fomites (materials contaminated with body secretions). Practitioners as well as the general public are issued reminders about infection controls and preventive measures against respiratory tract infections.

13 MARCH

China	The Health Minister agrees to a WHO mission to help find the cause of the Guangdong outbreak. Separately, the Ministry of Health writes to WHO requesting training for laboratory staff in the use of the micro-neutralization test for H5N1.
Viet Nam	The Ministry of Health forms an interdepartmental task force chaired by the Vice-Minister of Heath to address the outbreak.
Singapore	The Ministry of Health reports that the three cases of atypical pneumonia all stayed at the Metropole Hotel in Hong Kong. One checked in on 20 February; the other two on 21 February.
Canada	Mr TCK dies and other members of his family are now ill [see 7 March]. Health Canada is notified. A patient who was in the emergency department with Mr TCK on 7 March returns to the Scarborough Hospital after suffering a heart attack. By then, his contact with Mr TCK is known, but his illness is not thought to be compatible with atypical pneumonia. Health-care workers

use only standard infection-control procedures while treating the patient. He is transferred to York Central Hospital, north of Toronto, and passes on the virus to more than 50 people.[9]

14 MARCH

Canada

Toronto outbreak is reported

The Ontario Ministry of Health and Long-Term Care announces at a press conference that four members of a family in Toronto have atypical pneumonia, and two have died. The cases draw intense media interest.

Viet Nam

The WHO team, mobilized through GOARN, starts arriving.

Taiwan

First Taiwan case is reported

The wife of a 54-year-old man who was in Guangdong in late February and who was hospitalized on 8 March, is also admitted with respiratory symptoms [see Chapter 8]. The two cases are reported. The man passes on the virus to one other family member; only one hospital worker is infected. Over the next five weeks up to 21 April, only one more local transmission is identified, even though there will have been 24 confirmed SARS cases by then.

15 MARCH

Singapore

In Frankfurt, German authorities await the arrival of flight SQ25, which stops in transit from New York to Singapore; full protection against infection is ready. As soon as the plane lands they quarantine it and remove a 32-year-old physician who treated the two cases in Singapore's Tan Tock Seng Hospital at the start of the month, and developed symptoms while attending a medical conference in New York. Before he boards the plane home, he phones a colleague in Singapore saying that he is unwell and returning to Singapore. The colleague advises the Singapore authorities, who in turn advise the German authorities through WHO. As they thought, the physician has SARS. All the passengers and crew are followed up for signs of infection. The physician passes on the virus to his wife and mother-in-law, who were travelling with him, and to one crewmember. All recover. None of the other passengers or the participants at the medical conference develops infection.

WHO | **WHO issues emergency travel advisory and names the fatal illness**
Prompted by the SQ25 event, WHO issues a rare travel advisory as evidence mounts that the virus is spreading by air travel along international routes. WHO names the mysterious illness after its symptoms—severe acute respiratory syndrome (SARS)—and declares it "a worldwide health threat". WHO issues the first case definitions of suspect and probable cases of SARS,* and calls on all travellers and airlines to be aware of the signs and symptoms. [See Appendix 2 for the full text of the press release.]

China | **Widespread transmission occurs on flight CA112**
Flight CA112 leaves Hong Kong for Beijing. On the flight is 72-year-old Mr LSK, who is already very sick from SARS. He was infected while visiting his brother in ward 8A of Prince of Wales Hospital, where a 26-year-old pneumonia patient was being treated [see 4 March]. At least 22 of the 119 passengers and two of the eight crewmembers on that flight will develop SARS—the only event with widespread in-flight SARS transmission [see Chapter 15].[10] Mr LSK is also the second index case for Beijing, where at least 59 of his contacts develop SARS.[7]

Singapore | The Ministry of Health forms a task force to deal with the outbreak.

16 MARCH

WHO | **WHO releases list of "affected areas"**
WHO releases a list of areas where the health authority has reported local transmission of SARS. These are: Guangdong, Hanoi, Hong Kong, Singapore, Toronto, and Vancouver. [See Appendix 3 for WHO's list of areas that experienced local transmission of SARS from 16 November 2002 to 5 July 2003.]

WHO | WHO receives reports of over 150 suspect and probable cases of SARS. Most were in very close contact with other cases. More than 90% are health-care workers.

---

* The WHO case definition is based on fever and respiratory symptoms with "suspect" and "probable" case definitions [see Annex 2 for case definition]. There is no confirmed category, as no laboratory test is available as yet. The case definition is very broad and focuses on exposure to areas with known transmission, making it more challenging for these areas.

Philippines	Media reports, based on WHO information, wrongly include the Philippines on the list of affected areas. A suspect case—Mr JC's business associate who travelled with him to Hanoi—returned to the Philippines on 11 March and was isolated on 15 March. The associate did not have pneumonia and did not meet WHO case definitions.
China	WHO shares laboratory information from Hong Kong and Hanoi with the Ministry of Health, and encourages the Ministry to do the same.
Viet Nam	Active contact tracing of close contacts starts.
Canada	Mr P, who was exposed to Mr TCK in the emergency department of Scarborough Hospital, Grace division [see 7 March], returns to the hospital with respiratory symptoms and a fever. Mr P is isolated and then transferred to the intensive care unit (ICU). His wife, who accompanies him to the hospital, is not asked about her symptoms until he is in ICU. By then, she has passed on the virus to seven visitors to the emergency department, seven hospital staff, two patients, two paramedics, and a fire fighter.[9]

17 MARCH

WHO	**WHO says travel restrictions are not justified** WHO urges national health authorities to be vigilant, but does not advise restrictions in travel or trade.
WHO	WHO sets up a laboratory network (11 laboratories in nine countries) to share scientific information by telephone and on secure websites to identify the cause of the virus. Similar networks will be formed on 20 March to address clinical aspects (78 clinicians in nine countries) and on 28 March to deal with epidemiology (nine sites in nine countries).
WHO	The WHO Western Pacific Regional Office outbreak team organizes itself into the SARS Outbreak and Preparedness Response Team with a SARS Response Group for affected areas and a SARS Preparedness Group for countries not yet affected. There are several daily teleconferences between the Regional Office and the outbreak sites, as well as with WHO Headquarters [see Chapter 3].

WHO	The Regional Office also creates logistics bases and supply chains to ensure that protective equipment and medicines are available when needed.
China	The Ministry of Health submits a brief first report on the Guangdong outbreak to WHO. The outbreak is said to have tapered off. The first SARS press briefing is held at the WHO country office.
Singapore	SARS is made a notifiable disease under the Infectious Disease Act.

18 MARCH

WHO	WHO adds Taiwan, China, to its list of affected areas. WHO repeats its previous statement that no travel restrictions are necessary, as most cases of infection occurred in close contact with known cases.
Hong Kong	Because of staff shortages resulting from the high number of staff reporting ill, the Prince of Wales Hospital decides to suspend accident and emergency services from 19 to 21 March, pending a review. The department will eventually reopen on 30 March.
Canada	Health Canada issues a health advisory and screens patients arriving from Hong Kong.

19 MARCH

WHO	WHO removes Vancouver from its list of affected areas because there was no local transmission from the imported case.
WHO	WHO announces that research teams in Germany and Hong Kong have found particles of a paramyxovirus in SARS patients. Awareness of the disease is now very high throughout the world.
Hong Kong	**Link to the Metropole Hotel is identified** The Department of Health learns that seven cases can be traced to the 9th floor of the Metropole Hotel. Professor LJL is identified as the index case [see 21 February]. Meanwhile, Professor Sydney Chung, Dean of the Faculty of Medicine at The Chinese University of Hong Kong, writes to the Director of Health, asking

her to "urgently consider all possible measures including quarantine of patients and contact to contain the outbreak before it is too late".[11]

China
WHO receives a letter from the Ministry of Health that *Chlamydia* was found by electron microscopy in five SARS patients.

Taiwan
Officials report three "probable" SARS cases and seek inclusion in GOARN and support and advice from WHO

Viet Nam
The Ministry of Health disseminates guidance on SARS surveillance and control to all district Preventive Medicine Teams, provincial Preventive Medicine Centres, clinical services, and port health authorities.

20 MARCH

WHO
The WHO laboratory network works on clinical specimens to identify the pathogen; the research is focused on the paramyxovirus. Meanwhile, the Singapore laboratory identifies, under electron microscopy, coronavirus-like particles in the respiratory samples of the three Singapore patients.

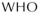

Coronavirus-like particles revealed in the respiratory samples of patients in Singapore.

WHO
WHO organizes two daily teleconferences to share first-hand experience in the management of SARS cases among clinicians in Asia, Europe, and North America.

Taiwan
The Department of Health protests the inclusion of Taiwan, China on the WHO list of affected areas.

Viet Nam
A 24-hour SARS reporting hot line is established.

21 MARCH

WHO
WHO updates clinical picture of SARS cases
WHO provides a more complete clinical picture of SARS, pooled from the findings of clinicians treating SARS patients in seven countries.[12] WHO also posts an advisory to guide the safe

discharge and follow-up of convalescent cases, and updates this on 28 March.[13]

China

There is increasing pressure from the media and embassies for more information. The WHO country office holds its second press briefing.

Singapore

The first WHO liaison officer arrives.

22 MARCH

China

In Hong Kong, WHO's Regional Director for the Western Pacific meets with the Health Minister of China to ask for more information on Guangdong Province, as well as clearance for a WHO team to visit the province.

Hong Kong

Amoy Gardens index case is hospitalized

Mr LTC, a 33-year-old with autoimmune kidney disease, arrives at Prince of Wales Hospital for scheduled dialysis; his condition worsens and he is admitted. Although Mr LTC lives and works in Guangdong, he visits Hong Kong twice a week for treatment. Each time he stays with his brother who lives in Block E of the Amoy Gardens housing complex. On 15 March, after spending the night with his brother, Mr LTC was treated in ward 8A of Prince of Wales Hospital for fever and diarrhoea. He will be diagnosed with SARS on 27 March.

Hong Kong

Coronavirus is identified as possible cause of SARS

The Hong Kong University announces that a coronavirus has been identified as the agent responsible for SARS and that a diagnostic test has been developed to detect antibodies in infected patients. Using electron microscopy, CDC in the United States of America also identifies an isolate from a SARS patient as coronavirus, and sends over sequences of the virus the next day for posting on the WHO website.*

---

* Over the next few weeks, other laboratories will support this finding. The virus will be found to be an entirely new, or until now undetected, member of the coronavirus family, and will be named SARS-CoV. It will be proven to be the cause of SARS [see 16 April].

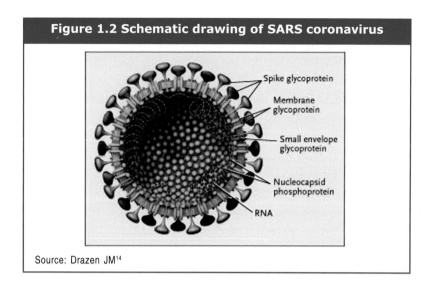

Figure 1.2 Schematic drawing of SARS coronavirus

Spike glycoprotein

Membrane glycoprotein

Small envelope glycoprotein

Nucleocapsid phosphoprotein

RNA

Source: Drazen JM[14]

| Singapore | Tan Tock Seng Hospital is designated as the only hospital to observe and isolate suspect cases and treat all cases. |

23 MARCH

| China | International experts arrive in Beijing and form a second WHO team with WHO China staff. The team will start work in Beijing and seek permission to travel to Guangdong. |

| Hong Kong | Students are asked to stay home for one week if they have relatives or contacts suffering from "atypical pneumonia". About 180 students will be affected. The Chief Executive of the Hospital Authority—a statutory and independent body that provides all public hospital services in Hong Kong—is hospitalized with SARS. |

| Canada | **Toronto hospital closes**
 The Scarborough Hospital, Grace division, in Toronto is closed to new patients and visitors. Employees are stopped from working in other hospitals. Anyone who was in the hospital after 16 March is asked to go on 10-day home quarantine. Health Canada reports 11 cases of SARS in Canada: 10 in Toronto and one in Vancouver [see 7 March].[9] |

24 MARCH

| WHO | WHO maintains that no travel restrictions to any destination are needed, and notes that there is no evidence to date of widespread SARS transmission during air travel. |

Hong Kong	Secretary for Health, Welfare and Food Dr Yeoh Eng-kiong, referring to doctors using a regime of ribavirin and steroids, says the results are encouraging, with 85% of patients on the regime showing improvement. Meanwhile, members of the public are urged to avoid visiting public hospitals unless necessary.
Singapore	**Health officials quarantine hundreds of people who may have been exposed to SARS** The Ministry of Health requires contacts of SARS cases to be quarantined at home for 10 days. More than 300 contacts have to be traced. The Ministry also bans hospital visits to SARS patients. Meanwhile, epidemiological tracking shows that only one of the first three cases led to other infections. This one case led to 22 other infections.

25 March

Hong Kong	**Cases infected on flight CA112 start to be identified** Nine SARS cases are found to have been on flight CA112. The Department of Health seeks to trace all passengers on this flight and reminds people who have respiratory symptoms to avoid travelling by plane. In total, 24 people were infected on the flight [see 15 March and Chapter 15].
Canada	The Ontario government designates SARS as a reportable, virulent, communicable disease under its Health Protection and Promotion Act. Health Canada recommends deferring travel to Hanoi, Hong Kong, Guangdong Province in China, and Singapore.

26 March

WHO	The WHO Clinical Network holds virtual "grand rounds" with 80 clinicians from 13 countries. The discussion focuses on presenting features, progression, treatment, prognostic indicators, and discharge criteria. The consensus findings, including the conclusion that no therapy has been proven to be effective, are disseminated.
China	The WHO team concludes that the Guangdong outbreak of "atypical pneumonia" was most likely SARS, and the origin of the multicountry outbreak.

| Hong Kong | **First patients from Amoy Gardens outbreak present** |
| | The Department of Health is notified that 15 residents of the Amoy Gardens apartments have been admitted to Union Church Hospital with suspected SARS, and immediately initiates an investigation [see Chapter 16]. |

Singapore   The Government orders the closure of all primary schools, secondary schools, junior colleges, and centralized institutes from 27 March to 6 April 2003. This is to allay public concern, although the risk of contracting SARS is limited to close contacts of cases showing symptoms.

Canada   The Premier of Ontario declares a province-wide SARS emergency. All hospitals in the Greater Toronto Area are placed on "Code Orange" and required to suspend nonessential services. Hospitals are also instructed to create isolation units, provide exposed staff members with protective clothing, and limit visitors. Hospital access will be further limited on 30 March.[9]

27 MARCH

WHO   **WHO issues new travel advice: recommends exit screening**
WHO issues more stringent advice to international travellers and airlines, and recommends that passengers from affected areas be interviewed for SARS symptoms or history of contact.

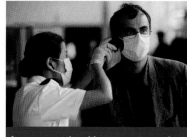
A passenger has his temperature taken prior to checking in for a flight at Hong Kong airport.

WHO   WHO adds Beijing and Shanxi Province, China, to its list of affected areas.

China   The Ministry of Health reports 792 cases (a third of them health workers) and 31 deaths from "atypical pneumonia" from 16 November 2002 to 28 February 2003 (it previously reported 305 cases and five deaths up to 9 February [see 11 February]).

Hong Kong   The Director of Health makes SARS a statutorily notifiable disease by revising the Quarantine and Prevention of Disease Ordinance. The amended ordinance provides the legal basis for mandating close contacts of SARS patients to report daily to one of four designated medical centres (to start operating from 31 March) for up to 10 days. Later, the ordinance will also be used to enable home quarantine of contacts. Meanwhile, the Government announces that all secondary and primary schools and preschools will be suspended for nine days, starting 29 March. The Rolling Stones cancel their Hong Kong concert.

28 March

China

The Ministry of Health agrees with the WHO team that the Guangdong outbreak was a SARS outbreak [see 26 March]. The WHO team emphasizes the need to visit Guangdong [see 23 March], but no agreement on the matter is reached. WHO China issues the statement: "This week, China has become, very clearly, part of the global network in dealing with the disease."[15] The Ministry of Health will provide WHO with regular, up-to-date reports from all provinces from 1 April.

Singapore

The fourth imported SARS case, who was infected on flight CA112 [see 15 March and Chapter 15], is reported.

Taiwan

There are six new cases, four of whom travelled on flight CA112. The Department of Health classifies SARS as a statutory communicable disease and requires visitors to fill out a health declaration form. Civil servants are banned from visiting China, Hong Kong, and Viet Nam.[16]

29 March

WHO

Dr Carlo Urbani dies of SARS in Thailand. Special tributes for his work in general, and especially his early alert about SARS, start to come in [see Chapter 18].

Dr Carlo Urbani

Hong Kong

All incoming passengers must fill out health declaration forms as part of the new screening procedures for SARS. Departing passengers are required to answer questions relating to SARS.

Australia

The Government warns citizens against travelling to Hong Kong, Singapore, China, and Viet Nam.

USA

The Government extends its travel advisories to China, Hanoi, Singapore, and Hong Kong.

30 March

Hong Kong
Among the residents of Amoy Gardens, 190 are now hospitalized with suspected SARS.

Canada
York Central Hospital is closed to new patients; employees are asked to quarantine themselves. Thousands of other Toronto residents face quarantine at home.

31 March

Hong Kong
Amoy Gardens residents are quarantined
The Director of Health issues an exceptional order to isolate all the residents of Block E for 10 days [see Chapters 7 and 16]. Of the 213 residents of Amoy Gardens that are hospitalized with suspected SARS, 107 come from Block E.

Singapore
Mr TSC, a 64-year-old vegetable seller, is infected when he visits his brother, Mr TKC, at the Singapore General hospital. Mr TSC will become the index case for a community and hospital outbreak [see Chapter 17]. Mr TKC is the index case of a hospital outbreak that will be recognized on 4 April.

Singapore
Nurses at Changi Airport begin visual screening of inbound passengers from affected areas.

1 April

China
China starts daily reporting
Health authorities begin daily reporting of probable SARS cases and deaths nationwide, and by province.

Hong Kong
Amoy Gardens residents are evacuated
As cases continue to increase and preliminary evidence suggests an environmental source, the Government evacuates all the quarantined residents of Block E of Amoy Gardens to two holiday camps to complete their 10-day quarantine. The block is then intensively investigated and disinfected.

2 April

Hong Kong, China
WHO issues travel advisory for Hong Kong and Guangdong
In response to the continuous export of virus from Hong Kong (in nine people since the global alert) and the community spread

at Amoy Gardens, WHO issues its most stringent travel advisory in its 55-year history: consider postponing all but essential travel to Hong Kong and Guangdong [see Table 1.1].

China   The Ministry of Health allows the WHO team to travel to Guangdong [see 23 March and 28 March]. The team visits Guangdong from 3 to 8 April. There is intense media interest in the visit; an information officer joins the team in Guangdong to help with media queries and interviews.

Singapore   Ngee Ann Polytechnic College is closed for three days following the discovery of a suspected SARS case among its students.

USA   The Government authorizes its nonessential diplomats and families to leave China and Hong Kong.

Table 1.1 Chronology of World Health Organization travel advisory notices

Date	Notice
2 April	Travel advisory issued for Hong Kong and Guangdong, China
23 April	Travel advisory issued for Beijing and Shanxi, China and for Toronto, Canada
29 April	Travel advisory lifted for Toronto
8 May	Travel advisory issued for Tianjin, Inner Mongolia, and Taipei, China
17 May	Travel advisory issued for Hubei, China
21 May	Travel advisory extended to all of Taiwan, China
23 May	Travel advisory lifted for Hong Kong and Guangdong
13 June	Travel advisory lifted for Hubei, Inner Mongolia, Shanxi, and Tianjin
17 June	Travel advisory lifted for Taiwan
24 June	Travel advisory lifted for Beijing

Source: Update 92: Chronology of travel recommendations, areas with local transmission. Geneva, World Health Organization, 2003 (http://www.who.int/csr/don/2003_07_01/en/index.html).

3 APRIL

Viet Nam   **New cluster of cases starts**
             Just as the local outbreak appears to be over, a new case (linked to the Hanoi-French Hospital) is found in another hospital in Ninh Binh Province. This case will transmit the virus to six others (including a physician), but there will be no further transmission of SARS in the country.

China   The Minister of Health addresses SARS-related issues on national television.

| Hong Kong | The Government announces that school suspensions, which began on 29 March, will be extended to 21 April. In public hospitals, a no-visiting policy is implemented in all acute wards and a restricted-visiting policy is enforced in convalescent and psychiatric wards. |
| Thailand | Officials announce that entire planeloads of visitors from high-risk countries will be quarantined for 14 days if anyone aboard is found with symptoms of SARS. |

4 APRIL

| Singapore | **Outbreak occurs at Singapore General Hospital**
Thirteen staff from two wards of Singapore General Hospital are discovered to have developed fever. Over the next two days, all the patients and staff are transferred to Tan Tock Seng Hospital. The index case, Mr TKC, did not have typical symptoms. He presented with bleeding from the gut [see 31 March], and is confirmed to have SARS only on 9 April, but has been isolated since 2 April. By then, 24 health-care workers, 15 patients, and 12 family members and visitors have been infected.[17] |
| USA | President George W. Bush orders SARS added to the list of communicable diseases. Anyone suspected of having SARS can be quarantined. |

5 APRIL

| China | **ILO official, infected on flight to Beijing, dies**
A 53-year-old Finnish staff member of the International Labour Organisation (ILO) dies of SARS in Beijing. On flight TG614 from Bangkok to Beijing on 23 March, he sat next to a symptomatic Chinese official who had been infected on 15 March on flight CA112 and had discharged himself from a hospital in Bangkok [see Chapter 15]. |

7 APRIL

| WHO | WHO reports that three types of tests for SARS are now available, but each one has important limitations. The enzyme linked immunosorbent assay (ELISA) detects antibodies but is reliably positive only 20 days after the onset of symptoms, so its results cannot be used to isolate and treat a patient, and to initiate |

public-health action. An immunofluorescence (IFA) assay detects antibodies reliably by the tenth day of infection, but is a demanding and comparatively slow test requiring the growth of the virus in cell culture. The polymerase chain reaction (PCR) test (detecting SARS virus genetic material) is more useful in the early stages of infection, but produces many false-negatives.

China

WHO team members and Guangdong Health Bureau officials brief the international consulates in Guangzhou on the team's findings. The international representatives are advised that SARS cases were still occurring, but a good surveillance system and isolation and infection control has been established and the outbreak is being contained, with fewer infections.

Taiwan

A Cabinet spokesperson says the foreign-worker policy towards Thailand might be reconsidered in retaliation for a Thai demand that Taiwanese visitors wear masks at all times while in Thailand.

8 APRIL

China

A military doctor sends a letter to journalists accusing the Government of concealing the number of SARS cases and deaths in Beijing. Underreporting by Beijing military hospitals fuels concerns that China is not reporting the real situation.

9 APRIL

China

The WHO team that visited Guangdong (3–8 April) meets with senior officials, including Vice-Premier Wu Yi. They state that Guangdong Province has responded well to the outbreak but that other provinces do not have the same capacity for response. The team expresses concern about reporting, contract tracing, and isolation practices in Beijing [see Chapter 6].

Singapore

The Roman Catholic Church suspends the hearing of confessions.

10 APRIL

Hong Kong

Officials announce that, effective immediately, all household contacts of SARS patients will be quarantined at home, with no visitors, for up to 10 days. To start with, around 150 persons in 70 to 80 households are subject to the new requirement.
Residents of Block E, Amoy Gardens, who were moved to holiday camps on 1 April, return to their homes.

| Singapore | A commercial security firm is hired by the Government to serve Home Quarantine Orders and to install "electronic picture cameras" in homes to ensure compliance. |

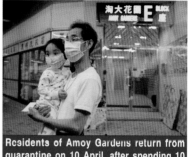

Residents of Amoy Gardens return from quarantine on 10 April, after spending 10 days in an isolated holiday camp.

| Taiwan | The international airport begins checking the temperature of every arriving passenger. |

11 APRIL

| Hong Kong | Officials announce that, from 14 April, close contacts of SARS patients will be barred from leaving Hong Kong during the quarantine period. |

| Singapore | The Ministry of Manpower imposes a 10-day quarantine on holders of Work Permits and Employment Passes who enter Singapore from SARS-affected countries. |

| South Africa | The first probable SARS case is reported. Cases in 19 countries on four continents have now been reported. |

12 APRIL

| WHO | WHO adds unspecified areas of the United States of America and London (United Kingdom of Great Britain and Northern Ireland) to its list of affected areas, noting that transmission has been limited.[*] |

| China | Premier Wen Jiabao concedes that the SARS outbreak in China is "grave" and pledges that the Government will "speak the truth" in disclosing information about the outbreak. |

| Mongolia | **Mongolia reports its first cases**
Five persons infected in Inner Mongolia, China, are isolated in an infectious disease hospital in Ulaanbaatar on 12 and 13 April. A |

---

[*] WHO will later announce that both countries have not had any local transmission. The case associated with local transmission in the United Kingdom will be discarded on 12 May 2003, as the clinical picture and laboratory findings are consistent with influenza. In the United States of America, the infection in one of two reported secondary cases more likely happened during travel, and the other case was later discarded. Very little information was made available about the details of the situation in the USA during the outbreak.

relative who did not travel to Inner Mongolia will develop symptoms on 15 April and be admitted to hospital on 19 April— the only case of local transmission in Mongolia [see Chapter 11].

13 APRIL

Philippines

Index case of the Philippines outbreak is isolated
Ms AC, a 46-year-old nursing attendant working in Canada, is isolated in San Lazaro Hospital in Manila. She will die early the next day. Ms AC arrived in the Philippines on 4 April, having been infected just before leaving Toronto. There will be eight other infections in the chain of transmission from Ms AC, all among family and hospital contacts. Extensive contact tracing does not identify any other cases [see Chapter 10].

14 APRIL

Canada, USA

SARS virus genome is sequenced
Laboratories in Canada and the United States of America announce that they have fully sequenced the SARS virus genome. The sequences are practically identical.

China

President Hu Jintao says on state television that he is "very worried" about SARS.[18]

15 APRIL

China

The WHO team in Beijing meets with the Mayor and Vice-Mayor. The team is allowed to visit two military hospitals, on the understanding that the findings will not be released to the public. Until the visits were granted, rumours about cases were rife but there was no way to verify them.

Singapore

SARS patients discharged from hospital are to be placed on 14-day home quarantine as an added precaution.

16 APRIL

WHO

A new form of a coronavirus never before seen in humans is confirmed as the cause of SARS
WHO announces that, thanks to extraordinary global collaboration, a new coronavirus is confirmed to be the cause of SARS, with Koch's postulates fulfilled. An initial suggestion is to name it the "Urbani virus", in recognition of Dr Urbani's contribution to its control. It is finally named SARS coronavirus (SARS-CoV).

China	A WHO team in Beijing Municipality attends a tumultuous and crowded media briefing from 11 to 15 March. The media are frustrated by the lack of information from the Government amid fears of a large outbreak in Beijing. Asked to estimate the number of cases, the team responds that "given the inadequate surveillance system, and the hospital practice of maintaining cases as 'under investigation' when they actually met the case definition for 'probable cases', there could be 100–200 probable cases (or 3–6 times more than ... reported). In addition to about a thousand cases still 'under investigation'." The team also uncovers serious lapses in hospital management and infection control. These concerns were shared earlier with the Ministry of Health.

17 APRIL

Hong Kong	The Department of Health announces the findings of an investigation into the Amoy Gardens outbreak. The report attributes the environmental transmission to an unusual combination of events affecting the sewage system [see Chapter 16]. Passengers departing from the international airport start to undergo temperature screening. Later in April and May, screening will be extended to transit and arriving passengers as well as to travellers at land and sea border control points.

18 APRIL

China	Leaders warn local officials against covering up reports on the spread of SARS. The WHO team in Beijing expresses strong concern over inadequate reporting of SARS cases in military hospitals as rumours of undisclosed cases mount.
Singapore	All public hospitals allow only one visitor per patient per day.
United Kingdom	Officials report that they have placed on 10-day quarantine about 150 boarding-school pupils returning from Asia.

19 APRIL

Viet Nam	Officials mark the first week with no new probable case of SARS. The 1,130-kilometre border with China, officials say, may be closed to prevent the risk of importation.
Canada	Toronto authorities investigate a cluster of 31 suspected and probable SARS cases among members of a charismatic religious

group, related to two large gatherings of the group on 28 and 29 March.

WHO	WHO adds Inner Mongolia to its list of affected areas.

20 APRIL

China **Chinese officials are fired for downplaying SARS**
Health Minister Zhang Wenkang and Beijing Mayor Meng Xuenong, both of whom were seen to have responded inadequately to the SARS crises, are removed from their posts. This marks a turning point in control efforts in China. Beijing starts more accurate daily reporting of cases, and reports 295 previously unreported cases (for a cumulative total of 339). By early May, Beijing will have reported more than 2,000 cases, and 100 new ones will be reported daily.

Singapore Officials close a large wholesale fruit and vegetable market after detecting a cluster of three cases linked to a 64-year-old vegetable seller [see 31 March and Chapter 17].

22 APRIL

Taiwan **Taiwan outbreak starts**
A cluster of six cases is reported from Hoping Hospital, Taipei. This is the start of a major outbreak in Taiwan [see Chapter 8].

China A WHO expert arrives to help develop measures to prevent the spread of SARS through travel during the May Day holidays. SARS has spread to some of the poorest provinces and regions, including western Guangxi, northern Gansu, and Inner Mongolia.

Hong Kong Senior secondary schools resume classes, with students required to wear masks and undergo daily temperature checks. Junior secondary schools will resume classes on April 28. Primary schools and other special schools will open on 19 May.

Singapore Doctors and nurses in private hospitals, working for private agencies, or self-employed are ordered to work in only one hospital. Patients can no longer be transferred between hospitals.

23 April

Canada, China	WHO extends its travel advisory to Toronto, Beijing, and Shanxi Province.
China	Beijing officials suspend all primary and secondary schools for two weeks.
Singapore	Authorities install thermal imaging scanners to check for fever at Changi Airport and at the two main border entry points with Malaysia—Woodlands and Tuas.

24 April

China	Health officials seal off the People's Hospital of Beijing University (directly across the street from the Ministry of Health building) and the People's Armed Police General Hospital, and put thousands of patients and medical workers under observation.
Hong Kong	The Department of Health announces that a WHO team from Health Canada will assist in its investigation of the environmental transmission of SARS at Amoy Gardens and other sites, including the Metropole Hotel. There is considerable public and media interest in the team, which will report on 16 May. Also, inbound passengers start to have their temperature screened in addition to filling out health declaration forms [see 29 March].
Canada	**Canada objects to WHO advisory against travel to Toronto** Canada writes a letter to WHO, objecting strongly to its inclusion in the travel advisory. The letter says: "There is no evidence of any casual transmission of SARS in Toronto and every case of SARS can be linked back to the original Canadian case."[19] Health Canada states: "Travel to any destination in Canada is safe."
Taiwan	Hoping Hospital is quarantined as the number of new cases continues to rise [see 22 April]. The number of potentially exposed persons is estimated at 10,000 patients and visitors, and 930 staff members. Home quarantine is also ordered for discharged patients and visitors who were at the hospital from 9 April.

26 APRIL

Malaysia

ASEAN + 3 Ministers of Health Special Meeting on SARS is held in Kuala Lumpur. In a joint statement, health ministers urge their heads of government to provide adequate resources to respond effectively to the epidemic.

China

The WHO team in Shanghai from 21 to 26 April concludes that there is no evidence of systematic underreporting of cases, and that the level of preparedness and response is good. In Beijing, officials order the closure of all the city's theatres, cinemas, Internet cafés, and other public entertainment places. The new mayor of Beijing discusses WHO support for SARS control in the city with WHO China. A WHO team visits the Center for Disease Control of Beijing and finds inadequate access to SARS data, which are kept by the Beijing Health Bureau.

28 APRIL

Viet Nam

WHO removes Viet Nam from its list of affected areas (the last case was isolated on 7 April), making it the first country to contain SARS successfully.

Singapore

Dozens of food markets are closed for mass cleaning. Thermal scanners are installed at the Singapore Cruise Centre and Tanah Merah Ferry Terminal. Checks with ear thermometers are conducted at Changi Ferry Terminal, Changi Immigration Checkpoint, West Coast Pier, and Clifford Pier. All shipmasters are directed to make a health declaration four hours before arrival.

29 APRIL

Thailand

Special ASEAN Leaders Meeting on SARS is held in Bangkok.

Singapore

All six public hospitals implement a "no visitor" rule.

Hong Kong

The Government announces that it has chartered an aircraft to Taipei to collect a tour group that was quarantined after one of its members was suspected of having SARS. This person is later found to not have SARS.

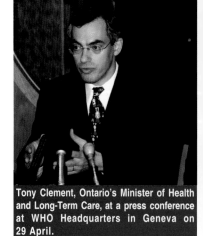

Tony Clement, Ontario's Minister of Health and Long-Term Care, at a press conference at WHO Headquarters in Geneva on 29 April.

30 April

WHO   **WHO lifts its travel warning against nonessential travel to Toronto**
                   WHO cites local measures to stop the spread of SARS. The affected area reported no new cases in the preceding 20 days.

China   Authorities institute travel screening for all modes of transport (boat, bus, train, plane). The screening is limited to temperature checks at exit points of areas with known transmission. It is later assumed that those with fever stopped travelling as a result. No recorded exports of SARS virus between provinces are recorded after this date.

Singapore   About 200,000 primary students are issued oral digital thermometers for their personal use.

1 May

WHO   WHO removes the United Kingdom and the United States of America from the list of affected areas, but adds Tianjin, China, and Ulaanbaatar City, Mongolia.

WHO   WHO updates its case definition for SARS to take into account the appropriate use of results from laboratory tests. [See Appendix 4 for the updated, and final, SARS case definition.]

China   Shanghai announces strict SARS measures, more stringent than those recommended by WHO, including a 14-day quarantine period for travellers arriving from affected areas and the setting up of traffic checkpoints for health screening.

2 May

WHO   In its daily updates, WHO starts using the term "areas with recent local transmission" instead of "affected areas"; it begins to classify the extent of local transmission in each area as low, medium, or high, depending on the extent of spread.

China   While Beijing reporting is complete and timely, WHO team members in Beijing call for better data. "The public needs to have more information on when and where infection is happening," the team says. "We don't know that right now."

Hong Kong	Authorities receive a distress call from a Malaysian cargo ship saying its sailors have SARS-like symptoms. The ship enters Hong Kong waters on 4 May and is allowed to anchor. Ten of its 24 crewmembers are rushed to hospital. All of them are later found to be SARS-free.
Singapore	The Chua Chu Kang, Yishun, Geylang, and Tampines polyclinics set up tents outside their buildings for screening and treating patients with fever.
Viet Nam	The last SARS case is discharged from the Institute for Clinical Research in Tropical Medicine, Bach Mai Hospital, Hanoi.

3 MAY

Taiwan	WHO staff start arriving to join the WHO team composed of CDC staff who have been there since the start of the outbreak.

4 MAY

WHO	WHO reports laboratory network data showing that the SARS virus can survive in urine and in faeces at room temperature for at least one to two days.[20]
Singapore	A 50-year-old man who disobeyed home quarantine orders becomes the first person to be publicly named and charged under the Infectious Diseases Act.

5 MAY

China	About 1,000 villagers surround a local government office in Xiandie in the coastal Zhejiang Province in a violent protest against the quarantine near their homes of suspected SARS patients. The villagers smash and overturn police and government cars, and demand that the patients be moved elsewhere. Meanwhile, a three-member WHO team arrives in Guangdong to review the SARS data of the province and hypothesize on the origins of human infection.
USA	The University of California at Berkeley announces that it will not accept summer students from those parts of Asia that are affected by the SARS virus.

6 MAY

Hong Kong   WHO staff members and Hong Kong officials hold a videoconference on the SARS situation. WHO issues the following statement: "The number of new cases (in the single digits for the last several days) has steadily declined, suggesting that the outbreak has peaked."

Belgium   European health ministers meet in Brussels to standardize anti-SARS measures across the continent.

7 MAY

WHO   WHO estimates the case fatality ratio to be less than 1% in persons up to 24 years old, 6% in those aged 25 to 44 years, 15% in those aged 45 to 64 years, and more than 50% in those who are at least 65 years old. WHO confirms its previous assessment that the maximum incubation period is 10 days.

Philippines   WHO adds the Philippines to the list of areas with recent local transmission, and categorizes the transmission in the country as medium because more than one generation of local transmission is involved. The WHO Representative clarifies in a press release that the risk of infection in the Philippines is negligible because there is no community transmission. This helps address the negative impact of the country's inclusion in the list of countries affected by SARS.

8 MAY

Philippines, Taiwan   WHO states that Manila is the only area with local transmission in the Philippines, and adds Taipei in Taiwan, China, to the list of areas with recent local transmission.

China   WHO extends its advisory discouraging all but essential travel to other parts of China: Tianjin, Inner Mongolia, and Taipei in Taiwan, saying, "The extent of local chains of transmission [and] the potential for spread beyond these areas were also major factors in the reasoning for this advice."

China   A joint team from the Ministry of Health and WHO visits Hebei Province (8–12 May). Joint teams will also visit the Guangxi Autonomous Region (12–16 May), Henan Province (14–18 May),

Anhui Province (18–22 May), Tianjin City (6–14 June), Shanxi Province (17–25 June), and the Inner Mongolia Autonomous Region (17–25 June).

9 MAY

Mongolia

Mongolia is declared "SARS-free"
WHO removes Mongolia from its list of countries with recent local transmission (the last and only case of local transmission was isolated on 19 April).

10 MAY

Philippines

The Government calls the WHO classification damaging and inaccurate
The Government complains in a letter to WHO that the country's inclusion in the WHO list of areas with recent local transmission gives a misleading impression of the risk in the country, citing the negative effects on its relations with other countries [see Chapter 10]. The small outbreak was brought under control by the end of April, the risk of transmission was significantly limited to close contacts, and all contacts were extensively traced.[21] WHO says in reply that it considers the outbreak to be "well contained. There appears to be no increased transmission risk in the Philippines. For these reasons, WHO does not recommend any restrictions on travel to the Philippines."[22]

WHO

WHO starts classifying the type of local transmission as "A", "B", or "C" and no longer as "low", "medium", or "high", while still retaining the same definitions for the categories [see 2 May and Chapter 10].

12 MAY

Singapore

The government-run resort Aloha is converted into alternative accommodation for people who want to spend their quarantine period away from home. The cottages and rooms are offered to those discharged from hospital, those who have been near SARS patients, and tourists issued quarantine orders.

13 MAY

WHO

WHO adds Hebei, Hubei, Jilin, Jiangsu, and Shaanxi provinces in China to the list of areas with recent local transmission.

WHO	WHO reports that SARS can be contained through case detection, patient isolation, and contact tracing.
Singapore	Twenty-four patients and six nurses from the Institute of Mental Health are suspected to have SARS (and are treated as SARS patients). Their infections are eventually found to be caused by the influenza B virus.

14 MAY

Canada	WHO removes Toronto from the list of areas with recent local transmission. But some undiagnosed chains of transmission continue.
China	The WHO team that visited Hebei (8–12 May) meets with senior officials, including Vice-Premier Wu Yi. They report that SARS has spread to nine of the province's 11 prefectures, that 40 of the cases in the province have been traced to migrant workers returning home from Beijing, and that infection controls in Hebei hospitals scrupulously follow the national guidelines.
USA	CDC calls on businesses and universities to continue plans for meetings and events that involve people from SARS-affected areas, and gives guidance on how to minimize risk.

15 MAY

WHO	WHO issues guidance for mass gatherings with persons from affected countries, as well as precautionary recommendations to address the theoretical risk that SARS might be transmitted through blood products.

16 MAY

Hong Kong	**WHO announces findings on environmental transmission at Amoy Gardens and the Metropole Hotel** The WHO team [see 24 April] releases its reports on the Amoy Gardens and Metropole Hotel outbreaks. The team confirms the findings of the Department of Health that a unique sequence of environmental (including the sewage system) and health events, which happened simultaneously, contributed to the SARS outbreak in Amoy Gardens [see 17 April and Chapter 16]. A large viral load outside room 911 of Metropole Hotel may explain the transmissions in the hotel [see Chapter 14].

| Taiwan | The Health Minister resigns over criticism of the authorities' handling of the SARS outbreak. The director of Taiwan's CDC also offer his resignation. |

17 MAY

| WHO | WHO extends its travel advisory to Hebei Province, China. WHO wraps up the first global consultation on SARS epidemiology in Geneva (16–17 May). More than 40 leading epidemiologists from 16 countries attend the meeting, which confirms that control measures recommended by WHO are supported by available evidence.[23] |

18 MAY

| China | The Media Centre of the Beijing Joint Working Team for SARS Prevention and Treatment opens. This is the culmination of WHO support to Beijing through a consultant who has been helping the authorities there for the past weeks. |

19 MAY

| WHO | **Analysis of in-flight transmissions finds low risk**
 A WHO analysis of 35 flights with a symptomatic SARS case among the passengers or crewmembers finds that only four were associated with the possible transmission of infection to fellow passengers or crewmembers. In only one flight, CA112 from Hong Kong to Beijing, was there widespread transmission [see Chapter 15]. |

| China | The WHO team that visited Guangxi reports that the area appears to be responding well to its relatively small SARS outbreak. |

20 MAY

| Philippines | **The Philippines is declared "SARS-free"**
 WHO removes the Philippines from its list of areas with recent local transmission of SARS. The Health Department's efficient surveillance and reporting system has helped prevent further transmission. |

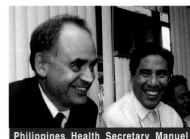

Philippines Health Secretary Manuel Dayrit (right) and World Health Organization Representative Jean-Marc Olivé during a press conference on SARS.

21 May

Taiwan

WHO includes all of Taiwan (and not just Taipei) in its list of areas with local transmission and in its travel advisory.

Singapore

The SARS Channel, a television station devoted exclusively to SARS, is launched.

22 May

China

Beijing students return to class.

USA

A CDC employee working with a WHO team in Taiwan, China, is suspected of having SARS. Testing will later disprove this.

23 May

Canada

A second outbreak in Toronto is reported
A cluster of five possible SARS cases associated with a single hospital in Toronto is reported to WHO. As a result, the United States of America reinstates a travel alert for Toronto.

A passenger passes a SARS information board at Pearson International Airport in Toronto.

Hong Kong, China

WHO removes its travel advisory for Hong Kong and Guangdong Province, which have successfully contained their outbreaks.

Hong Kong, China

Research teams announce the results of a joint study of wild animals from a market in southern China that sells such animals for food. The study detected several coronaviruses closely related genetically to the SARS-CoV in two of the animal species tested (masked palm civet and racoon dog). The study also found that one other species (Chinese ferret badger) showed antibodies against the SARS-CoV. These and other wild animals are traditionally considered delicacies and are sold for human consumption in markets throughout southern China. The study gives a first indication that the SARS virus exists outside a human host.

24 MAY

Canada

Health officials identify two clusters of possible SARS cases under investigation: five patients associated with St John's Rehabilitation Hospital in Toronto, and 26 cases, including 10 health-care workers, associated with North York General Hospital. One patient undergoing investigation is linked to both hospitals.

26 MAY

Canada

WHO puts Toronto back on the list of areas with recent local transmission of SARS.

Canada

Health Canada reports clusters of 26 suspected and eight probable cases of SARS linked to four Toronto hospitals. WHO does not recommend any travel restrictions to Toronto.

Taiwan

Taipei's health bureau chief Chiou Shu-ti resigns, making her the third official to step down because of the epidemic.

27 MAY

WHO

World Health Assembly passes a resolution on SARS
More than 190 countries participating in the World Health Assembly—the governing body of WHO—unanimously approve a resolution on SARS. Delegates also approve a resolution setting out procedures and a timetable for revising the International Health Regulations to strengthen WHO's management of future outbreaks.

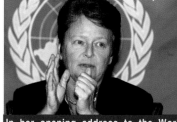

In her opening address to the World Health Assembly, WHO Director-General Gro Harlem Brundtland called for greater international cooperation in fighting emerging diseases such as SARS.

31 MAY

Singapore

Singapore is declared "SARS-free"
WHO removes Singapore from its list of areas with recent local transmission of SARS.

1 JUNE

Singapore

The "no visitors" rule at hospitals is lifted, except for suspected and probable SARS cases. Prime Minister Goh Chok Tong launches the OK Campaign for the Community to promote personal hygiene, environmental cleanliness, and public health.

4 JUNE

China   WHO is starting to feel that the outbreak can be contained. Meanwhile, a WHO training course in the laboratory diagnosis of SARS (27 May–4 June) ends.

Germany   A newly reported case, in a man recently returned from Taiwan, China, results in the quarantine of around 50 contacts. The man is hospitalized in isolation.

USA   CDC removes its travel alert for Singapore and downgrades its travel advisory for Hong Kong to a travel alert.

10 JUNE

ASEAN   **ASEAN officials declare the region SARS-free**
                     Health officials from the Association of Southeast Asian Nations, including representatives from China, Japan, and the Republic of Korea, declare the region "SARS-free" and urge countries that have issued travel advisories to lift them. The ministers also praise China for its "strong political commitment" to containing SARS.

11 JUNE

China   A WHO team from Headquarters and the Regional Office arrives for a three-day visit. The team will confirm that the outbreak is nearly under control and that effective public-health measures have been implemented.

Canada   Health authorities in Toronto go on high alert, and treat all hospital-associated clusters of patients with fever or respiratory symptoms as possible SARS cases until proven otherwise. Possible cases are immediately isolated. All contacts are being traced and, where warranted, quarantined at home. Infection-control measures are being followed in all affected facilities. WHO officials welcome the precautionary measures and say in a statement that they are "deeply concerned by the resurgence of SARS cases in Toronto" [see 23 May].

13 JUNE

China   **Most of China is declared "SARS-free"**
                     WHO lifts its travel advisory for Hebei, Inner Mongolia, Shanxi, and Tianjin, and drops Guangdong, Hebei, Hubei, Inner Mongolia, Jilin, Jiangsu, Shaanxi, Shanxi, and Tianjin from the

list of areas with recent local transmission. Only Beijing and Taiwan, China are still on both lists.

Canada | WHO upgrades Toronto's transmission category from "B" to "C" because a person not previously identified as a contact has developed the disease.

Taiwan | Taipei reports no new potential SARS cases for the first time in two months. Meanwhile, the Department of Health warns people about products that falsely claim to cure SARS. The Department reports that its investigation found such false claims in 193 instances, including ads about pineapples, bee propolis, tomato juice, teas, and vegetables.

17 JUNE

Taiwan | The WHO Regional Director for the Western Pacific announces that Taiwan, China, is no longer on WHO's list of areas to which all but essential travel is to be avoided. But WHO continues to discourage travel to Beijing.

Malaysia | **First global conference on SARS opens in Kuala Lumpur**
The two-day event, convened by WHO, is attended by more than 900 scientists and clinicians from 43 countries, including specialists who have been at the front line of SARS investigation and response since the start of the outbreak.

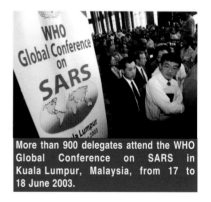

More than 900 delegates attend the WHO Global Conference on SARS in Kuala Lumpur, Malaysia, from 17 to 18 June 2003.

23 JUNE

Hong Kong | **Hong Kong is declared "SARS-free"**
WHO removes Hong Kong from its list of areas with recent local transmission of SARS.

24 JUNE

China | **Beijing is declared "SARS-free"**
The WHO Regional Director for the Western Pacific announces the lifting of WHO's travel advisory on Beijing, the last area still under a SARS-related travel advisory. WHO also removes the Chinese capital from the list of areas with recent local

transmission. At a press conference, the Regional Director says, "Today is a milestone in the fight against SARS, not only for China but for the world."

Malaysia   A four-day WHO investigation concludes that the country's five cases were infected in other countries. There has been no local transmission. The controls at the border with Singapore at Johor Baru, which were also investigated, are working well.

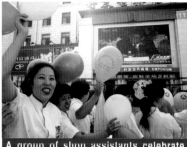

A group of shop assistants celebrate in Beijing, 24 June 2003, as they watch the WHO press conference live on a large television screen, with the announcement of the lifting of the travel advisory on Beijing.

25 JUNE

China   A 77-year-old woman who fell ill in Guangdong Province is reclassified as a probable case. She has been in isolation since 3 June. This is the first new case reported from Guangdong since 17 May. As she has been in isolation for over 20 days, there is no change in the status of Guangdong.

28 JUNE

Thailand   Health Ministers of the Asia-Pacific Economic Cooperation (APEC) forum meet in Bangkok to decide on common actions to contain the spread of SARS.

2 JULY

Canada   **Canada is declared "SARS-free"**
            WHO removes Toronto from its list of areas with recent local transmission of SARS. The last case was detected and isolated on 12 June.

5 JULY

Taiwan   **Taiwan, China, is declared "SARS-free", with no remaining chains of transmission**
            WHO removes Taiwan, China, from its list of areas with recent local transmission of SARS. The last case was detected and isolated on 15 June. This means that all known chains of person-to-person transmission of the SARS virus have now been broken.

SARS CASES AFTER THE 2002-2003 OUTBREAK

14 AUGUST 2003

Canada
Public-health officials report that 143 residents and staff of an aged-care facility in British Columbia have developed a respiratory illness. Initial testing suggests SARS. Laboratory analysis will later conclude that the virus responsible for the outbreak is not SARS coronavirus but another human coronavirus known as OC43, which causes the common cold.[24]

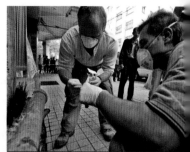

Two experts from WHO collect suspected SARS specimens at a wildlife restaurant in Guangzhou on 10 January 2004. China reported a suspected SARS case on 8 January of a waitress who worked at the restaurant.

10 SEPTEMBER 2003

Singapore
Health authorities report that a 27-year-old laboratory worker has developed SARS through accidental contamination in a microbiology laboratory in the National University of Singapore. Rapid identification and isolation prevent other infections.

17 DECEMBER 2003

Taiwan
Taipei health authorities report that a research scientist has been infected with SARS. He accidentally touched a culture with his bare hands while working in a high-security laboratory. No one else is infected.

26 DECEMBER 2003–31 JANUARY 2004

China
China reports four cases of SARS from Guangdong that do not appear to be epidemiologically linked: a television journalist, a waitress, a man, and a hospital director and practising physician from Guangzhou. Authorities say none of these patients' contacts or attendant health workers was infected. The virus is not traced conclusively to its source, but may have been of animal origin. However, only the waitress and physician have been exposed to an animal (a palm civet). Two WHO teams visit Guangzhou to investigate the outbreak. As part of the second team, two environmental health experts from Health Canada look for evidence of SARS-CoV in the palm civet cages at the restaurant and other sites.

22 April 2004

China   China reports two cases of SARS, with onset in late March and mid-April, among researchers at the National Institute of Virology in Beijing, where experiments using live and inactivated SARS coronavirus have been carried out. The Institute is closed the next day. One of the cases leads to the spread of the virus to nine other cases over three generations, but by 18 May, three weeks later, the outbreak will be declared contained with no further cases. Two further cases are identified retrospectively through blood tests. An official investigation later recommends major changes in procedure at the Institute.

REFERENCES

[1] Xu R-H et al. Epidemiologic clues to SARS origin in China. *Emerging Infectious Diseases*, 2004, 10(6):1030–1037.

[2] Zhong NS et al. Epidemiology and cause of severe acute respiratory syndrome (SARS) in Guangdong in February 2003. *The Lancet*, 25 October 2003, 362(9393):1353–1358.

[3] *Acute respiratory syndrome in China – Update 2*. Geneva, World Health Organization, 14 February 2003 (http://www.who.int/csr/don/2003_02_14/en/, accessed 1 April 2005).

[4] Acute respiratory syndrome, China. *Weekly Epidemiological Record*, 14 February 2003, 78 (7):41.

[5] *Influenza A(H5N1) in Hong Kong Special Administrative Region of China – Update*. Geneva, World Health Organization, 20 February 2003 (http://www.who.int/csr/don/2003_02_20/en/, accessed 1 April 2005).

[6] Enserink M. SARS in China: China's missed chance. *Science*, 2003, 301(5631):294–296.

[7] Liang W et al. Severe acute respiratory syndrome, Beijing, 2003. *Emerging Infectious Diseases*, 2004, 10(1):25–31.

[8] *Acute respiratory syndrome in Hong Kong Special Administrative Region of China/ Viet Nam*. Geneva, World Health Organization, 12 March 2003 (http://www.who.int/csr/don/2003_03_12/en/, accessed 1 April 2005).

[9] National Advisory Committee on SARS and Public Health. *Learning from SARS. Renewal of public health in Canada*. Ottawa, Health Canada, 2003.

[10] Olsen SJ et al. Transmission of the severe acute respiratory syndrome on aircraft. *New England Journal of Medicine*, 18 December 2003, 349(25):2416–2422.

[11] Hong Kong Legislative Council report.

[12] *Preliminary clinical description of severe acute respiratory syndrome.* Geneva, World Health Organization, 2003 (http://www.who.int/csr/sars/clinical/en/, accessed 1 April 2005).

[13] *WHO hospital discharge and follow-up policy for patients who have been diagnosed with severe acute respiratory syndrome (SARS).* Geneva, World Health Organization, 28 March 2003 (http://www.who.int/csr/sars/discharge/en/, accessed 1 April 2005).

[14] Drazen JM. SARS – Looking back over the first 100 days. *New England Journal of Medicine*, 2003, 349:319–320.

[15] Severe acute respiratory syndrome – Press briefing, Beijing, China. China, World Health Organization, 28 March 2003 (http://www.who.int/csr/sars/2003_03_28/en/, accessed 1 April 2005).

[16] Republic of China Government Information Office. DOH mandates increased measures against SARS. *Taipei Times*, 28 March 2003.

[17] Chow KY et al. Outbreak of severe acute respiratory syndrome in a tertiary hospital in Singapore, linked to a primary patient with atypical presentation: epidemiological study. *British Medical Journal,* 2004, 328:195–198.

[18] *Severe acute respiratory syndrome (SARS) – multicountry outbreak – Update 30.* Geneva, World Health Organization, 15 April 2003 (http://www.who.int/csr/don/2003_04_15/, accessed 1 April 2005).

[19] Broughton J. *Health Canada letter to the World Health Organization.* Ottawa, Population and Public Health Branch, Health Canada, 24 April 2003 (http://www.hc-sc.gc.ca/english/protection/warnings/sars/letter.html, accessed 1 April 2005).

[20] *First data on stability and resistance of SARS coronavirus compiled by members of WHO laboratory network.* Geneva, World Health Organization, 2003 (http://www.who.int/csr/sars/survival_2003_05_04/en/index.html, accessed 1 April 2005).

[21] World Health Organization. SARS outbreak in the Philippines. *Weekly Epidemiological Record*, 2003, 78:189–192.

[22] *Severe acute respiratory syndrome (SARS) – multicountry outbreak – Update 52.* Geneva, World Health Organization, 10 May 2003 (http://www.who.int/csr/don/2003_05_10/en/, accessed 1 April 2005).

[23] *Consensus document on the epidemiology of severe acute respiratory syndrome (SARS).* Geneva, World Health Organization, 2003 (WHO/CDS/CSR/GAR/2003.11).

[24] Acute Respiratory Disease in British Columbia, Canada. *EID Weekly Updates: Emerging and Reemerging Infectious Diseases Region of the Americas*, 2003, 1(8).

2 COORDINATING THE GLOBAL _____RESPONSE_____

When WHO alerted the world to SARS on 12 March 2003, next to nothing was known about the new disease. It didn't even have a name. But enough was known to cause alarm. And learning, as the world did on 15 March, that the virus appeared to travel on aircraft, did not help.

In its explosive spread the disease claimed hospital workers in large numbers. Many others fell critically ill and needed respirators. No treatments worked. Tests for all known causes of respiratory illness, including influenza, turned up negative. How the disease came to be and how it developed were unknown; what seemed inevitable was that there would be further spread.

Less than four months later, on 5 July, WHO could announce that all known chains of human-to-human transmission had been broken. An arduous battle waged in a few countries where the virus had spread had averted the first potential pandemic (global epidemic) of the 21st century—but only after 8,098 cases, with 774 deaths, had been reported in 29 countries and areas. This chapter describes the international mechanisms that contributed to this victory.

NEW MECHANISMS PUT TO A SEVERE TEST

The world rose to the challenge of SARS with unprecedented scientific collaboration and public-health determination. Several factors may help explain the intensity of the response. First, the clinical and epidemiological features of SARS made its threat particularly ominous. The disease required no vector, displayed no particular geographical affinity, mimicked the symptoms of many other diseases, took its heaviest toll on hospital staff, killed around 10% of those infected, and spread across borders with ease. SARS challenged the assumption that wealthy nations, with their well-equipped hospitals and rigorous standards of hygiene, would be shielded from its spread. Contrary to expectations, SARS spread most efficiently in sophisticated urban hospitals. Clearly, the disease could cause all countries great harm.

Second, conditions in a closely interdependent and highly mobile world favoured its spread. With airlines carrying about 1.6 billion passengers yearly, every country with an international airport was at risk of importing the disease. The social disruption and economic losses caused by SARS were way out of proportion to the number of cases and deaths, and went well beyond the outbreak sites. News about the disease jolted stock markets. Economic growth projections had to be lowered. Commerce

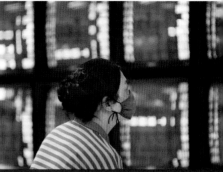

A masked investor watches the monitors showin the stocks index in Taipei on 13 May 2003. Shar prices dropped with reports of new SARS cases.

suffered in distant countries that depended on Asian goods and manufacturing capacity. Schools, hospitals, businesses, and some borders were closed. The public, made deeply aware of SARS through electronic communications and extensive media coverage, worried about its spread. Travel to affected areas plummeted, causing losses of about US$ 10 billion to airlines with Asian routes. These consequences, apparent early on, drew political support at the highest level for the fight against the disease and increased pressure to contain the outbreak quickly. They also highlighted the need to join forces against a common threat.

Third, another new disease—AIDS—had tragically shown what could happen when an emerging disease is allowed to spread around the world and become endemic. AIDS had also shattered expectations that vaccines and curative drugs could be developed fast enough to prevent a new disease from spreading. Having learned from these experiences, public-health authorities considered prevention: perhaps an all-out effort might stop an emerging disease from becoming established as yet another permanent threat to health.

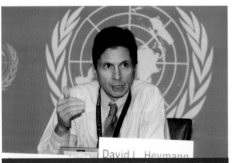

WHO's global response to SARS was coordinated by Dr David Heymann, Executive Director of Communicable Diseases at WHO Headquarters in Geneva from 1998 to 2004.

In coordinating the global response, WHO aimed at the outset to help contain transmission in affected countries, seal off opportunities for further international spread, and prevent SARS from becoming endemic. Although neither the cause nor the potential for the spread of the disease was known, WHO set these ambitious goals with some solid backing. Since 1996, the Organization had been developing and testing a system, supported by a range of new mechanisms, to strengthen international capacity to detect and contain outbreaks. These mechanisms, in turn, were an outgrowth of a previous crisis: the 1995 outbreak of Ebola haemorrhagic fever in Kikwit, the Republic of the Congo. That outbreak, which raged undetected for three months, caught the international community by surprise and showed the urgent need to improve capacity in several specific ways.

In 1995, the world was ill prepared to respond to emerging and epidemic-prone diseases on almost every level. The Congo was only one of many countries where the public-health surveillance system was at best rudimentary. Internationally, no back-up system gave early warning of unusual disease events to compensate for this critical weakness. Infrastructure for detecting and diagnosing unusual disease events had deteriorated worldwide. Laboratory capacity was inadequate: some of the few biosafety level IV facilities had been dismantled, and many laboratories no longer had the reagents to diagnose rare diseases. International stockpiles of protective equipment and supplies were either outdated or depleted, delaying and interrupting control measures. The highly publicized Ebola outbreak, which caused 310 laboratory-confirmed cases, 250 of them fatal, showed that the very foundations of infectious-disease control needed rebuilding. The urgency of the situation was formally acknowledged in May 1995 when the World Health Assembly, in its first resolution on emerging infections, asked WHO to draw up plans and strategies for improving world capacity to recognize and respond to new diseases.

SOLUTIONS TO LONG-STANDING PROBLEMS

In 1996, WHO began building up a system, and the supporting virtual architecture, to detect outbreaks earlier and respond to them more quickly and effectively. The Global Public Health Intelligence Network (GPHIN), developed and maintained for WHO by Health Canada, continuously scans the Internet for rumours and reports of suspicious disease events. This sensitive early-warning system introduced in 1997 far outpaced traditional systems that raise an alert only after local case reports filter to the national level and are passed on to WHO. GPHIN also

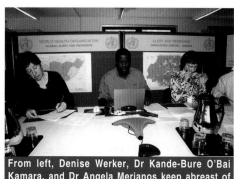

From left, Denise Werker, Dr Kande-Bure O'Bai Kamara, and Dr Angela Merianos keep abreast of new developments in the Alert and Response Operation Room at WHO Headquarters in Geneva.

helped compensate for the reluctance, motivated by economic concerns, of many national authorities to disclose outbreaks promptly and frankly.

To expand and formalize the response capacity, the Global Outbreak Alert and Response Network (GOARN) was set up in early 2000.[1] A "strike force" of specialized staff and technical resources could now be rapidly assembled and deployed for emergency investigations and on-the-spot assistance. This overarching network links, in real time, 120 networks and institutes having much of the data, laboratory capacity, specialized skills, and experienced personnel needed to act rapidly on many different fronts when outbreaks require international assistance. As GOARN partners have a broad geographical base and many have staff in countries often affected by outbreaks, the network formally complements GPHIN's "artificial intelligence" as a first-hand human source of early information about outbreaks.

The establishment of GOARN solved several long-standing problems. First, being able to draw on the resources and expertise of a broad range of technical partners made it unnecessary to maintain a permanent staff of dedicated experts— with all the associated expenses—in the face of a danger that was sporadic and unpredictable. Second, as outbreaks demand widely varying controls, GOARN brought much-needed flexibility and a surge capacity that could be tailored to outbreak needs. It also helped ensure frequent opportunities for experts from any single country to practise and sharpen their technical skills during international responses. Finally, GOARN introduced a formal mechanism for balancing national and international strategic interests, particularly when the response to an outbreak in one country affects the international community.

A new system of electronic communications was set up to make better use of a unique geographical and strategic resource: WHO's 141 country offices, concentrated in the developing world and located within or close to ministries of health. These offices became yet another channel for instant news about diseases within countries, and for GOARN resources to come to the aid of those countries. With all these systems drawing abundant rumours, WHO at the same time took a novel approach to verifying rumoured outbreaks, to rapidly determine which ones were of genuine international concern, and then translating the findings into action-oriented information and transmitting it electronically to its partners.

In other developments, a WHO surveillance network set up in 1947 to alert the world to new variants and novel strains of influenza viruses, especially those with pandemic potential, inspired similar electronically linked networks of experts and laboratories for other epidemic-prone diseases like dengue. All these developments drove sweeping changes in the International Health Regulations, which govern the reporting of epidemic-prone diseases worldwide and the application of measures to prevent their spread. The international response to SARS tested these new mechanisms simultaneously under the extreme conditions of a global public-health emergency.

Initial suspicions: a "fatal flu"?

In late November and early December 2002, GPHIN began picking up rumours of a major "flu outbreak" in mainland China, said to affect large numbers of schoolchildren. In investigating these rumours, WHO could rely on a new network of laboratories established in China to strengthen global capacity for influenza surveillance. On 12 December 2002, WHO received a detailed report on data collected at surveillance sites in Beijing and Guangdong. Laboratory analyses identified influenza B as the cause. The number of cases, compared with the number during the same period in 2001, supported the conclusion that influenza activity in both areas was normal for the season. Laboratories in the global influenza network independently verified the findings. The results were reassuring, also because they indicated that China's new influenza network was performing well.

Then on 10 February 2003, the WHO country office in Beijing received an email message describing a "strange contagious disease" that had "already left more than 100 people dead in Guangdong Province in the space of one week". GPHIN also picked up media reports of an unusual epidemic of fatal pneumonia-like illness in Guangdong. [See Chapter 1 for the subsequent events as WHO sought to obtain more information on this outbreak, which eventually led to the WHO alerts.]

Roll-out of new response mechanisms

On 15 March, WHO issued its second, stronger global alert, and quickly set in motion all international mechanisms for outbreak response. WHO issued case definitions and reporting requirements, as well as tools for their implementation, and began reporting cases as they developed and assessing the evolving situation daily on its website.

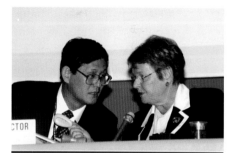

Dr Shigeru Omi (left), Regional Director for the Western Pacific, confers with Dr Gro Harlem Brundtland, then Director-General of WHO, at a SARS technical meeting on 27 May 2003 in Geneva.

The two alerts, widely carried by the international media, heightened the vigilance of clinicians worldwide, and prodded ministries of health to report suspected cases to WHO through country and regional offices, especially in the Western Pacific Region. Perhaps most important, hospitals that detected possible cases followed WHO advice, issued with the first alert, to isolate patients and manage them according to strict procedures of infection control. WHO staff members also began tracking and analysing the nearly 300 SARS-related rumours that GPHIN would retrieve from 83 countries during the four months of the international outbreak. Of these, well over a third proved substantive.

On 17 March, WHO used a secure website, teleconferences, and videoconferences to set up virtual networks of scientists, epidemiologists at the outbreak sites, and clinicians. Setting aside competition, these experts collaborated around the clock to identify the cause of SARS, develop diagnostic tests, define clinical features, and investigate modes of transmission, all in record time. Within a month, the laboratory network traced SARS to a previously unknown coronavirus. The network of epidemiologists confirmed that the virus was transmitted through close person-to-person contact, collected data on incubation periods and peak infectivity, checked for evidence of asymptomatic transmission, tracked the significance of "super-spreading events", and recommended control measures. The clinical network generated knowledge about the course of infection, the management of cases, and characteristic signs and symptoms seen at different outbreak sites.

SARS marked the first international outbreak in which information about a new disease was gathered and made public in real time, as the disease evolved. During the outbreak, WHO issued a score of guidelines and recommendations for responding to SARS. These ranged from advice on how to recognize and report cases, to instructions for performing diagnostic tests and guidelines for mass gatherings. To seal off further spread through international travel, travellers had to be given advice. Governments and a concerned public also had to be steered away from unsafe travel destinations. As the disease became better known, health officials gained confidence that the initially recommended control measures—case detection, contact tracing, isolation, and infection control—would eventually stop transmission.

In the evolution of SARS, the global alerts of mid-March drew a clear line between the earliest outbreaks in China, Hong Kong (China), Hanoi, Toronto, and Singapore—all severe—and the reported cases in all other areas. Outbreaks before the global alerts accounted for about 90% of all cases and 79% of all deaths worldwide. After the alerts, high vigilance and preparedness, and rapid advice on control measures, prevented further spread or minimized the number of secondary cases in all areas with imported cases.

On 5 July, WHO declared that all known chains of human-to-human transmission had been interrupted—a triumph of both political commitment and time-honoured control measures. The goal of preventing the new disease from becoming permanently established had been achieved.

References

1   Heymann DL, Rodier GR (WHO Operational Support Team to the Global Outbreak Alert and Response Network). Hot spots in a wired world: WHO surveillance of emerging and re-emerging infectious diseases. *Lancet Infectious Diseases*, 2001, 1(5):345–353.

3 RESPONSE OF THE WESTERN PACIFIC _REGIONAL OFFICE_

Like most other epidemics, SARS came unannounced and unexpected. As it spread from southern China, it exposed patchy surveillance systems, weak public-health infrastructures, skill shortages, and neglected infection-control practices.

SARS posed a challenge unlike any that WHO's Regional Office in Manila had ever faced. This chapter describes how the Regional Office responded through experts from around the world working as a team. Most of these people had never worked together before. Now they joined forces to fight a common enemy.

FIRST RESPONSE

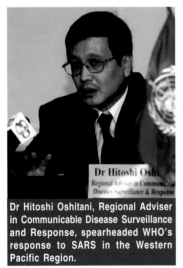

Dr Hitoshi Oshitani, Regional Adviser in Communicable Disease Surveillance and Response, spearheaded WHO's response to SARS in the Western Pacific Region.

News of an outbreak of atypical pneumonia in Guangdong reached the Regional Office on 10 February. Nine days later came reports of avian influenza (H5N1) in a family in Hong Kong (China) that had been in Fujian Province, China. The Regional Office went on heightened alert. As Regional Adviser in Communicable Disease Surveillance and Response (CSR), Dr Hitoshi Oshitani was used to dealing with a whole range of communicable disease issues, including outbreaks, in the 37 countries and areas of the Western Pacific Region. But aside from Dr Oshitani, there was only Dr Elizabeth Miranda (on a short-term assignment in rabies control) in CSR at the Regional Office, under Dr Brian Doberstyn, Director of the Division for Combating Communicable Disease. No response team stood ready to act at the first sign of a major outbreak.

By Friday, 7 March 2003, as the outbreak in Hanoi was rapidly evolving, it was clear that WHO needed more support. Dr Carlo Urbani, WHO Medical

Officer in Viet Nam, urgently emailed Drs Oshitani and Doberstyn in the afternoon: "Situation is scaling up. ... I request technical assistance."

The data from Viet Nam suggested that the outbreak was spreading to close contacts. Supplies such as masks and gowns, as well as technical assistance, would be needed to prevent the spread.

Dr Oshitani was in Beijing, tracking down information about the Guangdong outbreak and the H5N1 situation in Fujian. He had been in Beijing since 23 February and would go from there to Viet Nam on 10 March [see Chapter 5]. He would not be back in the Regional Office for another week.

Meanwhile, Dr Doberstyn formed an ad hoc emergency team in the Regional Office, and the task of obtaining supplies fell to the team's first recruit that Friday. Dr David Bell had been working on malaria tests. Over the next week he would have to master equipment specifications and sources.

A constant flow of email bloated the workload. "I called it the black wall," Dr Bell remembers. "I would go for coffee having cleared my email inbox, and on my return the screen had gone black again, full of unread email. But we knew we had to do all that we could to get the needed supplies to protect the health-care workers in Viet Nam—and, of course, for other countries if it spread."

For Dr Bell and others in the emergency team, the weekend of 8–9 March marked the end of normal life. Work took over nearly every waking hour, even on weekends. Little time was left for sleep.

"HOW SOON CAN YOU BE HERE?"

On Tuesday, 11 March, Dr Doberstyn called Dr Rob Condon, a communicable disease control specialist, in the WHO South Pacific office in Suva, Fiji.

"There's something happening in Viet Nam," Dr Doberstyn said. "It's already forced a hospital in Hanoi to close and we think it's just appeared in Hong Kong. We don't know what it is, we don't know how it's spreading, but HQ is putting out a global health alert tomorrow. We need you to get here as soon as you can—today if possible."

A cyclone was raging just south of Fiji. Suva airport was closed and all aircraft had been grounded. But at 5:30 the next morning, Dr Condon was on the first flight out of Suva, on his way to Manila.

Over the days and weeks to come, the same call to arms would be heard and answered around the world. Dr Keiji Fukuda, an influenza expert from the Centers for Disease Control and Prevention in Atlanta, just happened to be in the right place. He was in Hong Kong on 11 March, at the government's invitation, to review the avian influenza A (H5N1) cases reported on 19 February. He stayed for several weeks as WHO team leader in Hong Kong, working in close collaboration with the Hong Kong health authorities. He was also part of the WHO team in Beijing.

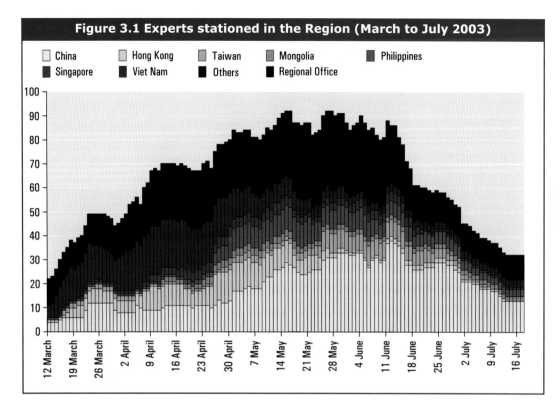

Figure 3.1 Experts stationed in the Region (March to July 2003)

Legend: China, Hong Kong, Taiwan, Mongolia, Philippines, Singapore, Viet Nam, Others, Regional Office

FIRST GLOBAL ALERT: QUESTIONS WITHOUT ANSWERS

On the morning of 13 March, the Manila emergency team met, tired and a little shaken by the recent events. The global alert from Geneva the night before had raised the stakes considerably. War had been declared on the new infectious disease. All the known cases were in the Western Pacific Region, so the Manila office would be in the front line.

The team knew that the index case in Hanoi had been evacuated to Hong Kong on 6 March and was already dead. Many of the doctors and nurses who had treated him in Hanoi were now showing signs of the same illness, as were health-care workers in Hong Kong. And Dr Urbani himself was under observation in the isolation ward of a hospital in Bangkok.

Were the cases in Hanoi and Hong Kong linked? How were they related to the Guangdong outbreak and the reported cases of avian influenza A (H5N1)? What were the odds of three unrelated outbreaks of respiratory illness occurring at the same time in neighbouring countries? Where would the disease strike next? Was this the start of what many experts thought to be overdue: the next influenza pandemic?

Or could a genetically manipulated agent of biological warfare have been released, by chance or on purpose? After all, had al-Qaeda not threatened to follow up the 11 September attacks on New York with targeted strikes on "unexpected places", using chemical, biological, and other weapons?

WHO experts had to answer these questions to help control the outbreaks in Hanoi and Hong Kong. They would also have to delve further into the situation in Guangdong, and help health officials in neighbouring countries prepare for the worst—the imminent arrival of an unknown disease with global implications.

SECOND ALERT: MOMENTUM BUILDS

By Saturday, 15 March, new cases had been identified in Singapore and Toronto, and on flight SQ25 from New York to Singapore. The disease could evidently travel by plane. Urgent teleconferences between the Regional Office, Singapore, and Geneva discussed flight SQ25 and the implications for global spread. That evening, WHO issued a second, more strongly worded, health alert.

It spelled out the agreed case definition and potential risks to international travellers, and urged heightened surveillance and the rapid isolation and appropriate management of suspected cases.[1] A new word was born: SARS.

By Monday, 17 March, the situation looked grim. Patients were not responding to the antibiotics or antiviral medications commonly used to treat atypical pneumonia. Up to one-fifth needed respirators. Not one had recovered; at least two had died, and more were likely to follow. And hospital workers were still prominent among the new cases.

But the actions needed to control the disease were clear. Infections in hospital had to be prevented, through the use of personal protective equipment. Cases had to be isolated as soon as possible; and contacts traced and followed up.

THE OPERATIONS ROOM

A room on the fourth floor opposite Dr Doberstyn's office, which had been used for training, became the operations room. At first, with only one telephone and one computer, team members dashed from one office to another as anxious colleagues in Geneva, Hanoi, and then Hong Kong sought to make contact.

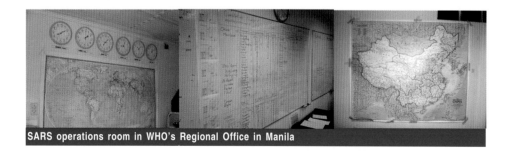

SARS operations room in WHO's Regional Office in Manila

The makeshift arrangement soon morphed into a full-fledged SARS operations room, with secretarial support, extra telephone lines, networked computers, whiteboards, and maps of Viet Nam and southern China on the walls.

The workday started when the sun rose over Fiji and ended when it set over the Americas. Workdays averaged between 12 and 16 hours, and in the early days, staff worked up to 20-hour days. Life revolved around regular meetings and teleconferences, interrupted only by hurried meals and occasional bouts of sleep [see Box 3.1].

The daily meetings kept everyone in the loop in the early days. New knowledge had to be shared, especially with new team members (some of them in transit to the field), who were arriving in a constant stream and needed to be briefed and assigned roles. But as information about SARS in medical journals began to outstrip the capacity of team members to keep up, the meetings became staff development and journal club sessions. These were often attended by visiting dignitaries and consultants as they entered or left the resource pool, by television crews, and often by the Regional Director.

Box 3.1 SARS team schedule

Daily

- Meeting of all team members at 8 a.m. and at 4 p.m.
- Meeting of the human-resource planning and logistics team to identify, recruit, and deploy consultants.
- Teleconference with all the country teams and Headquarters.

Weekly

- Two to three meetings with WHO teams in affected countries to share information, as well as challenges, victories, and disappointments.
- Two teleconferences with WHO Representatives in countries not directly affected-one with Pacific countries and a separate one with Asian countries.
- Meetings with three global groups of technical experts—epidemiological, clinical (including infection control), and laboratory—to share state-of-the-art knowledge, further data needs, and research priorities.
- Two teleconferences with senior WHO management at Headquarters and in the five other WHO regional offices at 10 p.m. or 11 p.m. (These were held daily at the start.)

When needed

- Media interviews and conferences.

A way was eventually found to sort out and coordinate the jumble of meetings and teleconferences. And the search for more specialists—epidemiologists, infection-control practitioners, laboratory experts, and logisticians—to join the team at the Regional Office or in the field went on [see Figure 3.1]. [Appendix 5 lists all the staff, consultants, and members of other organizations that were involved in the Region's response.]

PLAN OF ATTACK

The aim was to stop transmission and prevent the virus from becoming endemic. Therefore, the team had to help contain the outbreaks in affected areas and prevent the virus from spreading elsewhere. The SARS team organized itself into a SARS Response Group, to support the teams in the field in the affected areas, and a SARS Preparedness Group, to minimize the risks of importation into countries not yet affected by SARS, strengthen surveillance in those countries, and develop contingency plans for responding to a crisis [Figure 3.2].

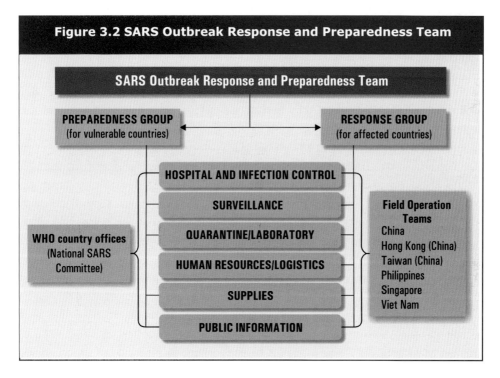

Figure 3.2 SARS Outbreak Response and Preparedness Team

As governments and health workers (and other people) fought the virus, WHO provided a range of support, a critical one being collecting, analysing, and sharing information [see Box 3.2 and Chapter 4].

WHO sent teams to China (including Hong Kong and Taiwan), and to Mongolia, the Philippines, Singapore, and Viet Nam. Public-health and infection-control experts also visited unaffected countries.

FINDING THE PEOPLE, AND MOVING THEM

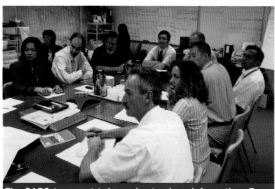

The SARS team met twice a day to share information. From left, Zenaida Cariaga, Dr Richard Nesbit, Dr Brian Doberstyn, Dr Hitoshi Oshitani, Dr Robert Condon, Dr Mahomed Patel, Dr Takeshi Kasai, Rosanne Muller, and Peter Vanquaille.

The fight against SARS needed experts in epidemiology, surveillance, public health, clinical diagnosis and infection control, animal health, laboratory diagnosis and biosafety, environmental health, data management, logistics, and media relations.

The Regional Office had to find the right people with the right skills who could also move at short notice. The Global Outbreak Alert and Response Network (GOARN) [see Chapter 2] and WHO Headquarters helped. But with most of GOARN's resources tied down in Europe and North America, the Regional Office itself had to do most of the finding.

Existing formal and informal networks within the Region were used and developed, particularly the Training in Epidemiology and Public Health Intervention Programs Network (TEPHINET), Field Epidemiology Training Programmes (FETPs), and academic institutions. The FETPs in Australia, Japan, and the Philippines were an excellent source of junior and senior epidemiologists.

Normal administrative procedures were neither responsive enough nor flexible enough to respond to large-scale emergencies. All aspects of administration—personnel, recruitment, finance, budgeting, and travel—had to change.

The Regional Office hired a logistician, Peter Vanquaille, to help find and recruit people. Setting aside other obligations, he travelled at short notice, arriving in Manila on 7 April. "I had been working in all kinds of emergencies before, in the field and in capitals around the world," he recalls. "I thought that I had previously reached the limits of the amount of work that I could do. But in Manila, with the SARS team, I went beyond those limits. Only sleep interrupted the work. But it was all worthwhile, not just because the task was an important one, but also because of a sense of partnership with the team."

WHO normally takes weeks to recruit consultants. With SARS, recruitment had to be fast-tracked down to a few days "Three days was the shortest time I managed to get a consultant on the plane, including all the paperwork done," Mr Vanquaille remembers. "The initial medical clearance was done over the phone while I was reading the medical history to the nurse. The consultant arrived at the airport before the ticket. So with one phone I was guiding the consultant, and with the other phone I was talking with the travel agent to get the ticket there. An hour later, the consultant was on the plane."

Box 3.2 Range of activities for WHO consultants and teams in countries, in coordination with governments

- Investigating possible cases and outbreaks, and exploring the dynamics and risk factors of transmission, and the effectiveness of control measures
- Adapting and implementing public-health, clinical, infection-control, and laboratory guidelines, and developing the knowledge and skills of clinicians, nurses, laboratory scientists, and other health-care staff
- Assessing the ongoing risk and minimizing the spread of SARS in health-care settings, laboratories, communities, airports and seaports, and all forms of public transport
- Assessing and helping strengthen the degree of prevention and preparedness (through training workshops and other means)
- Advancing and supporting immediate essential research to improve the understanding of SARS
- Communicating with the media
- Monitoring and mobilizing resources

Most of the consultants were recruited quickly, thanks to the personnel, medical, and administrative units of the Regional Office and their willingness to circumvent normal procedure. However, it was not always smooth going. With no clear operating procedures for emergencies, personalities could sometimes get in the way. Mr Vanquaille says, "Staying professional with that little, but important, personal touch of treating people with friendliness and equal respect, had an effect almost like magic."

SUPPLIES AND PROCUREMENT

On Sunday, 9 March, Peter King, Supplies Officer at the Regional Office, was enjoying the weekend when he got a telephone call from Dr Doberstyn. Supplies had been ordered for a preparedness kit a short time before. Dr Doberstyn wanted to know where the supplies were.

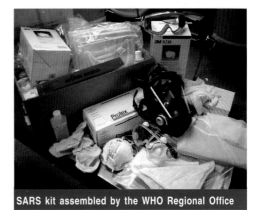

SARS kit assembled by the WHO Regional Office

"Did you indicate that the order was urgent?" Mr King replied. He quickly learnt that what had been routine was now urgently needed. Preparedness was now response. And it would be months before Mr King got another leisure day.

Both affected and unaffected countries needed various supplies—personal protective equipment, drugs like ribavirin (which at first was thought to help in treatment), supplies for collecting and shipping laboratory samples, and everything from respirator hoods to gum boots. Finding those supplies in the required volume, and then shipping them out rapidly, was the main challenge.

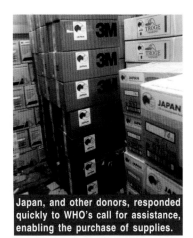
Japan, and other donors, responded quickly to WHO's call for assistance, enabling the purchase of supplies.

Procurement, especially when it has to be done over several time zones, was not a straightforward process.

Thanks to a good relationship between the Regional Office and the Government of Japan, US$ 3 million was immediately secured, through the Japan International Cooperation Agency (JICA). The swift response, as well as JICA's operating flexibility in the release of funds, helped the supplies team meet requirements even as these were constantly revised.

But all the money in the world cannot buy what is not available. There were general shortages in supplies (especially N-95 masks), aggravated by the Iraq War. Individual suppliers could also provide only a small fraction of what was needed. Mr King had to contact suppliers in many countries. And WHO had no system for doing this.

A special computer program had to be written to manage the new challenges of procuring and distributing these materials throughout the Region.

FUNDING SUPPORT

Besides funding support from Japan for supplies, other donors provided funds for the massive response implemented by the Regional Office, as well as directly to countries.

PREPAREDNESS IN UNAFFECTED COUNTRIES

From the outset, a major focus of control efforts was preventing SARS from reaching unaffected countries. In addition to preparing guidelines to help these countries, WHO dispatched consultants to give support.

Cambodia and the Lao People's Democratic Republic, with their poor public health infrastructure, were thought to be most at risk. Papua New Guinea and the other Pacific island countries and areas also benefited from rapid assessments of public-health and infection-control preparedness. One consultant island-hopped non-stop in eight weeks to assess 10 different areas (Fiji, Guam, Kiribati, Nauru, Tonga, Palau, Saipan, Samoa, Tuvalu, and Vanuatu).

In one country, a WHO consultant tested readiness by pretending to have SARS on arrival. She was pleased to find that the airport was well prepared, but news of her arrival had travelled to the hospital. When she arrived, she saw the last of the staff fleeing the premises.

WORKING WITH THE MEDIA

An early challenge for the SARS team was responding to the surging media interest. At the height of the crisis, WHO's three-person Public Information Office in Manila was fielding hundreds of phone calls a day. There were also live television and radio interviews (including regular late-night calls from radio stations as far away as Bolivia and Croatia) and requests for information from embassies, corporations, schools, and members of the public. Like the rest of the SARS team, the public information team spent practically every waking hour at work.

Peter Cordingley, a freelance journalist, had just been hired by the Regional Office for short-term editorial work entirely unrelated to communicable diseases. At the time, the position of Public Information Officer was vacant. When the calls started coming in, Mr Cordingley was catapulted into the hot seat as head of the media team.

"It was a challenge," he said. "I didn't know a lot about communicable diseases, but the truth is that none of us—the experts included—knew much about SARS. So we learned together: how the virus was spreading, how to spot it, and how

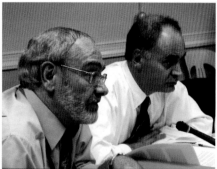

Peter Cordingley (left), Public Information Officer, at a press conference with Jean-Marc Olivé, WHO Representative in the Philippines.

to stop it. It was all a long way from what I had been hired to do, but, like everyone else on the team, I found it the experience of a lifetime."

Mr Cordingley's desk turned into a sea of yellow as Post-It notes from his assistants, Marilu Lingad and Teena Nery, tallied phone calls from journalists. "No matter how busy the day got, I tried to return each call," Mr Cordingley said, "even though I knew that in some cases it would be past the journalist's deadline. It seemed to me that the trust of the media was going to be an important element in the battle, and I didn't want to lose that. So I did my best to deliver what I knew from experience that all journalists need: an honest assessment of the situation, with no smokescreens or public-relations babble designed to throw them off the track."

As the disease spread in China, a series of media officers were appointed in Beijing. Bob Dietz, who was one of them, remembers, "I arrived in Beijing on a near-empty plane to find an almost deserted airport. The city, which I had grown to know after many visits over the years, was eerily empty. Not only were the customary traffic jams gone, but there were hardly any cars on the streets. My favourite restaurants, if they had managed to stay open, were deserted.

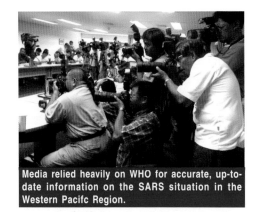
Media relied heavily on WHO for accurate, up-to-date information on the SARS situation in the Western Pacifc Region.

It was an indication of the fear SARS was causing—and a measure of the size of the job that awaited me."

The media officers in Geneva, Manila, Beijing, and Hanoi kept information flowing to the media almost round the clock. "We made mistakes," Mr Cordingley acknowledged later, "but I think it's fair to say we set some of the rules about how to respond to a public health crisis." The influential *South China Morning Post* in Hong Kong (China) agreed. In its issue of 25 February 2004, it cited the way Mr Cordingley had handled his public information responsibilities during the crisis as a prime example of how to communicate with the media.

For the media and everyone else, the Western Pacific Region's website became a one-stop guide to SARS—how national health services should prepare for the disease, which were the best masks to wear in a health-care setting, how to wash one's hands (a video offered on the site showed the correct way). This service, coupled with near-daily updates on the developing global situation and mountains of technical input on the website of WHO Headquarters, demonstrated the surging power of the Internet as a public-health tool.

Epilogue

The SARS outbreak highlighted the need to strengthen the weakest links in the outbreak surveillance and response chain, even as it tested new methods of collaboration. Improvements here should lead to generic improvements in other diagnostic, monitoring, and evaluation tools of public health.

Basic public-health principles defeated SARS. But the next virus may not be so easy to tame. The SARS response—rapid, effective, global as well as specific—must be the foundation for longer-term control of known diseases and emerging ones.

References

[1] *World Health Organization issues emergency travel advisory*. Geneva, World Health Organization, 15 March 2003 (http://www.who.int/csr/sarsarchive/2003_03_15/en/, accessed 1 April 2005).

—4 SURVEILLANCE—

The SARS outbreak had its origin and epicentre in the Western Pacific Region. By 5 July 2003, when all chains of transmission had been broken, 96% of cases had occurred here. It was therefore in this Region that surveillance was most critical—and where the epidemiological analysis of the surveillance data would be most informative.

To combat any disease, health authorities must know where the cases are, what sorts of people have caught the disease, and how it is spreading. These questions form the basis of a disease surveillance system.

In the case of SARS, its consequences, its unknown cause, and its emerging potential for rapid international spread made setting up a regionally coordinated surveillance system a matter of utmost urgency. The system would ultimately prove to be an essential element in the fight against SARS. It allowed WHO to assess which countries were affected or at imminent risk, to learn about patterns of transmission, and to prevent further local and international spread. In the gathering and sharing of information, the role of the Internet was unprecedented.

SETTING UP SURVEILLANCE

Surveillance is defined in the dictionaries as "close observation, especially of suspected persons". Disease surveillance, just like military surveillance, involves gathering and assessing intelligence from a variety of sources.

With SARS, as with any other outbreak, the first step in setting up a surveillance system was to establish standard case definitions. When WHO issued its second alert on 15 March 2003, the case definitions were very simple [see Box 4.1].

The case definition had to be very sensitive so that no cases would be missed. But that meant that it was also very non-specific, especially in areas with transmission, where travel history could not be used to exclude most cases. As fever and respiratory symptoms are very common, this created a considerable challenge.

More experience with the new disease allowed clinicians in the outbreak areas to define cases better (although atypical presentations would subsequently lead to chains of transmission in several areas).

Once the new coronavirus was confirmed as the cause of SARS and laboratory tests became available, the tests could verify the presence of the infection. On 1 May 2003, the case definitions were revised to include the use of laboratory

Clinical definition for suspect case

A person presenting with a history of:

- Fever (over 38°C)

AND

- One or more respiratory symptoms including cough, shortness of breath, difficulty breathing

AND

- Close contact* with a probable case

OR

- Recent history of travel (within 10 days) to Asia, especially in areas reporting cases of SARS

Clinical definition for probable case

A person meeting the suspect case definition together with severe progressive respiratory illness suggestive of atypical pneumonia or acute respiratory distress syndrome with no known cause

OR

A person with an unexplained acute respiratory illness resulting in death, with an autopsy examination demonstrating the pathology of acute respiratory distress syndrome with no known cause

* Close contact means having cared for, live with, or had face-to-face (within one metre) contact with, or having had direct contact with respiratory secretions and/or body fluids of a person with SARS.

Source: World Health Organization issues emergency travel advisory. Geneva, World Health Organization, 2003 (http://www.who.int/csr/sars/archive/2003_03_15/en/).

tests [see Appendix 4]. Unfortunately, frequent false-negative results early in the course of the illness, when control actions were most necessary, limited the usefulness of the laboratory tests.

WHO requested all affected countries to report daily on new cases that met the case definitions. The reports were to include the number of new cases and running totals of SARS cases and deaths. Daily reporting was requested, even when there were no new cases, to make sure that there were indeed no new cases and that a country had not simply neglected to send in its report on a given day. A standard reporting format was developed to help countries submit clear, consistent, readily analysable information. Throughout the reporting process, the Internet again proved invaluable, with many reports being submitted by email to the national level and on to WHO.

SURVEILLANCE INFORMATION

The SARS surveillance system transcended the usual mechanisms of public-health surveillance in two main respects: the level of detail and the speed of information gathering and dissemination. In-country teams needed more detail than conventional surveillance systems provide, to track down possible contacts and previously unrecognized routes of transmission. To allow authorities to control an emerging outbreak before it could spread, the information also had to be obtained very actively and very quickly.

The system gathered information through two channels: "official" (reports sent to WHO by ministries of health) and "unofficial" (unconfirmed rumours). These two types of information had to be handled very differently.

Official surveillance data

From the numbers of "probable" SARS cases in the daily case reports, the WHO team in the Western Pacific Regional Office plotted epidemic curves and distribution maps. In this way they could monitor the progress of local transmission and rapidly identify changes in the geographical distribution of cases. The Regional Office sent this information daily to WHO Headquarters in Geneva (for publication on the WHO website), to member countries, and to the media.

To assess transmission risk and guide travel advisories, it was important to know whether SARS in a particular country was spreading only among close contacts or more widely in the community. WHO devised a system for classifying SARS-affected countries according to their pattern of local transmission [see Appendix 3].

The WHO team paid special attention to cases associated with international air travel [see Chapter 15]. Seating and flight information was recorded so that any in-flight transmission (such as a passenger from a SARS-affected country developing symptoms after arriving in another country) could later be investigated.

These investigations directly influenced global policy for cross-border protection. Working with the International Civil Aviation Organization, the International Air Transport Authority, and national quarantine officials, WHO drew up exit-screening guidelines for passengers from SARS-affected countries, and airlines developed procedures for managing passengers with symptoms of SARS.

Some countries delayed the reporting of known SARS cases because of the economic implications. In other countries and areas, where information was openly shared, media coverage still outpaced government reporting. The official reporting therefore had to be supplemented, and rumour surveillance filled this need.

Rumour surveillance

Dictionaries commonly define rumour as "information, often a mixture of truth and untruth, told by one person to another" or "a story or statement widely spread, without proof as to facts".

Fear of this unknown disease that was spreading rapidly around the globe fed rumours in the print and electronic media and among the general public, especially early in the outbreak, when little was known about how the disease was transmitted. Government staff in affected countries and staff of international and nongovernmental organizations also forwarded rumours to WHO. Examples of the types of rumours that the team had to deal with daily are shown in Box 4.2.

An anonymous email sent directly to WHO by a member of the public:

I'm a foreign student ... doing an internship in XXX and I can confirm from a medical source that, last week, a hospital in the city ... admitted 5 people suffering from SARS. ... At least one of them is dead. Thank you for verifying and publishing this information. Good luck.

A rumour from the media:

SARS disclosed: A Corner Of The Iceberg Meltdown: Last year in October, all villagers in one village in XXX suffered from a mysterious disease and all died.

WHO played an important role in evaluating and responding to such rumours by seeking further investigation, clarification, and action, and guiding the countries in this matter at the national level. Figure 4.1 shows how the rumours were sifted and verified or dismissed. Two thirds of the rumours were later confirmed.

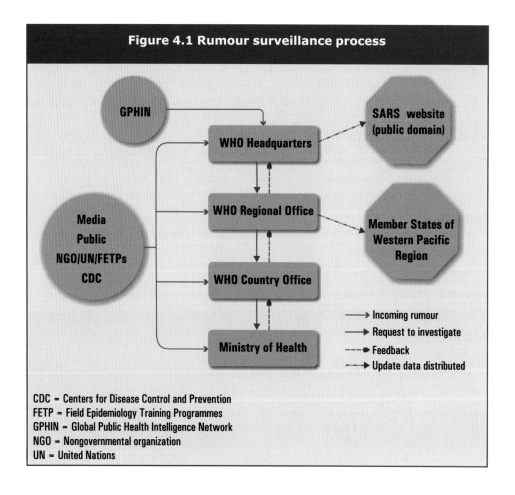

Figure 4.1 Rumour surveillance process

CDC = Centers for Disease Control and Prevention
FETP = Field Epidemiology Training Programmes
GPHIN = Global Public Health Intelligence Network
NGO = Nongovernmental organization
UN = United Nations

PART II: COUNTRY AND AREA PERSPECTIVES

5 CHINA: FROM DENIAL TO MASS ___MOBILIZATION___

The spring air in Beijing normally entices residents outdoors to the city's public places and parks. But in the spring of 2003, with the city in the grip of SARS, the air had never seemed so tainted. Some city residents were terrified to venture outdoors, fearing possible infection from the peripatetic movement of air and people.

By late April, quiet had fallen over the *hutongs,* or alleys, the lines at Bank of China branches had disappeared, bus and bicycle traffic had thinned, and tourism had come to a standstill. At Western Station, the main rail terminal, passenger traffic dropped by 75%. Normally a city teeming with 13 million people, Beijing seemed at times like a ghost town.

The SARS virus brought the public-health system to its knees while battering the country's political and economic front. The Asian Development Bank put the cost to Asian economies at about US$ 60 billion.[1] And China was at the epicentre of the escalating epidemic.

When the virus emerged in China, the public-health infrastructure was sadly underfunded and the country ill prepared to respond. China failed to issue a warning as the virus spread across the country and outside its borders.

During this difficult time, WHO approached China several times by way of telephone calls, letters, and face-to-face encounters, including a tense meeting in Hong Kong (China) on 22 March 2003, when WHO's Regional Director for the Western Pacific, Dr Shigeru Omi, pressed China's Minister of Health for more information and access to Guangdong Province.

The international community and the media also kept up the pressure to respond. Once China's central government realized that it needed to seriously tackle this new disease, the turnaround was impressive. By late April, China had started to mobilize its entire society in a "people's war" against SARS. Victory soon followed.

An incubator for viruses

Most newly emerging diseases come from animals. In southern China, the local penchant for exotic foods, the presence of unhygienic wet markets, high population density, and poor animal-husbandry practices—farm animals are often reared right beside pets and people—all favour the transfer of a virus from an animal to a human host.

Avian influenza

Guangdong has invited special attention from WHO disease-control experts because of concerns about avian influenza. In 1997, Hong Kong reported 18 cases of avian influenza A(H5N1) in humans, six of whom died. Countries feared that China was not reporting the real source of the disease. To provide some assurance that no outbreak of avian influenza was going undetected in China, a joint team from the Ministry of Health and WHO reviewed the animal and human disease surveillance and response system in the southern part of the country in January 1998. The team visited epidemiology units, hospitals, laboratories, and chicken-production facilities, and met with staff from both the animal and human health services. No evidence of an outbreak was found.

Animal markets

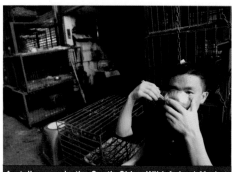

A stall owner in the South China Wild Animal Market in Guangzhou eating his breakfast next to empty cages that used to house raccoon dogs, civet cats and snakes sold for food.

Animal markets in the provincial capital, Guangzhou, offer a medley of live animals for culinary delicacies, such as civet cats, snakes, turtles, badgers, hedgehogs, and frogs, bringing rare viruses ever closer to humans. Outbreak experts, aware of the health risks these live markets present, keep a close watch on the area. Reports of a new disease in the area drew the immediate attention of Dr Hitoshi Oshitani, WHO's Regional Adviser for Communicable Disease Surveillance and Response.

First reports: WHO seeks epidemiological information

On 10 February, the first working day for many people after the weeklong Chinese New Year holiday, the WHO Representative in China, Dr Henk Bekedam, began receiving reports about an alarming outbreak in Guangdong Province. The son of a former WHO staff member sent this email to Alan Schnur, the Communicable Disease Team Leader of WHO China: "Am wondering if you would have information on the strange contagious disease (similar to pneumonia with invalidating effect on lung) which has already left more than 100 people dead in … Guangdong Province, in the space of 1 week. The outbreak is not allowed to be made known to the public via the media, but people are already aware of it (through hospital workers) and there is a 'panic' attitude, currently, where people are emptying pharmaceutical stocks of any medicine they think may protect them."

Mr Schnur forwarded the email at once to the Ministry of Health, and sought information. He added that the American embassy had passed on a similar rumour about a strange disease that was causing bleeding and many deaths in Guangzhou. Similar queries came from other embassies. Mr Schnur also told Dr Oshitani and WHO Headquarters about the reports. An official letter from WHO to the Ministry followed.

For the WHO office in China, such rumours were not unusual. Almost without exception, they were generally found to be false and based on some misunderstanding. An international event may have been cancelled without explanation, or the Government may have launched a vaccination drive without clearly informing the public that it merely sought to prevent and not to stop an epidemic. The new rumours therefore raised no great concern. But because they came from Guangdong, an area of risk for avian influenza, which could be reported as atypical pneumonia, the WHO office set aside its backlog of work and acted promptly on the rumours.

A senior local scientist maintained that chlamydiae bacteria had caused the outbreak. The theory was so prevailing that it proved inhibiting in a culture of deference to authority and seniority. When scientists in Beijing identified a new virus in late February, they chose not to say anything about it.[2]

WHO would continue to seek information from the Ministry of Health, while also urging that a WHO team be allowed to investigate the outbreak in Guangdong. That permission would not be given until 2 April. When the WHO team finally went to Guangdong, they found that the province was managing the outbreak well.

By that time, clusters of cases had already appeared in several cities near Guangzhou. The first case was found on 16 November 2002 in Foshan City and the second on 17 December in Heyuan City, in a chef dealing with exotic game animals.[3] Then, between 26 December and 20 January, 28 cases were recognized in Zhongshan City.[3] Two clusters, of several cases each, were also found in neighbouring Guangxi Province in December and January.

On 21 February, the virus travelled out of Guangdong to Hong Kong, where guests at a hotel would be infected and later carry the virus across the globe.

INFORMATION GRIDLOCK

Myths grew amid a dearth of information. An immediate response to the new disease was needed. China□s decentralized disease-surveillance system tended to limit information exchange between levels. Also, since SARS was a new disease, there was as yet no official reporting requirement for it.

SARS demonstrated the crucial need for accurate and timely information. Many questions arose and some answers—that smoking prevented SARS, for example—were incorrect. Some myths were downright dangerous. Boiling vinegar, supposedly to purify air, led to carbon monoxide poisoning from charcoal fires. How many were affected by this practice is not known.[4]

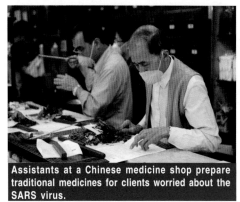

Assistants at a Chinese medicine shop prepare traditional medicines for clients worried about the SARS virus.

In early 2003, white vinegar and herbal medicines were selling briskly in some Guangdong cities. The air swirled with rumours about a contagious disease and locals were nervous. On 4 January, the *Heyuan News* ran a letter from the local disease-control centre calling for calm. Alarmed locals were stocking up on medicines such as *banlangen*, a traditional cold therapy made from the indigo tree. Provincial health authorities sent a team to investigate. The team□s head, Guangzhou respiratory specialist Dr Xiao Zhenglun, found the city in "chaos". In mid-January, residents of Zhongshan City were rushing to buy medicines, vinegar, and even food. Two months later, *banlangen* would also disappear from shelves in Beijing.

In China, disease outbreaks are investigated and controlled by local health officials, who typically refer outbreaks up the command chain only when they need help. Only a few diseases must be reported immediately to higher authorities, and even these have to be reported only after the source has been investigated and confirmed locally. This system worked well when people were much less mobile and stayed put in their counties or provinces. With rapid economic development and increased mobility, however, the old system could not respond fast enough to a new threat like SARS.

The disease was barely covered by the media, creating a fertile environment for the spread of rumours. Chinese journalists say they were dissuaded. At a press conference on 11 February, Guangdong health authorities announced that the outbreak of atypical pneumonia had started on 16 November 2002 and had affected 305 people, only five of whom had died. Then they quickly focussed attention on the National People□s Congress in Beijing in March, where a new president, premier, and Government would be chosen. Outsiders found the information that was filtering out of China hard to believe. They feared the outbreak was far worse.

The media turned to the WHO office for information that the Ministry of Health and Chinese Center for Disease Control and Prevention (China CDC) were unable or unwilling to provide. By the first week after the initial report on 10 February, the local media had identified the WHO office as a potential source of information on the new disease. It appeared that the potential spread of a new and deadly disease was of great concern to their readers and listeners.

An impromptu media briefing, the first on the outbreak, was held at the WHO Beijing office on Wednesday, 19 February. On that day, Mr Schnur was frantically networking with disease-surveillance staff, sending emails, and drafting queries to the Ministry of Health for more information. His receptionist alerted him that about 15 reporters were refusing to leave the reception area unless their questions were answered. But without official information from the Ministry of Health, there was little to add to what the media already knew. The media were

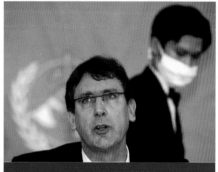

Dr Henk Bekedam, WHO Representative in China, speaks at a press briefing on 13 May in Beijing.

already working hard gathering information from Beijing and the provinces and in some cases they knew at least as much as the WHO staff did.

Yet this first impromptu press briefing was followed by even more calls from the media, encouraged perhaps by the quick and open response of the WHO office, led by Dr Bekedam.

After the rush of media interest, an office next to the WHO premises was rented for press briefings. WHO staff expected about 30 journalists at the first briefing, which took place before the WHO team visited Guangdong. After entering the room, the team was shocked to see more than 130 people crammed into the room, with journalists sitting on the floor with microphones just in front of the head table. There were more than 25 cameras from all the major news networks.

WHO TEAMS OF EXPERTS INVESTIGATE THE GUANGDONG OUTBREAK

The first WHO team of influenza experts arrived in China on Sunday, 23 February. This small team, drawn from Japan, the United States of America, and WHO, was very knowledgeable and had worked at length with respiratory diseases and disease surveillance. While this team sought to find out more about the disease in Guangdong, news of an outbreak in Viet Nam emerged.

After the departure of this first team, the Ministry of Health agreed to have a second group of experts visit Beijing and Guangdong and hold more detailed discussions with the Ministry of Health and China CDC. WHO was markedly increasingly its presence in China.

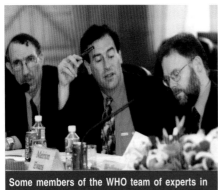
Some members of the WHO team of experts in China (from left): Alan Schnur, Dr Robert Breiman, and Dr Merion Evans.

In an unprecedented move that reflected its willingness to cooperate and the importance it gave to the work on SARS, the Government relaxed visa authorization procedures for the WHO experts. Normally it would have taken at least two weeks for the Government to issue a visa. Now visas became available at the airport on arrival. As the need for more experts grew, the Government started allowing the WHO office to fax visa authorizations within hours of receiving résumés. Experts could be on the plane to Beijing only a day after the Ministry of Health came to know about them. This cooperation between WHO and Ministry of Health was unprecedented and reflected the very high level of attention given to work by the Government.

Meetings between the second team and Beijing municipal health authorities were not encouraging. The team found many gaps in the information. The members doubted that the surveillance system was up to the task and that the municipal government knew enough about the disease to mount an adequate response.

The work in Guangdong started slowly, but picked up after a few days. WHO had developed a good working relationship with provincial health officials when the international influenza team had visited in 1998.

Discussions with Guangdong health and hospital officials were open and frank. Public-health workers had shown themselves to be extremely capable and courageous in identifying and tackling the new disease. The guidelines they developed in early February accurately assigned the case definition and advocated correct infection-control measures. Only slight revisions were needed in early March to reflect the need to stop visits to suspected SARS patients. These guidelines, with an emphasis on infection control and quarantine, would need to be relearnt in Beijing from experience.

The WHO team, together with the Guangdong Health Bureau, offered to hold a briefing session with representatives of all international consulates in Guangzhou. The briefing generated intense media interest. The team members reported their findings, taking note of the speed, accuracy, and quality of the actions taken by the Guangdong health authorities to set up a sensitive surveillance system and an extremely strict infection-control regimen. It was the first time that Bureau officials had spoken with consular officials. Both sides agreed that it wouldn't be the last.

After returning to Beijing, the WHO team visited many hospitals and districts from 11 to 15 April to see first-hand how things were. Far from being open and responsive, like their counterparts in Guangzhou, hospitals in Beijing were clearly withholding data, and some that were known to have SARS cases among their staff denied having a problem. Recommendations made by the team following the Guangdong visit were not yet being acted on in Beijing.

VIRUS SPREADS TO BEIJING

SARS had gone international with the WHO alerts of 12 and 15 March. The rest of the world responded to a degree never before seen for any health issue. China was still not releasing information about the substantial efforts being taken at the local level to control the new disease. That did not stop the virus from gaining hold in Beijing, where its impact would eventually be the greatest. On 2 and 15 March, two cases arrived in Beijing, both causing super-spreading events.[5]

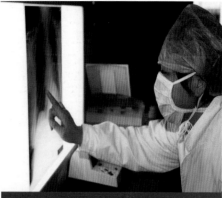

The chest X-ray of a patient showing symptoms of SARS is examined in Xiaotangshan Hospital, Beijing.

The first case was Ms YM, a 27-year-old woman who sold jewellery at a rented counter in a department store in Taiyuan, the capital of Shanxi Province. She developed symptoms on 22 February while on a business trip in Guangdong, and sought medical attention on her return to Taiyuan the next day. When her condition did not improve, she rented a car and drove to Beijing on 1 March. She was admitted to a military hospital on 2 March and transferred to another military hospital in the city on 5 March. Ms YM eventually recovered, but many of her close contacts developed SARS, including eight family members and friends, two doctors and a nurse in Taiyuan and at least 10 health workers at the two hospitals in Beijing. Both her parents died.

The second case was Mr LSK, a 72-year-old man from Beijing who was infected while visiting ward 8A of Prince of Wales Hospital in Hong Kong. He passed on the virus to at least 59 other people in Beijing after his arrival on 15 March (in addition to those infected on his flight, CA112 [see Chapter 15]).

By April, SARS was well established in Beijing, but only a few cases were being reported to WHO, even as the international media feasted on rumours of overflowing hospital wards and hidden cases.

On 9 April, a prominent surgeon and former director of a military hospital, Dr Jiang Yanyong, caused a sensation in the foreign media when he disputed the official count of 19 SARS patients. He cited at least 60 undisclosed cases in military hospitals. On 23 April, WHO issued a travel advisory for Beijing, thereby extending the travel advisory that was issued to Hong Kong and Guangdong on 2 April, and which would be extended to Tianjin and Inner Mongolia on 8 May.

WHO TEAMS ASSESS THE SARS SITUATION IN CHINA

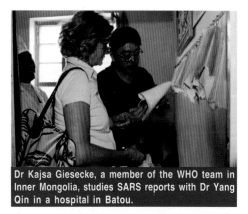

Dr Kajsa Giesecke, a member of the WHO team in Inner Mongolia, studies SARS reports with Dr Yang Qin in a hospital in Batou.

WHO expressed doubts over China's data, noting that military hospitals were not linked to the state medical system. "We have clearly told the Government the international community does not trust their figures," Dr Bekedam told a highly charged news conference on 16 April. With the WHO team that had visited Guangdong, he had just met for the first time with Madame Wu Yi, the Vice-Premier, to talk about their findings. Although generally satisfied with the control measures in Guangdong, Dr Bekedam and the team were concerned about Beijing's inadequate surveillance, reporting, and infection-control measures, as well as the medical fees that might discourage SARS cases from seeking treatment.

The media focused on underreporting of cases. Pushed to give a more precise estimate of the number of cases in Beijing, Mr Schnur said that there were probably between 100 and 200 cases, compared with the 34 reported by the local authorities.

WHO teams led by experts from top public-health institutions would later visit several other provinces. In all, around 80 experts from around the world were flown into China to assist WHO in its work.

On 20 April 2003, in a watershed event, China declared war on SARS, deeming it a "top priority". The country's leaders called for an accurate account of the epidemic from all levels and issued a strong warning against hiding cases. Following this, 295 previously unreported SARS cases in Beijing were disclosed, bringing the city's total to 339. Health Minister Zhang Wenkang and Beijing Mayor Meng Xuenong, both of whom were seen to have responded inadequately to SARS, were removed from their posts. Vice-Premier Wu, a highly respected woman in the Politburo, took charge of an ad hoc SARS committee.

WAS THE GENIE OUT OF THE BOTTLE?

But while China's leaders were now committed to battling SARS, the challenges ahead were enormous. China was short of data, capacity, resources—and time. The critical early period for containment, before April, had already passed. Experts feared it might be too late to put the brakes on SARS. By now the virus had crept into provinces with poor health infrastructures, such as Shanxi and Inner Mongolia. In Beijing, the numbers continued to climb. By early May, the city had over 2,000 cases, and 100 new cases were being reported daily.[5]

Half the probable cases reported no contact with SARS patients or health workers. The experts were baffled. Was the infection coming from unrecognized sources? Was there simply not enough time to look into contact histories? Or had officials, not daring to underreport, simply reported as SARS cases many that in fact were not? Control efforts, which used to be hampered by underreporting, now staggered under the number of new cases.

The May Day holiday threatened to shift the pace of the disease to a higher gear. Many rural migrant workers—the "floating population" in cities—return to their villages ahead of this holiday. There were fears that they would bring home the virus.

Could China cope? Hospitals lacked even essential equipment such as masks and gloves to undertake isolation needed for cases and suspect cases. Public health had been underfunded for years, as surveillance and rural health care were shunted aside in favour of revenue-earning services. SARS could overwhelm areas such as the "poverty province" of Guangxi, where most township clinics lack emergency medical supplies and basic laboratory equipment. Was the proverbial genie already out of the bottle? Was it too late to vanquish the virus before it became endemic?

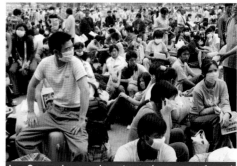

In Guangzhou, migrant workers are forced by worries over SARS to wait outside the train station on 2 May before returning home for the May Day holiday

There were two major concerns: did the hospitals have the capacity to treat and isolate all the cases and suspect cases? And could the virus be prevented from spreading out of the cities? To help address the first concern, a new 1,000 bed-hospital, built in a week in Xiaotangshan, Beijing, opened at the end of April. Unlike most other hospitals, it met disease-control requirements, with well-ventilated single rooms.

In early May, as WHO staff visited the Ministry of Health to discuss joint investigations in selected high-risk provinces, morale was at its lowest. The Ministry shared its cafeteria with the hospital staff of the quarantined People's Hospital and it was feared that some of the Ministry staff could have been infected. More than 100 new cases were still being reported daily; many provinces were reporting cases.

Some experts predicted the worst, and suggested that the best hope lay in suppressing and minimizing the disease. But WHO refused to concede defeat, reminding the world that other areas had contained and then eliminated their outbreaks. And, after all, this was China, where mobilizing the masses was something of an ancient art.

Mobilizing the masses

In Guangxi Province, minority groups sang folk songs on SARS. In Hohhot, the capital of Inner Mongolia, huge wall murals showing aspects of the SARS experience covered buildings in the city centre. In Beijing, revolutionary era-style banners spurred comrades on. On television, reports lauded the "white-coated warriors" and "angels in white".

President Hu Jintao declared a "people's war" against SARS. The Party's propaganda department worked feverishly to make SARS known to China's 1.3 billion people.

A desert of information gave way to a deluge. Finnish journalist Pekka Mykkanen remarked after observing SARS propaganda in a few provinces: "Once, there was nothing on SARS. Now, there is nothing but SARS."

From 30 April, people taking boats, buses, trains, and airplanes were having their temperature checked. As a result, after this date no exports of SARS virus between provinces was recorded. A WHO expert, Dr Sandy Cocksedge, helped develop and put in place the overall system for travel screening from the end of April. Unfortunately, these measures were not in place when about two million people left Beijing after the sacking of the Mayor.

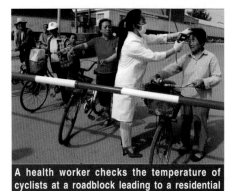

A health worker checks the temperature of cyclists at a roadblock leading to a residential area in Beijing on 8 June 2003.

In Beijing, authorities made good their leaders' pledge to act. They closed cinemas, karaoke bars, libraries, Internet cafés, and swimming pools, and quarantined entire buildings, including three university apartments and 27 SARS-designated hospitals. Schools were shut, and an online study service was set up for the 1.7 million students affected. As business vanished, restaurants voluntarily closed. The city emptied in "the most spectacular of disappearing acts," said *Time* magazine.[6] People stayed home, were quarantined, or tried to flee. Streets were empty, with traffic less than a quarter of the normal. Public life came to a standstill. And everywhere the smell of boiling vinegar pervaded.

In all, 30,000 people were quarantined in Beijing. Many more, perhaps as much as 20% to 30% of the population, isolated themselves. In Nanjing, 10,000 were quarantined in one stroke. Elsewhere, entire villages were sealed. In Guangxi, mass gatherings of more than 50 people were banned.

For this people's war, China developed "people's surveillance". Where China was lacking, it found ways to make do, using time-tested methods such as quarantine and thermometers. By mobilizing the entire population, China was able to rapidly identify the chains of transmission and isolate the cases. In this way, a situation that appeared to be rapidly growing out control was brought to heel within two months.

Old traditions were revived. Grassroots party structures gained new vigour, as people grew wary of outsiders. In Hebei, a province next to Beijing, villagers set up roadblocks at commuter entrances, their mini Great Walls. Vehicle wheels were sprayed with disinfectant, temperatures tested, and some cars turned back. Visitors from Beijing were especially unwelcome.

Other provinces also set up similar stop-spray-screen stations. Mr Mykkanen came across 20 such SARS stations in a four-hour drive from Datong, Shanxi, to Hohhot, Inner Mongolia. Yunnan Province even drove out tourists. Lijiang City closed all hotels in popular tourist spots.

Neighbourhood committees watched for SARS symptoms and returning migrants. One volunteer observed 10 households. Any new returnees were isolated for 15 days and had their temperature checked three times a day. Villagers also checked on one another, scrutinizing travel movements and possible symptoms.

"It's an intricate web of surveillance. It's like a fishing net," said Dr James Maguire, a member of the WHO team that visited Hebei. "It uses the traditional neighbourhood community unit so it is quite unique."

The impressive surveillance measures were matched by extreme measures to control the spread of SARS. Not all of these were rational. Some provoked fear. In Chagugang town, near the port of Tianjin, thousands rioted over plans to convert a school into a SARS ward. Two buildings were ransacked.[7]

Infection control was overdone at times. Procedures were unwieldy or unsustainable. Hospital staff made up for the lack of correctly designed protective gear by wearing whatever was available, in layers. In Guangxi, WHO experts found staff wearing three layers of gowns, gloves, and multilayered masks. Such clothing was oppressively hot—and unnecessary.

Dozens of fever clinics for SARS patients that were organized within Beijing hospitals were closed after reports of nosocomial infections. A study later found that visitors to these fever clinics were at high risk of contracting SARS because of inadequate separation of patients.[8]

Joint WHO–Ministry of Health teams, in their visits to the provinces, noted that cases were not widely dispersed and that the people had a remarkable level of knowledge of the disease. In one village in Hebei Province, the people had temporarily blocked a road to keep out visitors from Beijing. One of them said she was watching a roadblock on a side street to prevent the spread of SARS. Temperatures were being taken several times a day. Clearly, the nation was responding.

Slowly, the number of cases fell. By the second half of May, confidence was growing that SARS would be contained. Early case detection through the "people's surveillance" and large-scale quarantine, isolation, and infection control at designated SARS hospitals contributed to ending the epidemic. WHO lifted its travel advisory on Hong Kong and Guangdong on 23 May, followed by Inner Mongolia, Shanxi, and Tianjin on 13 June. At a press conference on 24 June, WHO lifted its travel advisory for Beijing and declared China SARS-free.

OLD LESSONS RELEARNT

SARS prompted the best and worst models of public-health responses, and exposed many of the weaknesses and strengths of the world's most populous nation.

The disease put infectious diseases firmly back on China's health agenda and highlighted critical cash-strapped areas of health provision. It served as a wake-up call. It demonstrated the need for a rapid-response capacity to combat changing disease situations. It showed how one nation's weak response could endanger the world's public-health security, and how a response drawing on unique local strengths—such as mass mobilization—could be effective.

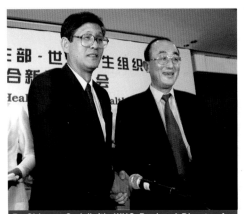

Dr Shigeru Omi (left), WHO Regional Director for the Western Pacific, shakes hands with Chinese Executive Vice Health Minister Gao Qiang after a press conference announcing the lifting of the travel advisory for Beijing, 24 June 2003.

China strengthened its disease-control fundamentals. On 9 May 2003, the State Council issued a new Regulation on Public Health Emergency Response to strengthen surveillance. The regulation covered future new disease outbreaks and improved reporting and response, including cooperation with technical agencies. In August 2004, the National Law on Communicable Diseases Prevention and Control was revised. Both of these changes were based on the experiences and lessons learnt from SARS.

The serious effects of delaying or blocking the exchange of public and scientific information are evident: rumours and myths replace facts and science. And once credibility is damaged, trust takes a long time to return.

In a country with great disparities in health care, where extensive computed tomography (CT) scans can be found in areas of low immunization coverage, SARS was also a timely reminder of the need for equity in health care—and the value of simple strategies over high technology.

This new disease, which spread on the wings of modernization, was ultimately beaten by some of the simplest and oldest tools of public health: contact tracing, quarantine, and isolation.

REFERENCES

[1] Assessing the impact and costs of SARS in developing Asia. In: *Asian Development Outlook 2003 Update*. Manila, Asian Development Bank, 2003.

[2] Enserink M. SARS in China: China's missed chance. *Science*, 2003, 301 (5631):294–296.

[3] Zhong et al. Epidemiology and cause of severe acute respiratory syndrome (SARS) in Guangdong in February 2003. *The Lancet*, 25 October 2003, 362(9393):1353–1358.

[4] Kong E. Two dead after boiling white vinegar. *South China Morning Post*, 13 February 2003.

[5] Liang W et al. Severe acute respiratory syndrome, Beijing, 2003. *Emerging Infectious Diseases*, 2004, 10(1):25–31.

[6] Beech H, Forney M. Control issues. *Time Magazine*, 5 May 2003.

[7] Mykkanen P, Eckholm E. Villagers in China riot over SARS. *New York Times*, 29 April 2003.

[8] Wu J et al. Risk factors for SARS among persons without known contact with SARS patients, Beijing, China. *Emerging Infectious Diseases*, 2004, 10(2): 210–216.

6 HONG KONG (CHINA): HOSPITALS ──UNDER SIEGE──

Twenty buses wound out of Block E of the Amoy Gardens residential complex in Kowloon in the dead of night on 1 April 2003. Picked out by the cold, white glare of TV camera lights, the men, women and children inside stared back in fear above their surgical masks. For the people of Hong Kong (China), this almost Dantesque scene seemed to be proof that the SARS outbreak had entered a new and altogether more frightening phase.

In fact, Amoy Gardens was to be the final big scare of the Hong Kong outbreak—but its effect was to linger for many months afterwards.

The sudden appearance of the virus in a housing block, with no clear indication at first of how or why it had infected so many people, changed everything.

From that day on, normal life in Hong Kong came to a standstill. People rarely ventured out of their homes without a mask. In a city where shopping is a mass activity, stores stood empty. Cinemas screened movies to nobody. And the normally bustling restaurants were silent.

International visitors stopped arriving, especially after 2 April, when WHO advised against all but essential travel to the territory. One by one, the aircraft of Hong Kong's No 1 airline, Cathay Pacific Airways, were mothballed at Chek Lap Kok airport. In the end, SARS cost Hong Kong billions of dollars in lost business, leaving the city teetering on the brink of its third recession in six years.

The nightmare was to last until 23 June 2003, when, 20 days after the last case was isolated, the outbreak was declared over [Figure 6.1]. By then the virus had infected 1,755 people, 299 of whom died. Health workers accounted for 386 cases (22% of the total). Four doctors, two health-care assistants, a nurse, and a ward attendant died.[1]

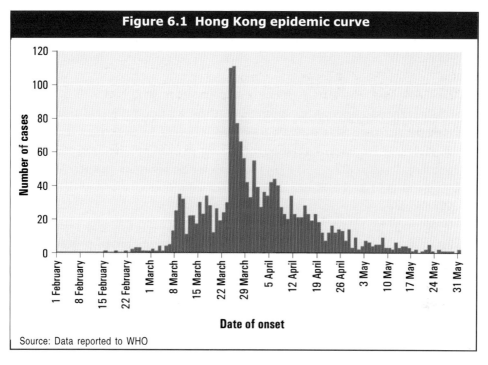

Figure 6.1 Hong Kong epidemic curve

Number of cases

Date of onset

Source: Data reported to WHO

OUTBREAK AT PRINCE OF WALES HOSPITAL

Before the Amoy Gardens outbreak, most SARS cases in Hong Kong had been limited to hospital settings. The first hospital to feel the full impact of the mysterious new virus from China had been the Prince of Wales. What happened there was the start of a crisis that would push Hong Kong's health-care system to the limit and make heroes of front-line hospital workers.

On 10 March 2003, seven doctors and four nurses from ward 8A of the Prince of Wales Hospital called in sick. Accounts of the cluster of infections appeared in a few Hong Kong Chinese newspapers the next day. Alerted by these reports, the Department of Health announced on 11 March that it was investigating hospital staff members who had developed "fever and upper respiratory infection".[2] The cases were reported to WHO. By the end of the day, 50 staff were on sick leave. All were recalled for medical examination; 23 were hospitalized and isolated.[1]

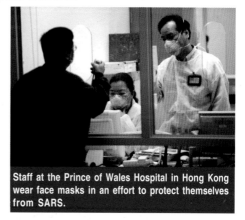

Staff at the Prince of Wales Hospital in Hong Kong wear face masks in an effort to protect themselves from SARS.

By 12 March, a preliminary investigation suggested an infection that was transmitted through droplets and fomites (materials contaminated with body secretions) with an incubation period of one to seven days.[1] The investigators used a case definition of fever and chills.

The index case was Mr CT, a Hong Kong resident who had visited a friend from San Francisco staying in room 906 at the Metropole Hotel from 18 to 23 February. To reach his friend's room, Mr CT had to walk past room 911, where Professor LJL, who had brought the virus from Guangdong, stayed on 21 February. Fever, chills, and rigors starting on 24 February pushed Mr CT to seek medical help at the Prince of Wales accident and emergency department on 28 February.

He returned four days later and was admitted to ward 8A with pneumonia. But his illness was not severe enough to trigger infection-control procedures or to prompt reporting to the Department of Health, which had instituted enhanced surveillance for severe community-acquired pneumonia on 12 February, following news of the Guangdong outbreak. Only on 13 March, when he was suspected of being the index case of the outbreak, was Mr CT isolated. By then his condition was already improving. The next day he was confirmed as the index case.[1]

SARS was subsequently diagnosed in 143 of Mr CT's contacts: 50 health workers, 17 medical students, 30 patients in ward 8A, 42 visitors to the ward, and four relatives who visited Mr CT in the ward.[1] One other person infected with SARS was not included in the tally, as his infection was diagnosed in Beijing: Mr LSK, the index case on flight CA112 [see Chapter 15].

Prince of Wales doctors attributed the super-spreading event involving Mr CT to failure to apply proper isolation precautions and use of a nebulized bronchodilator.[3] In all, 239 people fell ill sometime between 5 and 31 March during the Prince of Wales outbreak.

A HEALTH SYSTEM UNDER THREAT

Even as the Prince of Wales Hospital was grappling with the mystery outbreak among its health-care workers, other hospitals were fighting smaller fires.[1]

A sister-in-law of Mr CT developed symptoms on 10 March and was admitted to the private Baptist Hospital on 13 March. She stayed in two wards before being transferred to a public hospital. Four health workers from these wards became sick, and the hospital notified the Department of Health of the outbreak on 21 March. Contact tracing and medical surveillance eventually uncovered 25 transmissions in the Baptist Hospital: 10 hospital staff members, 11 patients (in the two wards), three visitors, and a visiting doctor. The visiting doctor passed on the virus to his wife and two of his patients. Five household contacts of the affected patients were also infected.

On 2 March, a 72-year-old Canadian tourist was admitted to the private St Paul's Hospital. He was infected during his stay in room 902 of the Metropole Hotel and passed on the virus to three health workers, five visitors, and one patient at St Paul's. Two family contacts of these cases were also infected. When the Canadian's condition worsened, he was transferred on 8 March to the intensive care unit of Queen Mary Hospital. As a result of adequate infection-control practices, no further transmissions were recorded.

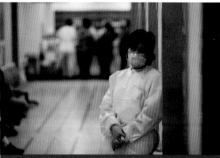

Fifty health workers, all contacts of the index case, fell ill during the Prince of Wales outbreak.

A frequent traveller to Guangzhou was admitted to Queen Elizabeth Hospital on 9 March and died from SARS on 30 March. A doctor and two nurses at the hospital developed pneumonia between 12 and 16 March. The wife of the index case and a relative of the patient in the next bed were also infected.

On 13 March, Pamela Youde Nethersole Eastern Hospital reported six health workers with atypical pneumonia to the Department of Health. The infection was traced to a middle-aged man who travelled frequently to southern China. After a trip to Zhongshan, Guangdong, on 22–23 February, he was admitted to the hospital on 2 March and died on 16 March. The outbreak affected 14 people: the index case, seven health workers, one patient, one visitor, and four close contacts of the affected health workers.

Patients who were not suspected of having SARS but were eventually found to have the disease sparked outbreaks in seven other hospitals. At Alice Ho Miu Ling Nethersole Hospital, 40 staff members, 75 patients, 17 visitors, and 24 close contacts were affected. Most hospital workers got the disease through direct contact with SARS patients in general wards who had unsuspected infection. At the time of contact, all hospital workers had used masks but not necessarily other protective devices.[4] The families of the affected hospital workers were not infected.

SARS patients also caused an outbreak, reported on 2 April, in the United Christian Hospital. Three patients with non-SARS diagnoses (including two residents of Amoy Gardens) were eventually identified as the cause. The outbreak affected 26 staff members, only five of whom worked in SARS wards. A distraught caller told a local radio show on 4 April that her son who worked at United Christian Hospital did not dare go home for fear of infecting his family. "I do not even know where he is," said the sobbing woman.[5]

SARS-DESIGNATED HOSPITAL

Princess Margaret Hospital, a 1,200-bed acute hospital serving 1.5 million people, was the only Hong Kong hospital with dedicated facilities for infectious disease (four isolation wards with 86 beds). On 26 March, it was chosen to be a designated hospital for SARS cases. At that time, it had been managing about 100 SARS patients but none of its staff had been infected.

To allow the hospital to focus on SARS cases, all the other patients were transferred to other hospitals from 29 March, and the accident and emergency department was closed. To become the SARS-designated hospital at the time of the Amoy Gardens outbreak was unfortunate timing for the Princess Margaret.

The hospital admitted 93 SARS transfers from other hospitals on 29 March. By the end of the week, 555 had been admitted, many of them from Amoy Gardens. The hospital was overwhelmed not only by the number of new patients but also by the critical condition of many of them.

The 593 cases treated at the Princess Margaret Hospital made up 34% of all SARS cases in Hong Kong—more than the number treated in any other hospital. Although the hospital managed at first to avoid infections among its staff, the outbreak took a heavy toll. A core team of intensive-care-unit doctors and nurses were infected in the first week of April. On 7 April alone, 12 Princess Margaret staff developed SARS. In total, 62 members of the staff were infected, 25 in the intensive care unit. This represented 16% of the total of 386 health workers who were infected with SARS during the outbreak.[6]

LEGAL BASE STRENGTHENED

The Quarantine and Prevention of Disease Ordinance, which was first enacted in 1936, had been revised from time to time. On 27 March 2003, the Director of Health added SARS to the list of infectious diseases, making it the 28th infectious disease listed, in addition to three "special" diseases—plague, yellow fever, and cholera. Medical practitioners were required to notify the Department of Health if they had reason to suspect the existence of SARS.

SARS was included in the ordinanace mainly to provide the legal basis to require all close contacts of SARS patients to report daily for up to 10 days to one of four designated medical centres. Contacts had to stay home and not go to work or school. The designated medical centres started operating from 31 March.

The move was a tough choice, acknowledged the Secretary for Health, Welfare and Food, Dr Yeoh Eng-kiong. "The ordinance [had] not been invoked for decades. And, internationally, it has rarely been invoked because everyone is worried that it may backfire."[7] Draconian measures such as compulsory quarantine were deliberately avoided initially because of concerns about driving SARS patients into hiding, issues of civil liberty and public acceptability, and uncertainty about effectiveness and the feasibility of enforcement.

The ordinance was later used to enable the quarantine of the residents of Block E, Amoy Gardens, on 31 March, and the evacuation of the block on 1 April, as evidence increasingly pointed to an environmental source for the virus [see Chapter 16]. On 17 April, the legislation was further amended to provide for temperature checks of travellers and to prevent SARS contacts from leaving Hong Kong.

TRACING HOUSEHOLDS BY ELECTRONIC MEANS

In the Amoy Gardens outbreak, the police were called in to trace households that had moved out of Block E before the isolation order on 31 March. By 4 April, the police had tracked down 55 of those 113 families.

On 6 April, the police began using its sophisticated Major Incident Investigation and Disaster Support System (MIIDSS) to assist the Department of Health in epidemiological investigations. The system allowed SARS investigators to validate addresses, map out their geographical distribution, reveal potential sources or routes of virus transmission, and show the connection between cases and contacts. By 7 April, the police said they had contacted all the other 58 families that had moved out of Block E.

Separately, the unprecedented speed and volume of cases swamped the paper-based disease-reporting system. The problem was resolved, under the leadership of Dr Yeoh, with the launch on 8 April of an electronic database (e-SARS) that enabled the Department of Health and the Hospital Authority to share and exchange information in real time. The collaborative application of e-SARS and MIIDSS significantly enhanced the swiftness and capacity of case investigation and contact tracing, thus reducing further spread of infection.

A REVIEW OF THE GOVERNMENT'S HANDLING OF SARS

To review how well the Government, including the Hospital Authority, had managed and controlled the outbreak, Chief Executive Tung Chee-hwa convened a SARS Expert Committee, composed of 11 international and local experts. The committee, reporting on 2 October 2003, declared that "overall, the epidemic in Hong Kong was handled well, although there were clearly significant shortcomings of system

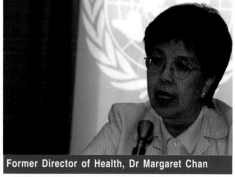
Former Director of Health, Dr Margaret Chan

performance during the early days of the epidemic when little was known about the disease or its cause. ... The committee has not found any individual deemed to be culpable of negligence, lack of diligence or maladministration."[1]

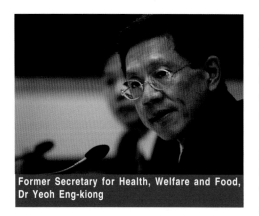

Former Secretary for Health, Welfare and Food, Dr Yeoh Eng-kiong

The committee also issued 46 recommendations to prepare the territory against a future outbreak. As a result, infection-control training for health-care workers was stepped up; a Centre for Health Protection (under the Department of Health) opened on 1 June 2004 to better focus on emergency preparedness; 1,400 isolation beds were made available in 14 public hospitals; and funds were sought for a new infectious disease centre at the Princess Margaret Hospital.

A separate review panel formed by the Hospital Authority to review the performance of the public hospital system during the crisis released its report to the public on 16 October 2003. The report did not seek to apportion blame but to make recommendations for future outbreaks. "We have emphasized the need for a strong and immediate response during crisis," the report stated. "Strong leadership and effective communication are essential."[6]

A third report, by a Legislative Council Select Committee, released on 5 July 2004,[8] was highly critical of the Government's response. In the end, the Secretary for Health, Welfare and Food and the Chairman of the Hospital Authority, Dr Leong Che-hong, resigned.

PAINFUL LESSONS LEARNT

SARS took Hong Kong, and indeed the world, by storm. When it struck Hong Kong in March 2003, little was known about the disease. The magnitude of the outbreak, the nonspecific nature of the symptoms, the lack of a quick diagnostic test for the syndrome, and the speed with which workload and cases increased had all contributed to the problems in managing the outbreak.

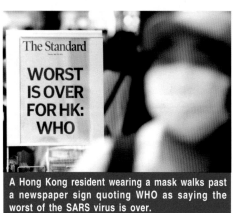

A Hong Kong resident wearing a mask walks past a newspaper sign quoting WHO as saying the worst of the SARS virus is over.

In the words of Dr David Heymann, Executive Director for Communicable Diseases of WHO at the time of the outbreak, Hong Kong's efforts to stem the spread of SARS were nothing less than "heroic". And Dr Jeffrey Koplan, former director of the American CDC, likened Hong Kong's well-established public-health system to a dam protecting its people from floods. For 50 years, it worked well. However, an unprecedented massive flood struck and the wall was found to be deficient; a higher wall had to be built. Hong Kong learnt painful lessons in the SARS epidemic and began taking proactive measures to strengthen the preparedness of its health system for public-health emergencies.

References

[1] *SARS in Hong Kong: from Experience to Action.* Report of the SARS Expert Committee, October 2003.

[2] *DH concerned about PWH Case.* Hong Kong Special Administrative Region of the People's Republic of China, Government Information Centre, 11 March 2003 (http://www.info.gov.hk/gia/general/200303/11/0311214.htm, accessed 1 April 2005).

[3] Wong R, Hui D. Index patient and SARS outbreak in Hong Kong. *Emerging Infectious Diseases*, 2004, 10(2):339-341.

[4] Ho AS, Sung JJY, Chan-Yeung M. An outbreak of severe acute respiratory syndrome among hospital workers in a community hospital in Hong Kong. *Annals of Internal Medicine*, 2003, 139(7):564–567.

[5] Reuters Health. Hong Kong police launch SARS manhunt, 4 April 2003.

[6] Report of the Hospital Authority Review Panel on the SARS Outbreak. Hong Kong (China), Hospital Authority, September 2003.

[7] Press conference on the latest measures to contain the spread of atypical pneumonia. Hong Kong Special Administrative Region of the People's Republic of China, Government Information Centre, 27 March 2003 (http://www.info.gov.hk/webbroadcast/pres279e.html, accessed 1 April 2005).

[8] *Report of the Legislative Council Select Committee to inquire into the handling of the Severe Acute Respiratory Syndrome outbreak by the Government and the Hospital Authority, July 2004.* Hong Kong Special Administrative Region of the People's Republic of China, Legislative Council, 2004 (http://www.legco.gov.hk/yr03-04/english/sc/sc_sars/reports/sars_rpt.htm, accessed 1 April 2005).

7 VIET NAM: TOUGH _DECISIONS PAY OFF_

FIRST ALERT

"There is something strange going on, but I am not sure exactly what it is," Dr Carlo Urbani, WHO's communicable disease specialist in Viet Nam, said on Monday, 3 March 2003. He had just been to the Hanoi-French Hospital and was telling WHO Representative Pascale Brudon about Mr JC, an American businessman who had recently arrived from Hong Kong (China) with atypical pneumonia.

By Wednesday afternoon, when four hospital staff were hospitalized and two more fell ill, it was clear that something was indeed happening. By the end of the day, seven hospital staff had been hospitalized. All of them had been in close contact with Mr JC.

An event of major public-health importance was definitely unfolding. Dr Urbani pressed for a reorganization of the Hanoi-French Hospital, and particularly for stronger infection controls. "But everything was very chaotic at that time," Ms Brudon recalled. "From the very start there was a sense of urgency. As soon as we heard about the first cases we informed the Ministry of Health. I also called the hospital's manager, who was then in France, to return to Viet Nam and deal with the impending crisis."

URGENT ACTION URGED

On Friday, 7 March, the situation was becoming more alarming, but there had been no response from the hospital management or the Ministry. Relying on a false-positive result, both believed that Mr JC was suffering from influenza B. Ms Brudon wrote to the Ministry of Health urging action to address this "potential public-health concern and international health hazard". She offered WHO's technical assistance and requested a speedier visa approval process for international experts. She also wrote to the manager of the Hanoi-French Hospital to emphasize the seriousness of the situation and the need to strengthen infection control. She recommended that all other patients be discharged or transferred, and that entry to the hospital be strictly limited to reduce the risk of exposure.

Twelve people had now been hospitalized in the Hanoi-French Hospital and many more were falling sick, adding a greater sense of urgency. "You absolutely must arrange a meeting with the Ministry of Health this weekend," Dr Urbani told Ms Brudon. The virus—or whatever it was—was spreading at such dramatic speed, he said, that no time could be lost.

A 9 a.m. meeting with the Vice-Minister of Health on Sunday, 9 March, would prove to be decisive. Dr Urbani and Ms Brudon argued at length for immediate action against the

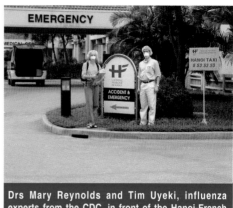

Drs Mary Reynolds and Tim Uyeki, influenza experts from the CDC, in front of the Hanoi-French Hospital.

dangerous and contagious new illness. Eventually, the Vice-Minister was convinced. He assigned a local team to review the situation at the Hanoi-French Hospital that same day. The key decision was agreeing to bring in experts to help investigate and control the outbreak. Dr Hitoshi Oshitani, WHO's Regional Adviser for Communicable Disease Surveillance and Response, arrived on 10 March to head the WHO team. Dr Tim Uyeki, an influenza expert from the Centers for Disease Control and Prevention (CDC), United States of America, flew in on 11 March.

WHO held an emergency meeting with the Vice-Minister of Health and the director of the National Institute of Hygiene and Epidemiology on 12 March. Drs Oshitani and Uyeki called the situation grave and, with support from Ms Brudon, explained why. Dr Uyeki, the influenza expert, said that a new pathogen, and not influenza, was the probable cause.

These conclusions, according to Dr Uyeki, were based on the preliminary epidemiology, clinical features, and estimated incubation period of the early Hanoi cases—information provided by Dr Urbani. "He is the hero of SARS for describing these so meticulously, for trying to implement control measures, and for notifying the world about the outbreak. Everyone else contributed to what Dr Urbani started," Dr Uyeki later said. Dr Uyeki recommended immediate implementation of control measures to prevent further transmission in hospital and surveillance for new cases, including contact tracing.

Dr Oshitani offered the help of WHO reference laboratories in providing the required laboratory confirmation. This was a public-health problem of regional and global significance, he said. The Ministry of Health should therefore take over the control and management of the Hanoi-French Hospital and draw on international assistance in carrying out research on the disease and the clinical management of hospitalized cases. The Vice-Minister agreed to most of the recommendations of the WHO team, but balked at the suggested takeover of the Hanoi-French Hospital because it was a private hospital.

Urgent action implemented

As WHO had recommended, the Hanoi-French Hospital discharged all its other patients on 12 March and stopped admitting new patients other than staff members who were believed to be infected. All other suspected cases were thereafter admitted to special wards at the National Institute for Clinical Research in Tropical Medicine at Bach Mai Hospital. Urgent technical issues—case definition, case management, and treatment guidelines—were discussed in a telephone conference with WHO Headquarters in Geneva. On 14 March, the Prime Minister, who had been informed about the evolving situation, responded by creating an interministerial steering committee. The Ministry of Health had agreed to WHO's suggestion and formed a Task Force the day before to manage the outbreak.

As soon as the WHO office in Viet Nam had an agreed strategy, Dr Oshitani returned to Manila to manage the regional response. On 16 March, Professor Aileen Plant took over as WHO team leader for the next 11 weeks. By then, a nine-person international team to help investigate and control the outbreak was in place at the WHO Viet Nam office. In all, 25 international experts and six local staff members would join the WHO SARS team in Viet Nam.

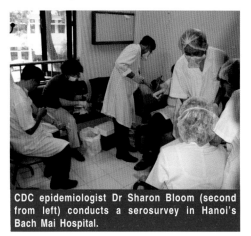

CDC epidemiologist Dr Sharon Bloom (second from left) conducts a serosurvey in Hanoi's Bach Mai Hospital.

Professor Plant quickly divided the team into groups looking after tasks such as epidemiology, rumour surveillance, laboratory testing, infection control and contact tracing, always working with counterparts in the Ministry of Health. She recalled, "The team [was] extraordinary—[the members] did whatever was asked of them, whenever it needed to be done. For instance one team member had been married only three weeks and left her husband; one had a gravely ill wife that he left behind. Everywhere people did whatever they could. The nurses and doctors at the French Hospital were just amazing; we will never know what they went through. Imagine going to work each day, watching your colleagues get ill and die with a new disease, and at the same time [feeling] the [diseases] beginning … in [you]—it is just un-imaginable. Yet, to my knowledge, not one doctor, not one nurse, in Viet Nam refused to look after people with SARS."

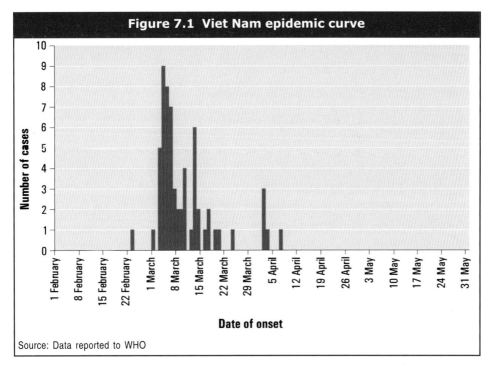

Figure 7.1 Viet Nam epidemic curve

Number of cases (y-axis)
Date of onset (x-axis)

Source: Data reported to WHO

DEALING WITH RUMOURS AND AIR TRAVEL

To combat SARS, Viet Nam also had to combat rumours. The local WHO office had to contend with intense pressure not only from the local and international press but also from a very worried international community. A call from Ho Chi Minh City reporting a suspicious illness and fever in an American child roused Ms Brudon from sleep early in the morning of 18 March. It later proved to be a false alarm. Still, WHO team members had to be sent hurriedly to Ho Chi Minh City, and the child had to be evacuated to Taiwan, China, at a time when charter airlines were not keen to perform such a service, even for non-SARS cases.

On 15 March, in an effort to avert the spread of the disease through international travel, Ms Brudon sought to have a public announcement aired on all flights out of Viet Nam. The message would describe the SARS symptoms and advise any passengers with those symptoms to notify the medical authorities. The managers of the international airlines swiftly shot down the request. "They couldn't read a notice like that on flights," Ms Brudon recalls being told. "People would be terrified." But after some discussion, airlines allowed the distribution of pamphlets in English, French, and Vietnamese describing the symptoms and the ongoing outbreak in Hanoi. Once the airport authorities knew what to look for, they were able to help screen passengers. A doctor from the Hanoi-French Hospital who was unwell was stopped from boarding his international flight. He was later found to have SARS. Soon after on the same day, WHO Headquarters issued its travel advisory as evidence mounted that the disease was spreading by air travel along international routes. Another doctor, who had also been infected at the Hanoi-French Hospital, wasn't stopped. He boarded flight AF171 on 22 March to Paris even though he was already unwell [see Chapter 15]. Two passengers on that flight were infected, as was the manager of the hotel in Hanoi where the doctor had stayed.[1]

A tragic incident around that time was a grim reminder of the risk of international travel. On 11 March, Dr Urbani called Ms Brudon from Hanoi airport on his way to a conference in Bangkok that had been planned for months. "He said he didn't feel well, and at first, I didn't think much of it," she told others later. "I told him to go, that we could handle things in Viet Nam without him." Then remembering that Dr Urbani had been shivering when they had last met in her office, she called Dr Brian Doberstyn, Director of Communicable Disease Control at WHO's Manila office. "I told him I thought Carlo might be sick," she said. As the two decided, Dr Urbani was met at the Bangkok airport and, because he had symptoms, was quickly isolated at a hospital. Less than three weeks later, on 29 March 2003, the doctor who first alerted the world to the existence of SARS died of the very disease he had helped to identify. His death, just when the Viet Nam office was working overtime to contain the outbreak, was a harsh blow for WHO. "We were all working insanely to try and stop SARS," said Ms Brudon. "And when Carlo died, it made the fight even more difficult." It was inspiring, however, to see the WHO office overflowing with beautiful flowers as locals and foreigners mourned Dr Urbani.

But Dr Urbani's efforts were paying off. The outbreak appeared to be coming to an end without spreading to the community. Strengthening infection control at Bach Mai Hospital became a high priority. When infection-control experts from Médecins Sans Frontières joined the WHO team, they were assigned to work with the hospital staff to ensure that internationally agreed protocols were understood and followed.

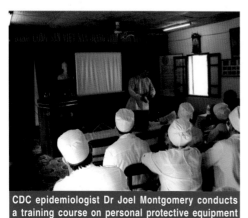

CDC epidemiologist Dr Joel Montgomery conducts a training course on personal protective equipment in Ninh Binh Province.

Before Viet Nam could declare the outbreak ended, however, rumours of a cluster of cases in Ninh Binh Province, about 90 kilometres south-east of Hanoi, were received at the start of April. A new case found in the province on 3 April was linked to the Hanoi-French Hospital. Six other people in the cluster were infected, but these were the last transmissions in Viet Nam. Prompt action had limited the outbreak in the country to only 63 people, most of these falling ill in the early days when tighter infection controls and surveillance still had to be set up.

First country to interrupt transmission

On 28 April 2003, about two months after its first case was recorded and 20 days after its last case, Viet Nam became the first country with an outbreak to be removed from the WHO list of areas with recent transmission of SARS. WHO and the Ministry of Health hosted a dinner to celebrate the occasion. "It was a very big day for us," Ms Brudon said, adding that, amid the toasts, there was awareness of the continued need for surveillance. "Even as we were drinking champagne, we were still looking for rumours. We weren't exactly nervous, but we couldn't let our guard down just yet." But the SARS outbreak in Viet Nam had indeed been successfully contained, and no further cases were detected. Said an exultant Ms Brudon, "It was a triumph both for WHO and for Viet Nam."

Why the success?

So why was Viet Nam able to control SARS? The early alert and actions of Dr Urbani were clearly vital. So was Viet Nam's willingness to address the outbreak rapidly and vigorously. In a collaboration based on trust, the Vietnamese Government made hard choices and made them quickly, following the advice of WHO and its team of international experts in Hanoi.

One of the earliest measures had been to set up a high-level SARS Task Force within the Ministry of Health, which met every day, and a national intersectoral Steering Committee for SARS Control. A special budget was allocated to the Ministry of Health for supplies, training and support for health staff working with SARS patients.

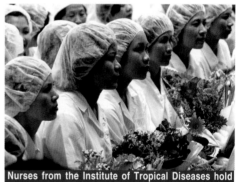

Nurses from the Institute of Tropical Diseases hold flowers at a ceremony on 2 May 2003 marking the release of the last SARS patients from the institute in Hanoi.

The Government also designated hospitals for suspected SARS cases and strengthened infection-control measures. It set up quarantine areas and isolation rooms at border crossings, airports, and seaports. Provincial governments were alerted in early March, at which time provincial steering committees for SARS control were created, local medical staff were trained, and guidelines were issued. Public-information campaigns helped prevent panic in the population.

"Immediate political commitment and leadership at the highest level were vital," said Ms Brudon. "A developing country—hit by an especially severe outbreak—can triumph over a disease when reporting is prompt and open, when WHO assistance is quickly requested and fully supported, and when rapid case detection, immediate isolation, infection control, and vigorous contact tracing are put in place."

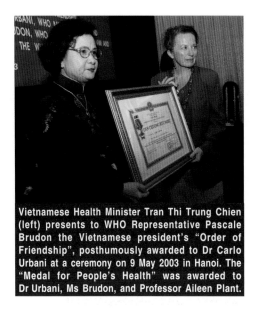
Vietnamese Health Minister Tran Thi Trung Chien (left) presents to WHO Representative Pascale Brudon the Vietnamese president's "Order of Friendship", posthumously awarded to Dr Carlo Urbani at a ceremony on 9 May 2003 in Hanoi. The "Medal for People's Health" was awarded to Dr Urbani, Ms Brudon, and Professor Aileen Plant.

In the final analysis, perhaps the most important factor was luck. There was only one super-spreading event—the index case. Dr Urbani's alert may have made infection control for all subsequent cases much more effective, as some would argue, but infection control was never perfect, perhaps just good enough, and luck kept the lapses from leading to further spread. As the experience in other countries showed, super-spreading events could quickly arise from cases that were missed. Nevertheless, rapid recognition of the outbreak and rapid implementation of control measures were exactly what were needed.

But the last word on the outbreak must be reserved for Dr Carlo Urbani. He did what was needed, knowing he was risking his life to save others. Recognizing his contribution to the world and Viet Nam in the control of SARS, the Vietnamese Government posthumously awarded Dr Urbani the Medal for People's Health, as well as the Order of Friendship, the highest honour given to foreigners.

REFERENCES

[1] Desenclos JC et al. Introduction of SARS in France, March–April, 2003. *Emerging Infectious Diseases*, 2004, 10(2):195–200.

8 SINGAPORE: WAVES _OF TRANSMISSION_

Picture this scene from a horror movie. The monster has been slain after an epic struggle. But just as the heroes exhale deeply and savour their victory, the monster rises again, changed but undefeated. Fighting SARS in Singapore was like being in one of those horror movies.

Recurrent waves of virus transmission, each with a new type of super-spreading event, alternated with rapid, heroic attempts by the Ministry of Health, the Government as a whole, and the people to halt further transmission. The fact that only five patients accounted for 103 of the 205 probable SARS cases in Singapore,[1] and that the vast majority of patients infected no one else, showed how devastating super-spreading events could be.[2]

INDEX CASES

As in other places outside China with substantial local outbreaks, individuals who had stayed at the Metropole Hotel [see Chapter 14] imported the first cases of SARS into Singapore. Shortly after returning to Singapore, three persons with pneumonia were admitted to hospital from 1 to 3 March. The Ministry of Health was notified of these cases on 6 March, and advised immediate isolation.[3] Until then, they had been nursed in an open ward, without barrier infection-control measures.[4] One of them, 22-year-old Ms EM, went on to seed an outbreak at Tan Tock Seng Hospital, with 22 of her contacts developing SARS.

The Ministry of Health kept in close contact with WHO about early cases, and immediately advised the body that a Singaporean physician who had treated the cases at Tan Tock Seng Hospital was boarding a plane in New York, bound for Frankfurt, Germany, with symptoms [see 15 March in Chapter 1]. This information was a key piece in the puzzle that led WHO to issue an unprecedented second global alert, only three days after the first.

INITIAL CONTROL MEASURES

To show how seriously they took the emerging threat, the Ministry of Health and the Government quickly responded with a comprehensive set of measures to contain the outbreak.

- Cases were identified early, and isolated promptly at Tan Tock Seng Hospital.
- Hospitals improved their infection controls. They limited visitors, screened patients in the emergency department, and made efforts to locate surplus isolation beds in anticipation of a wider outbreak.
- Contacts and sources of identified cases were traced.
- Travel to places with SARS outbreaks was discouraged.
- Campaigns were launched to educate and inform the public. The Government issued regular press releases and held press conferences (often daily) chaired by Health Minister Lim Hng Kiang.
- Ministerial and bureaucratic task forces were formed to respond to the growing threat.
- The Infectious Diseases Act was amended to allow the Government to compel contacts of suspected SARS cases to be quarantined at home, and provide for fines for those who refused to comply.

FIRST THREE WAVES OF SPREAD

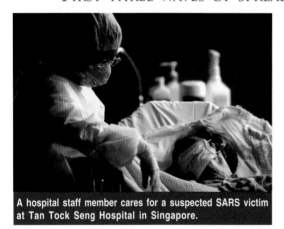

A hospital staff member cares for a suspected SARS victim at Tan Tock Seng Hospital in Singapore.

Despite these early measures, the SARS virus would not be so easily contained. One reason was the extent to which the virus had already spread, with many episodes of transmission by 12 March 2003, when WHO issued its first alert. By this date, this first wave of secondary cases already had symptoms, the virus had spread to the next wave of cases, and the third wave had started.

The second wave of spread was mostly from Ms AB, a 27-year-old Filipino nurse who was infected while caring for Ms EM at Tan Tock Seng Hospital. Ms AB was admitted to Tan Tock Seng Hospital on 10 March and isolated three days later. Twenty-two of her contacts in the ward (staff members, visitors, and other patients) were infected during those three days. Her husband may have been infected before she was admitted. One of the other patients infected was 53-year-old Ms PA, with diabetes and Gram-negative sepsis, who was admitted on the same day as Ms AB. She developed respiratory symptoms, and on 12 March she was transferred to the coronary care unit (CCU) as her symptoms were initially thought to be due to heart failure. Her presence in CCU resulted in a new round of virus transmission.

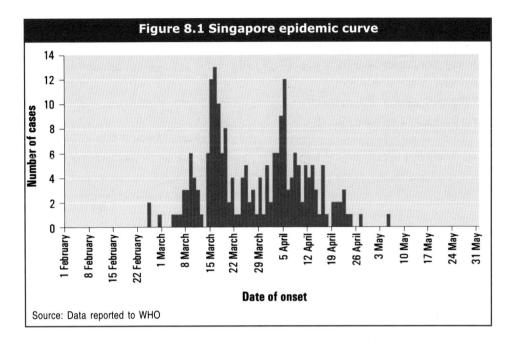

Figure 8.1 Singapore epidemic curve

Date of onset

Source: Data reported to WHO

These three generations of spread were confined to Tan Tock Seng Hospital and close contacts of cases. With effective hospital infection control in case treatment and follow-up of contacts, the Singapore outbreak was slowing down towards the end of March. There were no more episodes of hospital transmission in Tan Tock Seng Hospital, and no more cases were appearing in the community.

SPREAD FROM ATYPICAL CASES

But just when it seemed the outbreak was about to end, two patients who were infected at Tan Tock Seng Hospital, but missed because of atypical symptoms, were spreading the virus in the community and at other hospitals. The first was a 90-year-old resident of Orange Valley Nursing Home with multiple medical conditions.[5] She had been admitted to the Tan Tock Seng Hospital geriatric department on 7 March 2003 with pneumonia and urinary tract infection. She improved with antibiotics and was returned to the nursing home on 20 March, free of fever. In the following days, her breathing became progressively more laboured, and she was admitted on 25 March to Changi General Hospital, where she died on 30 March. Seven secondary cases, all in exposed family members and health-care workers at the nursing home and Changi General Hospital, were identified the week after.

The second cluster of cases to emerge from Tan Tock Seng Hospital would have more dramatic implications. Mr TKC, a 59-year-old man with multiple medical conditions (including ischemic heart disease with atrial fibrillation, a previous stroke with epilepsy, diabetes mellitus with kidney damage, and peripheral vascular disease) was treated as an in-patient at Tan Tock Seng Hospital from 5 to 20 March for diabetic kidney disease.[6] On 24 March he presented to Singapore General Hospital with gastrointestinal bleeding and a low-grade fever. Since his chest X-rays were normal, the source of his fever was ascribed to the *E.coli* bacteria found in his blood, and the fever responded to treatment with an antibiotic, as expected. It was only as the Singapore General Hospital outbreak was being controlled that he was identified as the index case.[7]

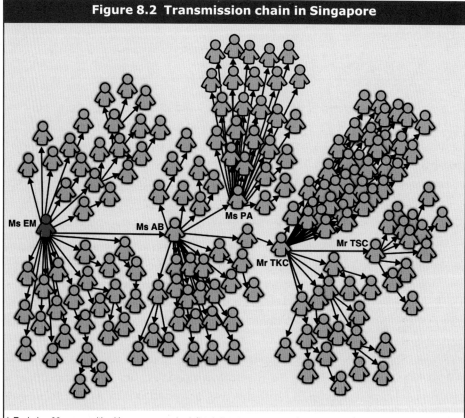

Figure 8.2 Transmission chain in Singapore

Ms EM

Ms AB

Ms PA

Mr TKC

Mr TSC

* Excludes 22 cases with either no or poorly defined direct contacts or who were cases translocated to Singapore and the seven contacts of one of these cases.

Source: Centers for Disease Control and Prevention, *Morbidity and Mortality Weekly Report*, 9 May 2003, 52(18):405–411.

The lessons from these episodes were clear: despite stringent controls, the virus would exploit every opportunity to evade detection and continue infecting people; super-spreading events were unforgiving; and the search for SARS cases had to be sensitive enough to catch atypical cases. The Singapore General Hospital outbreak led to a small cluster of seven cases in a social group that included workers from the hospital. The brother of the Singapore General Hospital index case set off a cluster at Pasir Panjang Wholesale Market [see Chapter 17] and infected several health-care workers and visitors to the National University Hospital, where he was first admitted.

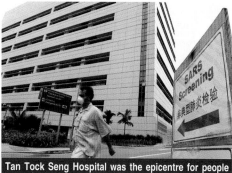

Tan Tock Seng Hospital was the epicentre for people experiencing symptoms of SARS in Singapore. As such, the Government designated it as an official SARS hospital.

CONTROL STRATEGIES

The successive waves of SARS infection from atypical cases and the devastation wreaked on the health-care system and on the people led to incremental improvements in control strategies. The key strategies that eventually led to containment were the following:[1]

HOSPITALS AND HEALTH-CARE FACILITIES

- Designation of Tan Tock Seng Hospital as a SARS hospital;
- Strict temperature surveillance of all staff and patients, isolation of staff, and identification of "fever clusters";
- Enforced use of fit-tested N95 masks and other protective equipment;
- Strict limits on hospital access for visitors and the general public;
- Establishment of peripheral "fever clinics" to take pressure off Tan Tock Seng Hospital, and properly assess and treat individuals with fever; and
- Infection control and isolation at primary health-care facilities.

COMMUNITY CONTROL

- Extensive, precise surveillance;
- Rapid tracing of sources and contacts, with personnel from the armed services and other sources ready to help when needed;
- Mandatory home quarantine up to 10 days from contact, with appropriate social support, as well as telephone and video surveillance and the threat of monetary fines and detention, to ensure compliance;

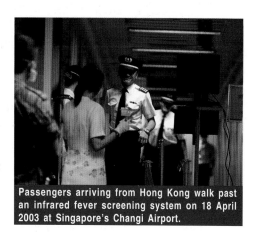

Passengers arriving from Hong Kong walk past an infrared fever screening system on 18 April 2003 at Singapore's Changi Airport.

- Ubiquitous temperature checks in schools, workplaces, and the community;
- A dedicated ambulance service to Tan Tock Seng Hospital; and
- Fever screening for incoming and outgoing passengers at Changi Airport and other entry points.

As might be expected, the use of very sensitive surveillance tools generated extra work and some false alarms. Other countries, fairly or unfairly, linked suspected SARS cases to individuals only in transit at Changi International Airport. A "fever" outbreak at the Institute of Mental Health, thought at first to be SARS, turned out to be due to the influenza B virus, but many inpatients and staff members had already been isolated or quarantined by the time the laboratory results were released.

A FIRM GOVERNMENT

In the Singapore Government's view, the community had a right to expect that all efforts would be made to limit further spread of the virus. By strictly enforcing quarantine orders, the Government showed that it was serious about doing all in its power to protect its citizens from being infected with SARS.

In an open letter to all Singaporeans on 22 April, Prime Minister Goh Chok Tong called for community cooperation, but made it clear the Government was not afraid to act firmly to stop the outbreak.[8] "For the wider good, we now have to take a tougher approach in enforcing Home Quarantine Orders," he said. "We simply cannot afford to have those on home quarantine breach it, and run the risk of going undetected for SARS, or worse, infecting others."

The purpose of these actions was clear. "These measures may be harsh," the Prime Minister added, "but they are necessary. Taking a lenient attitude will not help us break the cycle of infection. Instead, it may undermine the stringent infection controls we have painstakingly put in place to protect Singaporeans from SARS."

Early cooperation from Singapore provided essential information that helped in the global control of the SARS outbreak. All sectors cooperated, including the Ministry of Health, clinicians who cared for SARS patients, and laboratory experts who supported the hunt for the SARS virus and the development of early diagnostic tests. One of the most important early lessons was that proper infection-control practices, like those used in Tan Tock Seng Hospital, could quickly halt hospital transmission.

Success ... at last

The difficult measures paid off. On 31 May, after a number of false starts, the city-state was removed from the WHO list of areas with recent local transmission.

WHO called Singapore's handling of the crisis "exemplary" and said, "This is an inspiring victory that should make all of us optimistic that SARS can be contained everywhere."[9]

The WHO statement went on, "In a few cases, SARS transmission occurred in

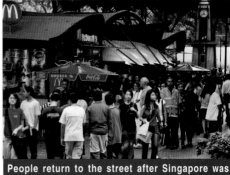
People return to the street after Singapore was removed from the WHO list of areas with recent local transmissions.

situations, such as taxis, elevators, and hospital corridors, where exposure may have been through a route other than face-to-face contact with infected droplets. This unusual pattern necessitated an expanded policy for contact tracing and home quarantine. Health authorities responded to all these challenges with extraordinary measures, adjusting strategies as each new problem emerged."

Characteristic of Singapore's vigilance, the Ministry of Health used the announcement by WHO not to congratulate itself, but rather to call for increased efforts to combat SARS. "There will be no pause in our efforts to maintain and further enhance all our existing measures to isolate and contain the disease and to prevent any export of the disease beyond our shores," the Ministry said.

"The possibility of a future imported case sparking off clusters of SARS cases in Singapore cannot be discounted. We must therefore continue to maintain the highest level of vigilance. ... So long as there are SARS-affected areas in the region and the world, we cannot afford to let our guard down."[10]

References

1 Tan CC. National response to SARS: Singapore. World Health Organization Global Conference on Severe Acute Respiratory Syndrome (SARS), 17–18 June 2003 (http://www.who.int/csr/sars/conference/june_2003/materials/presentations/en/sarssingapore170603.pdf, accessed on 1 April 2005).

2 Severe acute respiratory syndrome – Singapore, 2003. *Morbidity and Mortality Weekly Report*, 2003, 52(18):405-411.

3 Severe acute respiratory syndrome – Singapore, 2003. *Weekly Epidemiological Record*, 2003, 78:157–162.

4 Hsu L-Y et al. Severe acute respiratory syndrome (SARS) in Singapore: clinical features of index patient and initial contacts. *Emerging Infectious Diseases*, 2003, 9:713–717.

[5] Tee AKH et al. Atypical SARS in geriatric patient. *Emerging Infectious Diseases*, 2004, 10:261–264.

[6] Tan TT et al. Atypical SARS and *Escherichia coli* bacteremia. *Emerging Infectious Diseases*, 2004, 10:349–352.

[7] Chow KY et al. Outbreak of severe acute respiratory syndrome in a tertiary hospital in Singapore, linked to a primary patient with atypical presentation: epidemiological study. *British Medical Journal*, 2004, 328:195–198.

[8] *Fighting SARS together: A letter from Prime Minister Goh Chok Tong*. Singapore, Ministry of Information, Communications and the Arts, 22 April 2003 (http://www.sars.gov.sg/archive/PM Goh - Fighting SARS Together.htm, accessed 1 April 2005).

[9] *Singapore removed from list of areas with local SARS transmission, Update 70*. Geneva, World Health Organization, 30 May 2003 (http://www.who.int/csr/don/2003_05_30a/en/, accessed 1 April 2005).

[10] *WHO removes Singapore from list of areas with recent local transmission of SARS*. Singapore, Ministry of Health, 30 May 2003 (http://app10.internet.gov.sg/Scripts/moh/sars/news/update_details.asp?id=1&mid=7481).

9 TAIWAN, CHINA: FROM CONTROL TO ___OUTBREAK___

It is mid-June 2003 in Fu'an middle school in Taipei. The 175 graduates gather one last time as the principal gives out the awards. There is music, dancing, and laughter. As the ceremony closes, lanterns made by the graduates are lit. "Friendship Forever," says one; others shine forth good wishes. But some proclaim a less frivolous message: "Beat SARS, Taiwan!"

Only weeks earlier, that earnest rallying cry would have been dismissed as so much whistling in the dark. Yes, beat SARS, but how?

IMPORTATIONS APPEAR CONTROLLED

Taiwan, China, reported its first cases of SARS on 14 March 2003, just two days after the first WHO alert. A 54-year-old businessman had returned on 25 February from Guangdong Province, China, and developed a fever on 29 February. He was hospitalized on 8 March, and his wife, who had not gone with him on the trip, on 14 March. No special infection-control procedures were put in place until 14 March.[1] But the only hospital transmission was on 17 March, to a doctor who helped intubate the wife. Although the doctor wore protective equipment, his N-95 mask may not have been properly fitted. The couple also transmitted the virus to a family member.

Despite these incidents, by 21 April, Taiwan, China, appeared to be successfully controlling SARS. While many SARS cases had come in from Guangdong and Hong Kong (China), local transmission seemed limited to only one more family contact of another case (in addition to the three described above).[2] At this time a total of 29 probable cases and no deaths had been reported by Taiwan, China, to WHO.

But the virus in fact had been spreading.

HIDDEN SPREAD

Ms MLC, a 47-year-old unemployed construction worker, presented to the emergency department of Hoping Hospital on 9 April, after three days of fever and respiratory symptoms. Her chest X-rays showed that she had bilateral pneumonia. So although she was not known to have travelled anywhere or come in contact with a known SARS case, she was isolated in a negative-pressure room. This was the first local case without a clear source of infection, so there was some question as to whether the initial laboratory confirmation was a false-positive result.

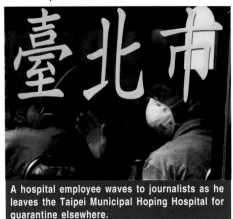

A hospital employee waves to journalists as he leaves the Taipei Municipal Hoping Hospital for quarantine elsewhere.

What was disclosed only weeks later, when Ms MLC came off the respirator, was that she had been on a train to Taichung on 28 March. On the same train was an infected resident of Hong Kong's Amoy Gardens [see Chapter 16], who was on his way to celebrate a traditional festival with his family. As she was three carriages away and had no obvious contact with the man, it remains uncertain how the transmission occurred. No one else was infected on the train. The man's brother would be the first to die from SARS in Taiwan, China.

Once the virus got into Hoping Hospital, it spread rapidly. It had taken two hours to isolate Ms MLC. That delay was enough to allow transmission of the virus. Hospital staff who had been in the area that she had passed through were infected. Of those infected, only the radiology technician who took her X-ray had direct contact with her, suggesting environmental contamination.

One of those infected was Mr CSL, a 42-year-old laundry worker at the hospital. He complained of fever and diarrhoea at the emergency department on 12 April, and returned twice with the same complaint, but continued working in the laundry. He was admitted to ward B8 on 16 April when his symptoms had worsened and treated with antibiotics for presumed Salmonella infection. On 18 April, his breathing grew laboured and he was moved to an isolation room in the intensive care unit. He tested positive for SARS on 22 April, and died on 29 April. Ward B8 has 24 staff; 15 were infected—the highest attack rate in the hospital (62%).

Outbreak

On 22 April, six Hoping Hospital staff were reported to have SARS. A rapidly increasing number of cases was reported every day. Just among the hospital staff, 23 nurses, eight members of the support service staff, five technicians, four nursing aides, and three doctors were later confirmed to have the disease.

An emergency task force met on 23 April and hastily sealed off the hospital on 24 April. The number of potentially exposed persons was placed at 10,000 patients and visitors, and 930 staff members.[2] Patients and visitors who had been at the hospital between 9 and 24 April were quarantined at home. Hospital staff were moved to designated government housing. SARS patients and suspect cases were isolated; some needed to be transferred to other designated hospitals when Hoping Hospital no longer had room for them.

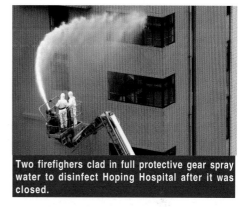

Two firefighers clad in full protective gear spray water to disinfect Hoping Hospital after it was closed.

But before the Hoping Hospital outbreak was recognized, infected patients had already been discharged into the community or transferred to other health-care facilities. Visitors to the hospital as well as other Hoping Hospital staff had also been infected, and were passing the virus on. Jen Chih Hospital, a small hospital a few blocks away, reported three cases on 30 April. The source of the outbreak was not clear.

A 52-year-old haemodialysis patient, treated at Jen Chih Hospital, sought treatment at Chang Gung Memorial Hospital in Kaohsiung, more than 300 kilometres south, on 28 April. Her low-grade fever was hardly noticed. At least 19 cases—11 nurses and 8 patients—at Chang Gung Memorial Hospital were later traced to this patient.

After struggling, vainly, for two weeks to contain the infection, Chang Gung Memorial Hospital was shut down on 15 May. Jen Chih Hospital was also closed and did not reopen until July. Outbreaks in five other hospitals could be traced back to patients who had been discharged from Hoping Hospital or Jen Chih Hospital before these were sealed off.

Newspaper headlines in early- to mid-May made much of a few cases of infection in the community. A taxi driver who routinely picked up passengers in front of Hoping Hospital died. Other reported cases included a street vendor, a cashier in a department store, a beautician, and various homeless people. But for all the attention these cases received in the media, they did not contribute substantially to the spread of SARS. Inadequate hospital infection control, exacerbated by delayed recognition of cases, was the major factor.

Confirmed cases peaked twice: from 22 to 28 April, during the Hoping Hospital outbreak, and around 12 May, during the Chang Gung Memorial Hospital outbreak [see Figure 9.1]. But the number of cases reported daily continued to rise. From 19 to 21 May, close to 90 cases were reported daily. Many were not genuine SARS cases, as there was a fear of missing cases. As well as creating additional work, the false cases heightened negative feelings among the local population and the international community.

The public's fears were slow to be contained. Paranoia thrived amid a perceived dearth of reliable information and failed attempts at concealment by public officials. Of those people polled in May, one in five felt they might be infected, and most thought the Government was not doing enough.

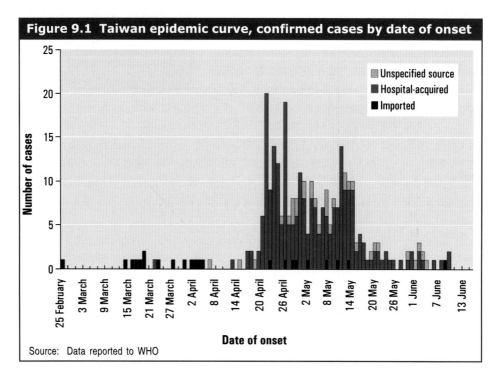

Figure 9.1 Taiwan epidemic curve, confirmed cases by date of onset

Source: Data reported to WHO

IMPACT OF THE EPIDEMIC

The outbreak in Taiwan, China, eventually became the world's third largest, after those on the mainland and in Hong Kong. By 5 July, 682 cases and 84 deaths had been reported to WHO. Laboratory tests from the start of September eventually confirmed 346 cases: 126 had a positive serology, 100 had positive PCR, and 120 others had both sets of positive results. Half (36 out of 73) of those who died were reported to have died from a pre-existing medical condition rather than SARS.

The youngest person to die from SARS was a 23-year-old on a community-service stint, assisting in the transport of patients in lieu of military service. Four foreign workers, all under 35 and hired as private nursing aides, also died from SARS.

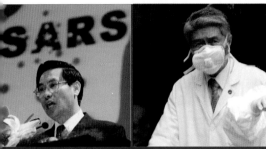

(Left) Twu Shiing-jer, Health Minister for Taiwan, China, resigned over his handling of the SARS crisis. (Right) Former Hoping Hospital superintendent Wu Kang-wen was accused of covering up an outbreak of SARS.

The outbreak also wounded the economy. The economic loss was estimated at US$ 820 million to US$ 1,300 million. During the SARS outbreak, hotels, restaurants, cinemas, shops, and markets stood empty. Idle taxis cruised abandoned streets, as people shunned public places and large gatherings. Those who had to venture outdoors for work and other duties wore masks. A play at the National Theatre in Taipei was allowed to proceed on 8 May. The consensus was, "The show must go on, but we all have to wear masks."

The crisis also claimed political casualties. Blamed by the media for the lax infection controls in hospitals, the Health Minister and the Director of the Center for Disease Control resigned from their posts. The superintendents of Hoping Hospital and Jen Chih Hospital, who had delayed reporting cases, faced criminal charges for professional negligence.

CONTROL MEASURES DURING THE EPIDEMIC

An emergency meeting of infectious disease specialists was held at the Taiwan Center for Disease Control on Sunday, 16 March. It turned out to be the first of the daily meetings of the SARS Expert Committee that formulated the control strategies. The committee also reviewed all reported cases and classified them as probable or suspect, or ruled out SARS if another diagnosis was appropriate.

At the request of the Ministry of Health, two epidemiologists from the Centers for Disease Control and Prevention, United States of

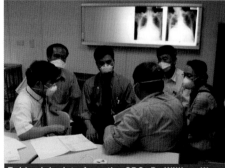

Epidemiologists from the CDC, Dr William Wong (third from left) and Dr Sarah Park (far right), with staff from the Chang Gung Memorial Hospital in Kaohsiung.

America (CDC), were present at the first meeting. Their participation was organized by the WHO Global Outbreak Alert and Response Network [see Chapter 2], and continued until the end of the epidemic in June. WHO staff joined the team on 3 May, and also stayed through to the end of the outbreak.

On 28 March, SARS was listed as a reportable infectious disease in the revised public-health code, giving teeth to the enforcement of isolation, quarantine, and other control measures. Those who violated quarantine could be fined up to NT$ 60,000 (~ US$ 1,800). A total of 131,132 persons—50,319 close contacts of suspected and probable SARS patients, and 80,813 travellers from areas identified by WHO to have been affected by SARS—were placed in quarantine.[3] But enforcement was difficult; and many skipped quarantine.

Hospital infection control was the focus of containment efforts. Patients were isolated in negative-pressure rooms. More of these were built during the outbreak so that by the end, more than 2,000 negative-pressure rooms were available. But the major failure was delay in recognizing cases, allowing SARS to spread in hospitals.[4] Other control measures included public-awareness campaigns, a dedicated fever advice hotline, and active surveillance for clusters of fever cases in health-care facilities.

As it did elsewhere, the SARS outbreak revealed weaknesses in hospital infection control, disease surveillance, and public health infrastructure in Taiwan, China. As the epidemic abated and the frenzy wound down, Taiwan-CDC put forward a comprehensive plan, including a massive overhaul of the public-health system, to prevent the spread of SARS, should it return.[5]

REFERENCES

[1] Chen Y-C et al. Infection control and SARS transmission among healthcare workers, Taiwan. *Emerging Infectious Diseases*, 2004, 10(5):895–898.

[2] Severe acute respiratory syndrome – Taiwan, 2003. *Morbidity and Mortality Weekly Report*, 2003, 52(20):461–466.

[3] Use of quarantine to prevent transmission of severe acute respiratory syndrome, Taiwan, 2003. *Morbidity and Mortality Weekly Report*, 2003, 52(29):680–683.

[4] Hsieh Y-H et al. SARS outbreak, Taiwan, 2003. *Emerging Infectious Diseases*, 2004, 10(2):201–206.

[5] Ho MS, Su IJ. Preparing to prevent severe acute respiratory syndrome and other respiratory infections. *Lancet Infectious Diseases*, 2004, 4(11):684–689.

10 THE PHILIPPINES: HOW CONTACT _TRACING WORKED_

HOLY WEEK 2003: IN SEARCH OF COMMUNITY TRANSMISSION

Easter is an important holiday in the predominantly Catholic Philippines. To celebrate it, families return in droves to their hometowns the week before. On Monday, 14 April 2003, as the traditional exodus out of Metro Manila* began, a drama was being played out. An intense search for an imported case of SARS was unfolding.

INDEX CASE

Ms AC, a 46-year-old Filipino nursing attendant in Toronto, Canada, had come home for the Easter holidays with a special mission: to find a faith healer for her father, who had cancer. She had given a goodbye hug to her housemate's mother before leaving Toronto on 2 April. The mother was feeling ill, and would be hospitalized with SARS by the time Ms AC arrived in the Philippines, late on 4 April.

Ms AC was met by relatives at the airport early Saturday morning, 5 April, and they drove north to their home village in Alcala, Pangasinan province (five or six hours' drive from Manila).

Ms AC started feeling ill and achy on 6 April, and developed fever, diarrhoea, and abdominal pains the next day. But she ignored her symptoms and tried to treat them herself. Intent on her quest for a faith healer for her father, she continued travelling with him over much of the northern provinces. On 11 April she started coughing. Worried relatives took her the next day to a private hospital in a nearby town, where she was admitted. On 13 April her condition worsened: she could hardly breathe. Only then did she mention that she might have been in

---

* Metro Manila is the metropolitan area that contains the City of Manila, the capital of the Philippines, plus 16 neighbouring cities and municipalities. Metro Manila is often simply referred to as Manila, especially by non-residents.

contact with a possible SARS case in Toronto. Her relatives transferred her at once to San Lazaro Hospital in Manila, the national referral hospital for infectious diseases as well as one of two SARS referral hospitals in Metro Manila. In rapid decline, Ms AC was intubated. At 4:10 a.m. on Monday, 14 April, just as the rest of the country was settling in for the Easter holidays, she died.

SEARCH FOR CONTACTS

Notified by San Lorenzo Hospital about Ms AC's admission and subsequent death, the National Epidemiology Center (NEC) of the Department of Health under the leadership of the Secretary for Health, Dr Manuel Dayrit, started mobilizing its network of "diseases detectives".[1] All of Ms AC's contacts from the time her fever had started on 7 April up to her admission and isolation at San Lazaro Hospital had to be identified. That week, Ms AC had travelled with her father and other relatives to nine cities and towns in four provinces and to Metro Manila [see Figure 10.1].

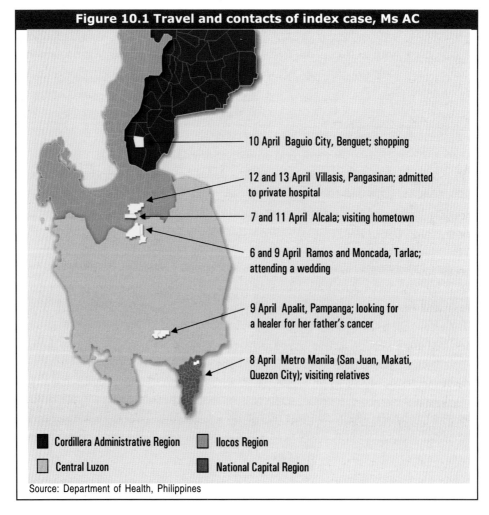

Figure 10.1 Travel and contacts of index case, Ms AC

10 April Baguio City, Benguet; shopping

12 and 13 April Villasis, Pangasinan; admitted to private hospital

7 and 11 April Alcala; visiting hometown

6 and 9 April Ramos and Moncada, Tarlac; attending a wedding

9 April Apalit, Pampanga; looking for a healer for her father's cancer

8 April Metro Manila (San Juan, Makati, Quezon City); visiting relatives

■ Cordillera Administrative Region   ■ Ilocos Region

□ Central Luzon   ■ National Capital Region

Source: Department of Health, Philippines

A massive, weeklong contact-tracing operation, unprecedented in scale, began. Fellows of the NEC's Field Epidemiology Training Programme (FETP) were placed on 24-hour rotation. They had been trained in SARS surveillance using investigation guidelines drawn up a month earlier and had also traced the contacts of previous suspected imported cases. A war room, with hotlines and other communication facilities, was set up at the NEC Epidemiology Surveillance Units (ESUs) in the field, particularly in the Ilocos region and Tarlac province, were contacted to support the investigation.

Epidemiologists hurriedly searched for contacts that week, while most Filipinos were on vacation in the provinces. From a handful of contacts on Tuesday, 15 April, the list on the war room whiteboard had grown to 54 by the next day. Those who had been at a wedding with Ms AC in nearby Tarlac province were included in the search. Photographs helped in tracking down the wedding party. In three days, about 200 contacts were added to the list, bringing the total by Easter Sunday to more than 250 family members and friends, and nine staff members at the hospital in Pangasinan province where Ms AC had first been admitted.

Close family members were quarantined at the Research Institute for Tropical Medicine (RITM) in Muntinlupa City, Metro Manila's other SARS referral hospital. All other contacts, including the residents in three zones in Ms AC's home village, were quarantined at home. Epidemiologists and health workers closely monitored these contacts and recorded their temperature and symptoms for 10 days after their last encounter with Ms AC.

WHOLE AREAS OF VILLAGE QUARANTINED

In Ms AC's home village, the epidemiologists identified two close contacts and 14 social contacts through a spot map they had drawn of all households. To prevent the disease from spreading around the village, they quarantined the three zones where these contacts lived. Food was brought in for 800 or so residents, who were not allowed to leave the zones. Only medical and surveillance teams from the Department of Health and the local government, and policemen on patrol, could enter these areas. A handful of journalists and TV crews, who had been in the area

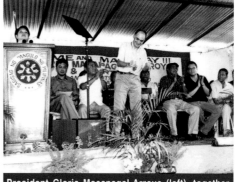

President Gloria Macapagal-Arroyo (left), together with government officials and Dr Jean-Marc Olivé, WHO Representative for the Philippines (centre), announces the lifting of the quarantine.

researching a story on the outbreak, had to be quarantined as well.

Already fearful of contamination with the deadly virus, the residents also had to endure discrimination. They could not sell their main crop, tobacco. Emotions understandably ran high. To remove the stigma and hasten the return to normal life once the village was cleared, the President of the Philippines, the Secretary of Health, and other top government officials, as well as the WHO Representative, visited the village on 2 May to declare the quarantine over.

THE OUTBREAK

Ms MDB, a 39-year-old radiology technician, had taken Ms AC's chest X-rays on admission to San Lazaro Hospital on 13 April. To take the X-rays, Ms MDB had to be in very close contact with Ms MC, who was in very poor health by then. Ms MDB apparently had not worn goggles and had worn her N95 mask over her surgical mask, resulting in a loose fit. She developed fever and malaise on 17 April, but was not isolated until 21 April, when she was hospitalized with pneumonia.[2]

Eight close family contacts of Ms AC were isolated in RITM on 18 and 19 April. Though her 73-year-old father (Mr MC) was feverish on admission, his temperature was just under 38°C because he was taking paracetamol to relieve the pain from cancer. He had no respiratory symptoms and his chest X-rays were normal. Only when his condition rapidly deteriorated, on 21 April, was he recognized as a SARS case. By then he had hypoxaemia and his chest X-rays showed bilateral diffuse infiltrates. He was intubated on 22 April, and died a few hours later. The 35-year-old nurse (Mr LA) and the 32-year-old doctor (Ms EM) who intubated him both developed SARS but were likewise not isolated until after the onset of symptoms.

Mr MC2, a brother-in-law of Ms AC, was with her from the time of her arrival and had carried the coughing woman into San Lorenzo Hospital. He became feverish and was admitted to hospital the next day but showed no further symptoms. His chest X-ray remained normal. But he tested positive for SARS-CoV.

Aside from Mr MC2, three of Ms AC's immediate family members developed SARS because of inadequate isolation during their hospital quarantine. Her 29-year-old niece, Ms JC, took care of Ms AC's father (Mr MC) up to the time of his death and may have been infected in the process. Ms JC probably passed on the virus to Ms AC's 71-year-old mother (Ms PC) and 52-year-old brother (Mr RC).

Mr RC was the last SARS case in this outbreak to show symptoms (on 3 May). There were no other transmissions. Nearly 60 contacts of the three infected health workers (Ms MDB, Mr LA, and Ms EM) were identified and monitored for fever. None developed symptoms.

In all, the outbreak involved nine people, including Ms AC [see Figure 10.2]. Transmissions after 22 April were limited to quarantined family members. Thus, when the Philippines was placed on the WHO list of countries with recent transmission on 7 May, there was no longer any risk of transmission, except in the isolation ward of that one hospital. Contacts who might have been infected at that time were being closely monitored for symptoms.

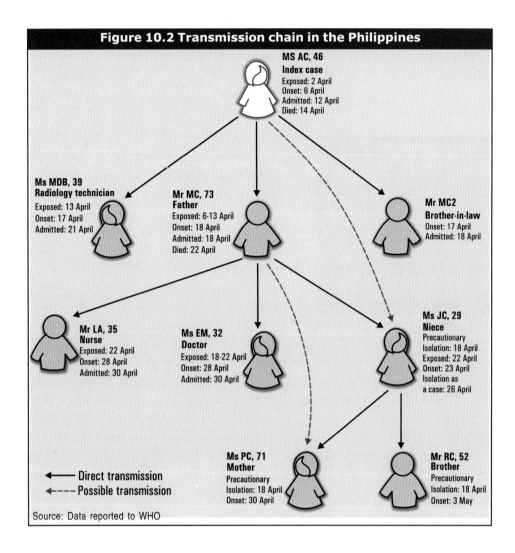

Figure 10.2 Transmission chain in the Philippines

MS AC, 46
Index case
Exposed: 2 April
Onset: 6 April
Admitted: 12 April
Died: 14 April

Ms MDB, 39
Radiology technician
Exposed: 13 April
Onset: 17 April
Admitted: 21 April

Mr MC, 73
Father
Exposed: 6-13 April
Onset: 18 April
Admitted: 18 April
Died: 22 April

Mr MC2
Brother-in-law
Onset: 17 April
Admitted: 18 April

Mr LA, 35
Nurse
Exposed: 22 April
Onset: 28 April
Admitted: 30 April

Ms EM, 32
Doctor
Exposed: 18-22 April
Onset: 28 April
Admitted: 30 April

Ms JC, 29
Niece
Precautionary
Isolation: 18 April
Exposed: 22 April
Onset: 23 April
Isolation as
a case: 26 April

◄——— Direct transmission
◄----- Possible transmission

Ms PC, 71
Mother
Precautionary
Isolation: 18 April
Onset: 30 April

Mr RC, 52
Brother
Precautionary
Isolation: 18 April
Onset: 3 May

Source: Data reported to WHO

Risk of infection in contacts

Excluding the three family members who were infected while in quarantine, only two of Ms AC's many contacts in the community (her father and brother-in-law) were infected, for an attack rate of less than 1%. On the other hand, the three health workers infected in the outbreak represented about 10% of health workers who had been in contact with the cases. This much higher risk of infection among health workers parallels the findings in other countries with larger outbreaks.

In retrospect, the community contacts had to be traced to prove that the virus had spread no further. If a single case had been missed, it could have generated many other chains of transmission.

Another interesting aspect is that three of the family members became infected while in hospital quarantine as isolation procedures were still being strengthened.

It is sometimes assumed that suspected cases could be quarantined together. This outbreak shows the danger of isolating people as a group, as anyone with the virus can spread it to the others.

CONTACT TRACING FOR OTHER CASES IN THE PHILIPPINES

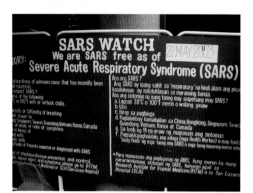

On 15 March, the Philippines learned from the WHO office in Viet Nam that a close contact (Mr RT) of Mr JC (the Hanoi index case) had returned to the Philippines from Viet Nam on 11 March. The Secretary of Health advised hospital quarantine. Mr RT was first admitted to a SARS reference hospital, and then released to home confinement. He had diarrhoea but did not develop respiratory symptoms.

Besides the cluster of nine cases that included the index case from Toronto, the Philippines reported four other probable SARS cases. The first was announced by President Gloria Macapagal-Arroyo on national television from the war room in Malacañang Palace on 11 April 2003. Although the four cases were not proven to be SARS cases, they led investigators to 100 contacts. Eighty other suspected cases where the probability of SARS was ruled out were linked to 400 contacts. All these contacts were identified and followed up to ensure that none developed symptoms. A panel of infectious disease, pulmonary, radiology and epidemiology experts formed by the Health Department met regularly during this time to review admitted cases of SARS. The recommendations of this panel guided Health Secretary Dayrit in choosing appropriate control measures.

In May, the United Kingdom notified the Philippines that a British-Filipino couple infected at the Metropole Hotel [see Chapter 14] and hospitalized with pneumonia in the Philippines in early March had tested positive for SARS when they returned to the United Kingdom. NEC searched for SARS transmissions among the contacts of this couple during their stay in the Philippines. Of the 115 contacts found, 80 had been in close contact with the couple, but none developed fever subsequently.[3]

IMPACT ON FILIPINOS WORKING OVERSEAS

SARS and the possibility of its spread terrified Filipinos. They shunned those who returned home from working overseas, for fear that they might be bringing back the virus with them. Worse news awaited these overseas Filipino workers and others wishing to join their ranks. On 7 May 2003 WHO classified the Philippine pattern of transmission as "medium" because more than one generation of spread was involved. As a result, several countries refused to admit anyone from the Philippines or banned the entry of Filipino workers, with huge personal and economic consequences for the country.

On 10 May, the Philippine Government complained in a letter to WHO that the "medium' categorization was misleading since the outbreak had been limited to hospital and family contacts. As a result, WHO changed the categories from "low", "medium", and "high" to "A", "B", and "C". But the definitions stayed the same, and so did the impact on the Philippines.

The small outbreak was contained by the end of April. Risk had been limited to close contacts, and all contacts had been traced. WHO's Regional and country offices tried to rectify the harm caused by the inclusion of the Philippines among the countries with SARS transmission, and to develop a more rational assessment of epidemiological risk.

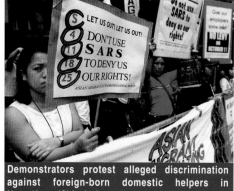

Demonstrators protest alleged discrimination against foreign-born domestic helpers in Hong Kong (China). A small group, mostly domestic helpers from the Philippines and Indonesia, claimed that, because of the SARS virus, employers refused to allow their helpers to take their days off.

REFERENCES

[1] Gepte TD, Daluro ATM. A race against a virus: a report of contact tracing conducted during the Philippines SARS outbreak. Manila, Department of Health, 2003. [Unpublished].

[2] Aumentado CP, Mapue MC. Narrative report of a SARS suspected case at San Lazaro Hospital. Manila, National Epidemiology Center, Department of Health, 25 April 2003.

[3] Lopez J et al. Investigation on Philippines contacts of United Kingdom SARS couple from X Hotel, Hong Kong. Manila, Department of Health, 21 October 2003.

11 MONGOLIA: A SMALL OUTBREAK _WITH A BIG IMPACT_

The independent country of Mongolia borders the northern Chinese autonomous region of Inner Mongolia. The shared name meant that tourists stayed away from Mongolia when WHO added Inner Mongolia to the list of affected areas and then advised against all but essential travel. Transmission in Inner Mongolia also led to a small SARS outbreak in Mongolia. The impact of this small outbreak, which involved a single local transmission, was profound. Among other effects, marketplaces and entertainment houses closed, and international travel was curtailed.

ORIGIN OF OUTBREAK

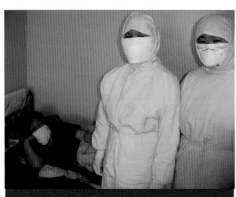

Ms NS (left) is considered to be the index case for the outbreak in Mongolia. She and five others were treated in the isolation unit at the National Center for Communicable Diseases in Ulaanbataar and recovered.

SARS transmission started in Inner Mongolia, China, after two flight attendants who were infected on flight CA112 returned home in late March [see Chapter 15]. They were admitted to a hospital in Hohhot City, the capital of Inner Mongolia, consequently setting off an unrecognized transmission of the virus.

The SARS virus was brought into Mongolia by five people from three local families. They had been infected while seeking medical treatment in Inner Mongolia in March.

A husband (63), wife (60), and daughter (32) in family A, a woman (57) in family B, and another woman (59) in family C, all spent time in the same hospital room in Hohhot City.

Family A

The 60-year-old woman, Ms NS, was the first to develop symptoms. On 29 March, she developed a fever and cough while being treated in a hospital in Hohhot. She was discharged from the hospital on 1 April, and returned to Ulaanbaatar by train on 4 April with her husband, daughter, and grandchild in the same cabin. As it was five to seven days before symptoms showed in any of the others, she is likely to be the index case for the outbreak.

The 63-year-old husband, Mr DU, accompanied his wife to Inner Mongolia and visited her in the hospital. He developed symptoms on 5 April. The 32-year-old daughter, Ms UB, cared for her mother in the hospital and slept in her room. She developed a fever on 7 April and a cough on 12 April.

Family B

The 57-year-old woman, Ms DTs, stayed in the hospital's hotel for three days and then was admitted. She was assigned to the same room as Ms NS and her daughter. Ms DTs flew to Ulaanbaatar on 4 April and, on the following day, developed a fever, cough, and headache.

Family C

The 59-year-old woman, Ms TsD, was admitted to the same Hohhot hospital on 18 March and shared a room with the other women until 24 March. She returned to Mongolia on 4 April on the same flight as Ms DTs. She developed symptoms on 7 April.

In early April, these five infected persons were referred to the National Center for Communicable Diseases and isolated in the infectious disease hospital on 12 and 13 April. Laboratory analysis of blood and chest X-rays was conducted. The five were kept in isolation with initial diagnosis of suspected SARS. Clinical specimens of serum, nasopharyngeal aspirate, and throat swab were sent for confirmation to a WHO Regional Reference Laboratory in Japan.

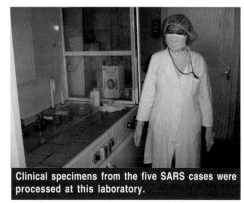

Clinical specimens from the five SARS cases were processed at this laboratory.

The Ministry of Health issued a Health Alert Notice for all visitors to Mongolia. Travellers were advised to observe their health for at least 10 days and to consult a physician or call the National Center for Communicable Diseases if they developed fever.

Local transmission

The impact of these five SARS cases was made much more serious by the fact that they led to one local transmission in Mongolia. Ms OZ, the 28-year-old daughter of Ms DTs who did not travel to Inner Mongolia, developed symptoms

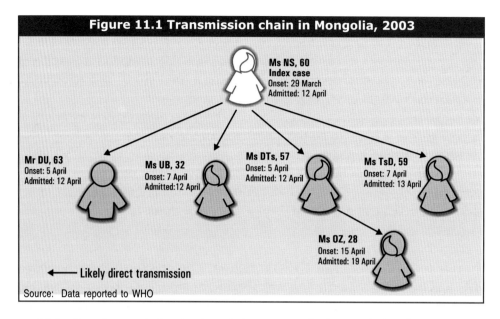

Figure 11.1 Transmission chain in Mongolia, 2003

Ms NS, 60
Index case
Onset: 29 March
Admitted: 12 April

Mr DU, 63
Onset: 5 April
Admitted: 12 April

Ms UB, 32
Onset: 7 April
Admitted:12 April

Ms DTs, 57
Onset: 5 April
Admitted: 12 April

Ms TsD, 59
Onset: 7 April
Admitted: 13 April

Ms OZ, 28
Onset: 15 April
Admitted: 19 April

◄─── Likely direct transmission

Source: Data reported to WHO

on 15 April and was admitted to hospital on 19 April. This single local transmission pushed Ulaanbaatar, Mongolia, onto WHO's list of affected areas.

Three more imported cases of SARS were identified in students returning from Beijing. They were isolated between 26 April and 2 May. All nine SARS cases in Mongolia recovered. And although intensive medical care services were provided to all probable and suspected SARS cases, no medical personnel were affected by SARS in the country.

From 12 April to 25 June 2003, 1,529 close contacts of the nine people with SARS were identified and quarantined in their home under the observation of their family doctor. None developed SARS. And neither did any of the 61,109 people who had been screened at the Mongolia–China border by 25 June, including 15 who were isolated at local hospitals in the south of the country.

CONTROL MEASURES

On 13 April, the Government of Mongolia responded to the impending crisis by issuing a decree specifying various control measures. Many of the activities had been recommended by WHO; others were even more stringent. Through the decree, the Government:

- closed 12 land border points between Mongolia and China, and from 23 April carried out strict entry screening and the disinfection of all cars, trains, and planes on entry;
- advised officials and workers not to travel to countries with local transmission;
- closed all big marketplaces, first for two weeks and later for another two;
- postponed public performances (e.g. cultural shows, circus shows) to reduce the chance of disease transmission;

- prepared health institutions to identify and manage suspected SARS cases, and set up isolation facilities in Dornogobi Province in the south, including five beds in the railway hospital in Zamyn-Uud district at the border with China and a 50-bed isolation ward in Sain-Shand, the provincial capital; and
- created four groups of experts to undertake surveillance and control of SARS together with city health-department workers, railway-station officials, and airport control authorities.

The Government set aside a substantial part of the national budget to support these measures, and coordinated with donors for additional funding. More than US$ 150,000 was allocated for the procurement of medical equipment and supplies that were not available in Mongolia, including personal protective equipment, respirator machines, laboratory equipment, and essential antiviral drugs. There were no in-hospital transmissions, partly thanks to the adequate supply of protective equipment for hospital staff, including masks, provided by Japan International Cooperation Agency and the Asian Development Bank (through WHO's Regional Office).

WHO dispatched international experts to Mongolia to help with infection control and case management. A SARS preparedness assessment was conducted with technical support from WHO, following the training of 650 health-care workers on barrier nursing techniques, case management, and infection control.

OUTBREAK CONTAINED

On 9 May 2003, WHO announced that Mongolia had been removed from its list of areas with recent local transmission. The last and only case of local transmission was isolated on 19 April.

Mongolia's small outbreak had a big impact on tourism. The year 2003 had been designated "Visit to Mongolia" year and the Government was hoping that the number of foreign tourists would increase to 230,000. However, tourist arrivals fell substantially in May; restaurants, the entertainment industry, and hotels lost revenue during the one month of emergency conditions in the capital city.

SARS also affected the transportation sector. According to MIAT Mongolian Airlines, the number of international flights

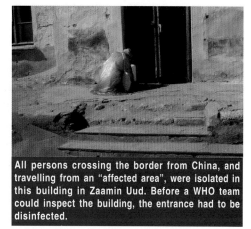

All persons crossing the border from China, and travelling from an "affected area", were isolated in this building in Zaamin Uud. Before a WHO team could inspect the building, the entrance had to be disinfected.

for the April–June period declined from 89 to 38. The Mongolian Railway Authority estimated that it lost more than 1 billion togrog (~US$ 1 million) in revenue due to SARS.

12 CANADA: HOW A __HOSPITAL COPED__

New glass walls went up in the intensive care unit of Scarborough Hospital in the winter of 2003. The floor-to-ceiling enclosures barricade each bed, separating one patient from another, keeping the sick from the healthy. If every war has its monument, these walls now stand as a symbolic victory to the only goal that mattered the winter that SARS hit Canada: containment.

Before the battle, Scarborough's multisite facility in Toronto's east end was known best for its two acute-care community hospitals, where women delivered babies, the elderly recovered from falls, and doctors performed surgeries. But after SARS appeared unannounced at Scarborough's Grace division in March 2003, the hospital earned a less enviable reputation as the epicentre of an outbreak that crippled Canada's largest city.

SARS killed 38 men and women in the Toronto area over a four-month period, 44 in all. More than 250 fell sick and around 10,000 were forced into quarantine. Local public health officials, like those in the rest of the world, knew little about their new microbial enemy when it hit. But what precious intelligence they did gather came largely from the devastation it wreaked first at Scarborough Hospital, the epidemiological root of nearly all of Toronto's cases.

The virus struck Scarborough Hospital twice, first at its Grace division and then in a demoralizing second wave at its General site. In all, 100 staff members fell ill, many of them seriously, forcing the hospital to close and plunging those left standing into the surreal horror of caring for sick colleagues, working under quarantine, worrying for themselves and their families, and all the while serving the patients who remained in their wards.

Paul Caulford, Scarborough Hospital's chief of family medicine and community services, said the experience represented the greatest challenge of their professional careers, but at the same time offered profound lessons about solidarity. "I always wondered how you can be in a war and the guy in front of you gets shot and somehow the next guy just steps up and keeps going," he said. "But we had a common enemy, we didn't panic. Everyone worked, under incredible strain, from the administration to the cleaners, who would scrub one area and a little while later come back and scrub it again."

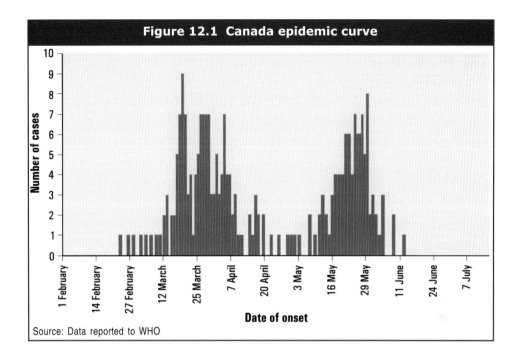

Figure 12.1 Canada epidemic curve

Source: Data reported to WHO

INDEX CASE

It had been a true ambush. Hospital and medical staff were unsuspecting and unprepared. The index patient, 44-year-old Mr TCK, arrived at the Grace emergency department on the evening of 7 March 2003 with symptoms that jam emergency rooms across the city every winter. His coughing, fever, and shortness of breath sounded like a routine flu or community-acquired pneumonia. But in fact, Mr TCK had contracted SARS—a mysterious disease that had not yet been named. His mother had been unknowingly infected during a recent trip to Hong Kong (China) and upon her return, passed the virus to her family before dying in her Toronto home on 5 March.[*]

Hospital staff, working with the city's public health officials and infectious disease experts, connected Mr TCK's case to the atypical pneumonia spreading in parts of Asia. Email alerts sent on 20 and 21 February had warned doctors, infection-control specialists and public-health authorities to look out for influenza-like symptoms in travellers returning from China. On 12 March, WHO issued a global alert regarding the mystery illness.

Mr TCK, who died on 13 March, had passed the virus to a 76-year-old patient who would become the source of another SARS cluster.[**] Six health workers contracted the disease in a single effort to intubate him and from 18 March

---

[*] For more information on the link between the outbreaks in Hong Kong and Toronto, see Chapter 14: Solving The Metropole Hotel Mystery.

[**] The patient was transferred to York Central Hospital, north of Toronto, where more than 50 of his contacts developed SARS.

onward, at least one staff member developed SARS every day for the next week—nurses in coronary care, ICU, emergency. Hospital rooms were soon filled with health-care workers.

"We were compiling list after list on staffing and patients, timings and shifts and points of contact, and who was taking care of which patients, and phone numbers and the names of all the families and families who visited," said Louise Leblanc, director of patient care for the emergency departments at Scarborough's Grace and General sites.

IMPACT ON HEALTH WORKERS AND SERVICES

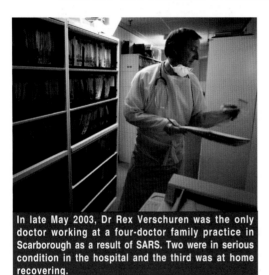

In late May 2003, Dr Rex Verschuren was the only doctor working at a four-doctor family practice in Scarborough as a result of SARS. Two were in serious condition in the hospital and the third was at home recovering.

Sandy Finkelstein, later chief of medicine at Scarborough's Grace site, was then director of its intensive care unit. Watching the disease spread to the staff as he struggled to find ways to treat the patients and control the infection "increased stress levels dramatically," he said. Yet there were no medical references to point to the best course of treatment. Nor was there space for the steadily growing caseload at the Grace site, which then had just four separate rooms and one negative-air-pressure chamber. On 23 March, 14 sick staff members had to be transferred to isolation units at the West Park Healthcare Centre, a former TB sanatorium in west Toronto.

Dr Finkelstein brought yo-yos and chocolates to his colleagues at West Park, many of whom were relying on respirators to breathe. "Seeing my staff there, sick, some of whom I know well, and some of them were really sick, was horrible," he said. "Some of them suffered chest scarring. Some of them will never come back."

Ontario's provincial health officials ordered the Grace site closed on 25 March. Few members of the staff were healthy enough at that point to even work the emergency department, one of the busiest in the city, with 40,000 visits a year.

Dr Finkelstein recalled the disturbing image of the yellow police tape that blocked off the Grace site hospital entrance as though it were a crime scene. Ambulances were diverted. Pregnant women were directed elsewhere. All appointments and procedures, including all cancer-related surgeries, were cancelled—a catastrophic setback for a public-health system already notorious for its dangerous delays and waiting lists. "The system is so tight that taking one hospital out of service was devastating," Dr Finkelstein said. "There was no coordinated effort to deal with the patients who had nowhere to go." Meanwhile, he said, there were doctors and surgeons around who had nothing to do for weeks.

Yet people continued to get sick. "You could not build a rabbit-proof fence," said Dr Caulford. "The elderly will still fall and have lacerations, there will still be people who need somewhere to go." But emergency services at the General site had also been curtailed as a preventive measure, and, as Dr Caulford saw it, support for the front-line family doctors in the community had been overlooked.

"The irony is that the only doctor to die in the outbreak was a family doctor in the community," he said. "It became apparent that family doctors weren't being given any instructions—or supplies."

Dr Caulford, who heads the area's Family Practitioners Group, received a flood of frantic calls from colleagues in those early days asking, "Should we take everyone's temperature? How would we know the (epidemiological) link? Where are the masks?" Dr Caulford ordered 6,000 masks to be distributed among them.

Inside the Grace site, a skeleton staff settled into a gruelling routine to keep the battered hospital running. Day after day, they started their shifts shivering in the cold, damp parking lot, waiting to have their temperatures taken to make sure they were SARS-free. Many arrived by 7 a.m. and worked late into the night. Some did not leave at all. Some were so worried they might infect family members they bunked at the hospital—including a nurse with a newborn at home, and another who had an elderly mother to care for. "Staff were scared. They were terrified for themselves and their families," said Dr Finkelstein.

But still they worked, in gowns, gloves, and, of course, the outbreak's trademark clammy and cumbersome N-95 masks.

No one was immune to anxiety. "We all wanted guarantees that we weren't going to be ill," said Ms Leblanc. Some questioned why certain staff members were quarantined in the comfort of their homes while others had to remain on duty during the 10-day period of isolation. Others grew frustrated and mistrustful of changing policies and protocols as authorities tinkered with infection-control procedures. Still others wondered why they had to work in the designated SARS ward, where patients had to wear television headsets to shut out the drone of the new negative-air-pressure units and where, naturally, the personal health risks were considered most daunting.

"Emotions ran very high, some positive, some negative," said Ms Leblanc. "There was anger at times. I think it was the fear of the unknown, yet we still had patients and they still had to work, and so we had the compliance of staff, and an acceptance of the situation."

Dr Finkelstein marvelled at how initial complaints from the staff simply melted away into the demands of a very demanding job: "People kept coming to work, not protesting. Emergency staff took care of their own until, literally, there was no one left standing," he said. "I gained a great deal of respect for many of my colleagues. They did a truly remarkable job, and all through it, people wore their feelings on their sleeves."

Ms Leblanc felt the staff survived because even the "little milestones" could lift spirits. "Every day there were no new cases, people had hope, so you never felt like giving up."

Despite their own concerns and hardships, staff members were deeply saddened to see patients suddenly finding themselves sicker and lonelier than they had ever imagined. While most patients had been evacuated when the Grace division closed, at least 30 remained in the building, as some were just too sick to be moved. It was heart-wrenching to have to deny them visitors, Ms Leblanc said.

"Every morning we made a list of patients who could have a single visitor, but it had to be the same visitor every time," she said, as she went on to describe a patient's delight at seeing his dog, whom a neighbour had brought to the hospital grounds.

Worse too, many of the patients were elderly, and had already also suffered heart attacks and strokes. "That was my difficulty," Dr Finkelstein said. "The patients."

Plans were under way to create additional isolation rooms at the General site for patients from the Grace division, where 44 nurses, technicians, and doctors were infected during the outbreak. The General, however, soon needed these rooms for its own staff. A patient transferred to the General in mid-May from an area nursing home turned out to be incubating the virus, which he had picked up at another hospital. But by the time the patient's symptoms appeared, the chain of infection had already been unleashed.

Although no one who had worn protective gear caring for the patient became infected, everyone had to be quarantined, some for the second time. In the end, nearly five dozen health workers at the General developed SARS, and some of them would still need respirators six months later.

Dr Caulford, who holds office at the General, feared then that the virus would defeat them. "Staffing was a nightmare in a system already bled dry," he said. "When I heard that Toronto had several thousand people in isolation, that people were also breaking their quarantine, and that Toronto Public Health didn't have enough staff to do proper fast-tracking of people, … I never believed for one minute that we would stop this thing."

But he discovered that no one allowed his or her worst fears to triumph. As they had done at the Grace site, staff members continued to clock in and camp out. "I never saw them in better form," Dr Caulford said. "The illness of colleagues heightened the resolve to work. It made us more cautious, reminding ourselves and each other about our precautions.

The long days were packed with meetings—conference calls between senior staff members and government health officials, administration and management meetings, nursing meetings, general meetings (but always in smallish groups, since large gatherings were to be avoided). There was a fevered swap of questions and issues. Dr Caulford said, "People wanted to know, 'What's the virus doing?' 'Who's sick?' 'How are we staffing this unit or that?' 'Can we transfer anyone?'"

He went on, "Sure, there was a lot of rancorous discussion about what we should do, about what was best. But these were constructive discussions. We had war rooms, bunkers, command centres."

What amazed him during this most stressful stretch was the sense of camaraderie, cooperation, and genuine concern among colleagues. "These were people who were ready to knock your kneecaps off two weeks before if their programme didn't get funded. ... You end up with a hell of a lot of admiration for people you work with."

In 48 hours Dr Caulford managed to recruit enough staff members to run a provincially ordered SARS assessment clinic that was hastily built in the General's parking lot on 2 June. The tented structure,

Several hundred health-care workers gathered outside Scarborough Hospital on 4 June 2003 for a rally aimed at the provincial government regarding the re-emergence of SARS and the conditions hospital staff found themselves working in since the outbreak.

outfitted with $500,000 in medical equipment, popped up overnight. The wind blew through it, there was no running water, but nurses and doctors stood guard inside until 31 July 2003, when, at long last, there were no more SARS cases left to catch.

But the public was hardly disposed to look kindly on Scarborough Hospital during these trying months. As SARS ruined businesses, closed schools, and curtailed medical services across the province, some people viewed the east-end facility much as they did the local Chinatown—with suspicion, and outright accusation.

Ms Leblanc recounted how motorists driving past the assessment clinic tent would roll down their windows and shout at the staff inside. "They were profanely abused for the state of the system, for the economy, for the mess SARS had left things in," she said. "When you are tired and frustrated, and you're working 16-hour days and more, hearing those comments drove many to tears." Within 24 hours a wall went up between the roadside and the clinic.

Dr Finkelstein blamed some media reports for the sense that "Scarborough was, 'oooh, a dirty place.'" He said, "From the inside, I thought people were quite heroic. Here we did backflips trying to care for the patients, treating people with a disease that you had no history on. You didn't know most people with fevers would go on to develop chest syndrome, and so on. All of this you learned as you went along."

At the end of May, provincial health authorities carried out an intense audit of the Grace hospital site based on 34 items. With no new cases in more than

10 days and evidence that the hospital had instituted strict measures to screen patients, control infection, and limit visitor access, the Grace slowly reopened. Obstetrics was the first unit to accept new patients. Beds in long-term care filled up once more, followed by the intensive care unit and coronary care. Then, on 3 June, the yellow tape was at last removed from the emergency department entrance.

An independent review by Justice Archie Campbell of the handling of the Toronto outbreak did not blame any one hospital for the spread of SARS in the region. Released in April 2004, the report said that Ontario's public health system had proved to be fractured, underfunded, poorly staffed, and poorly led during the SARS crisis. In fact, the Campbell review concluded that only the "heroic" efforts of dedicated health-care workers had prevented the wider spread of the virus in the community.

Epilogue

A year after the outbreak, there were clear signs of change at Scarborough Hospital. The Grace site had twice as many isolation rooms, and six negative-air-pressure chambers. Renovations were under way at the General division. Staff in the emergency departments—where visits were down nearly 10%—treated everyone who walked in, particularly those with respiratory problems, as suspicious and possibly contagious. And, of course, there were the glass walls in the intensive care unit.

Ms Leblanc compares the "new normal" to the changes that followed the emergence of HIV in the 1980s. No health worker would ever again work in any way with blood or bodily fluids without wearing gloves, she said. So now, in the post-SARS world, hospitals will greet every potential patient with face masks, walls, and intensive screening.

It must be this way, Ms Leblanc said, if hospitals are to defeat the next threat from the microbial world. For her, the hospital's closure was a low point of the outbreak. Hospitals have to remain up and functioning during outbreaks, she said. They are the battlegrounds. "If we are going to close them when these things happen, you feel like a failure."

Though buoyed by "a sense of 'wow, we did it'", the nursing staff at Scarborough Hospital, she said, is fragile. A few nurses have left their jobs. Others have chosen assignments outside the front-line emergency department.

"A lot of people have re-evaluated their lives professionally," said Dr Caulford, admitting the SARS experience has made the annual physical "a little less exciting". "This was extreme medicine, but it was the most purposeful work as a physician that I've ever done."

Dr Caulford mused, "It was a messy war, so how do you judge people? Is it enough to say that more things were done right than were done wrong? For all our human frailties, we won. And I never thought we would."

PART III: OUTBREAKS

13 THE FIRST SUPER-
_ SPREADING EVENT_

INDEX CASE

Mr ZZF, a 44-year-old seafood seller from the Fangcun suburbs of Guangzhou, in Southern China, had been troubled for five days by a cough and fever. On 30 January 2003, he decided to seek medical treatment at the No. 2 Affiliated Hospital of Zhongshan Medical University (also called Sun Yatsen Memorial Hospital) in Guangzhou. As his chest X-rays had patchy shadows in the upper right lung, he was admitted with a diagnosis of pneumonia. On 1 February, his condition worsened and he was transferred to the designated hospital for cases of atypical pneumonia: No. 3 Affiliated Hospital of Zhongshan Medical University. Medical staff began an emergency intubation down his throat. They had no idea that he would be so infectious, and that this procedure would be dangerous for them.

TRANSMISSIONS AT NO. 2 HOSPITAL

The impact of Mr ZZF's two-day stay at No. 2 Hospital was explosive. The SARS working group at the hospital linked 96 infections to his brief admission: 90 health workers, five family members, and one patient.[1] Their symptoms started appearing up to 20 days after contact with Mr ZZF, suggesting that some of them were not directly infected (as SARS generally has a maximum incubation period of 10 days). Another report on this super-spreading event states that 30 health workers were infected from contact with Mr ZZF in No. 2 Hospital, and that at least 50 hospital workers and 19 family members in all were infected.[2]

Perhaps the most important transmission chain was to Professor LJL, who worked at No. 2 Hospital [see next chapter]. His symptoms started on 15 February (that is, 15 days after the last time he might have been in contact with Mr ZZF), so he was most likely infected by a hospital worker who had been infected by Mr ZZF.

Further transmissions

During Mr ZZF's transfer to No. 3 Hospital, the ambulance driver, two doctors, and two nurses were infected. This ambulance driver may have been one of the first health-care workers to die from SARS. Within the next eight days, 20 more members of the medical staff at No. 3 Hospital were also infected. Nineteen members of Mr ZZF's family also developed SARS.

Mr ZZF also infected staff members at Guangzhou No. 8 People's Hospital, where he finally recovered. The hospital's president, Tang Xiaoping, recalled in a television interview: "Doctors and nurses complained. ... Why should such a critically ill patient be transferred to our hospital?

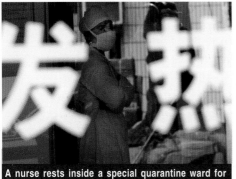

A nurse rests inside a special quarantine ward for fever patients at a hospital in Guangzhou.

"We gave the so-called 'virus king' the most meticulous care. We didn't wear masks or goggles then. We later found that secretions can be infectious if they contact the eyes. We had never encountered such a highly infectious disease."[3]

The source of Mr ZZF's infection is not known. A retrospective study has confirmed that SARS first appeared in Foshan municipality in Guangdong Province on 16 November 2002.[4] There were only sporadic cases until late January, when the number of cases spiked. Mr ZZF's contacts added to that increase in early February, after which the number of cases in Guangdong tapered off and was already declining by the time of the global alert. The relative role of this super-spreading event (from Mr ZZF) in the overall epidemic has not been defined, but was clearly substantial.

What causes a super-spreading event?

Early on, it was noted that there were "super spreaders" who passed the virus to many other people. This term emphasizes the role of the host (person infected) above that of the agent (nature of the virus) and the environment in accounting for the phenomenon; hence the preference for the term "super-spreading event". A super-spreading event is likely to derive from the classical explanatory triad of host, agent, and environment. However, the mechanism of highly efficient transmission of most of the super-spreading events is still largely unknown.

Table 13.1 Selected super-spreading events[a]

Name	Age	Event or location (corresponding chapter)	Exposure	Onset	Admit	No	Place
			Infection event dates			**Number and place of transmissions**	
Mr ZZF	44	Guangdong (13)	ND	26 Jan	30 Jan	>69	Probably all in hospitals
Mr LJL[b]	64	Hong Kong, Metropole Hotel (14)	ND	15 Feb	21 Feb	21	Most in hotel; effective infection control in hospital
Mr CT	26	Hong Kong, Prince of Wales Hospital (7)	21 Feb	24 Feb	4 Mar	144	Probably all in hospital; neublization helped spread
Mr LTC[b]	33	Hong Kong, Amoy Gardens (16)	ND	14 Mar	22 Mar	ND	329 through sewage; none while in hospital.
Ms YM	27	Taiyuan & Beijing (6)	ND	22 Feb	2 Mar	21	Most in hospital; believed to be family and friends in the community
Mr LSK	72	Flight CA112 & Beijing (15)	4-9 Mar	11 Mar	16 Mar	83	24 on the plane; at least 59 in Beijing hospital
Mr JC[b]	48	Hanoi (18)	21 Feb	23 Feb	26 Feb	>20	All in hospital, no hospital transmissions in Hong Kong (effective infection control)
Ms EM	22	Singapore (9)	21 Feb	25 Feb	1 Mar	22	All in hospital; isolated after 6 days; no further transmissions
Ms AB	27	Singapore (9)	1-6 Mar	7 Mar	10 Mar	21	All, except perhaps one, in hospital (10 staff, 7 visitors, 3 patients and 1 family member)
Ms PA[c]	53	Singapore (9)	10 Mar	12 Mar	10 Mar	26	All in hospital (19 staff, 13 patients, 6 visitors and 2 family members)
Mr TKC[c]	59	Singapore (9)	3-20 Mar	24 Mar	24 Mar	40	All in hospital
Mr TSC	64	Singapore (17)	31 Mar	5 Apr	8 Apr	15	In the community and hospital; before isolation (3 co-workers, 2 taxi drivers, 2 family members, 3 health-care workers, 4 patients and 1 visitor)
Ms MLC	47	Taiwan (8)	28 Mar	6 Apr	9 Apr	ND	All in hospital, despite infection control
Mr CSL[bc]	42	Taiwan (8)	9 Apr	12 Apr	16 Apr	ND	Hospital worker; transmissions not clear

ND, not determined

[a] Events selected based on available data

[b] Patients who died

[c] Patients with pre-existing medical conditions; all presented with atypical symptoms, except Mr LTC

The environment must, first of all, allow transmission. Early isolation and appropriate infection control can prevent this. But even supposedly good infection control did not stop all transmissions. Presumably, viral loads in some patients were high enough to exploit a minor lapse in infection control.

In all super-spreading events, infection control was lacking. There was no hospital spread from the index cases of the Metropole Hotel and Amoy Gardens outbreaks, except for the nurses who did not protect themselves around the time of admission of these cases. The Hanoi index case did not transmit any infections when he returned to Hong Kong. These cases suggest that with good infection control, even highly infectious individuals can be prevented from transmitting virus.

But lack of infection control alone does not explain super-spreading events. Many more cases with little or no infection control were associated with very little or no spread.

Super-spreading events are likely to be related to either a high viral load in the patient or increased efficiency in transmission (e.g. through nebulization) or both. What causes a high viral load? Host factors (e.g. old age and pre-existing medical conditions) were present in some. But three others in Table 13.1 were in their 20s and had no known pre-existing medical conditions. Viral factors could also explain it, and perhaps super-spreading could be associated with specific lineages of the virus. An analysis in China found two distinct lineages.[5] Most of the super-spreading can probably be traced to a chain of transmission that starts with the first super-spreading event in Guangzhou [Figure 13.1]. But most of the people infected by that virus did not go on to spread infection to any others.

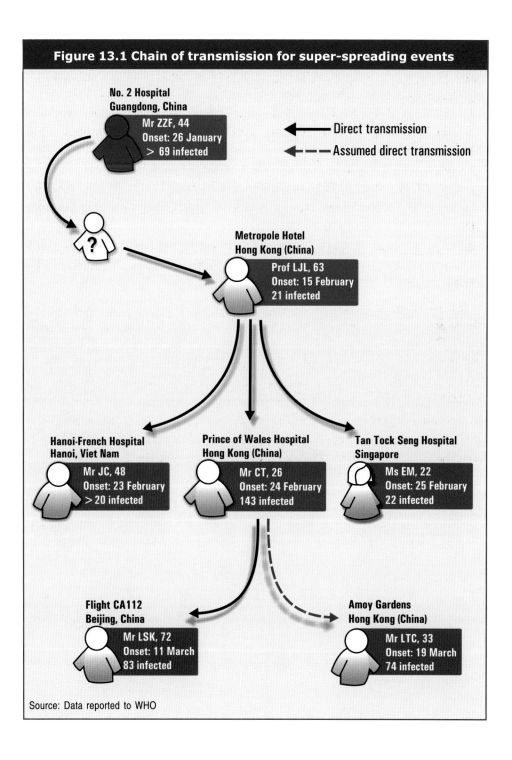

Figure 13.1 Chain of transmission for super-spreading events

No. 2 Hospital
Guangdong, China

Mr ZZF, 44
Onset: 26 January
> 69 infected

← Direct transmission

◄---- Assumed direct transmission

?

Metropole Hotel
Hong Kong (China)

Prof LJL, 63
Onset: 15 February
21 infected

Hanoi-French Hospital
Hanoi, Viet Nam

Mr JC, 48
Onset: 23 February
> 20 infected

Prince of Wales Hospital
Hong Kong (China)

Mr CT, 26
Onset: 24 February
143 infected

Tan Tock Seng Hospital
Singapore

Ms EM, 22
Onset: 25 February
22 infected

Flight CA112
Beijing, China

Mr LSK, 72
Onset: 11 March
83 infected

Amoy Gardens
Hong Kong (China)

Mr LTC, 33
Onset: 19 March
74 infected

Source: Data reported to WHO

REFERENCES

[1] Wu W et al. A hospital outbreak of severe acute respiratory syndrome in Guangzhou, China. *Chinese Medical Journal*, 2003, 116(6):811–818.

[2] Zhong NS et al. Epidemiology and cause of sever acute respiratory syndrome (SARS) in Guangdong in February 2003. *The Lancet*, 25 October 2003, 362(9393):1353–1358.

[3] Interview with Tang Xiaoping, president of No.8 People's Hospital, on China Today. *CCTV*, May 2003 (http://www.cctv.com/lm/124/31/86426.html).

[4] Xu RH et al. Epidemiologic clues to SARS origin in China. *Emerging Infectious Diseases*, 2004, 10(6): 1030–1037.

[5] Breiman RF et al. Role of China in the quest to define and control severe acute respiratory syndrome. *Emerging Infectious Diseases*, 2003, 9(9):1037–1041.

14 SOLVING THE METROPOLE HOTEL MYSTERY

INDEX CASE

Professor LJL was a doctor at the No. 2 Affiliated Hospital of Zhongshan Medical University in Guangzhou City, Guangdong Province, China. Mr ZZF had brought the virus into that hospital on 30 January [see Chapter 13].

In mid-February 2003, the 64-year-old physician was working late nights caring for patients who had developed a strange new form of pneumonia. Like other doctors fighting the disease, he wore a mask and gloves. But despite his precautions, he became ill on 15 February.

He was feeling better when he decided to attend a wedding in Hong Kong (China), as previously arranged. On 21 February, he and his wife took the three-hour bus ride south from Guangdong Province to Hong Kong.

There he checked into room 911 of the Metropole Hotel, one of the countless three-star hotels that line the roads of the tourist district in Kowloon. He felt well enough to go shopping later that day. But the next morning, the elderly doctor woke with a high fever. Instead of going to the wedding he walked to the nearest hospital, the Kwong Wah Hospital, and was admitted. Professor LJL told the hospital staff that Guangzhou had many patients with atypical pneumonia and that he had treated some of them in the outpatient clinic. But his illness was different, he insisted. He was wrong.

On 4 March, Professor LJL died of what would later be called SARS. During his one-night stay at the Metropole Hotel, the SARS virus had passed to at least 16 other guests and one visitor at the hotel. The virus then spread around the world, leading to outbreaks in other countries. But in early March, none of this was known.

Metropole identified as source of multicountry outbreak

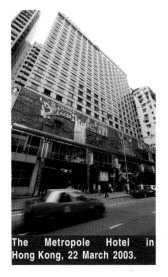

The Metropole Hotel in Hong Kong, 22 March 2003.

Less than a month later, Professor LJL's stay at the Metropole Hotel would be recognized as a key event. SARS outbreaks in Canada, Hong Kong, Singapore, and Viet Nam were all linked to the 9th floor of the hotel.[1] What had happened there?

On 24 February, the Hong Kong Department of Health was notified of Professor LJL's case of severe community-acquired pneumonia and started an investigation. The Department knew that Professor LJL had stayed at the Metropole, but did not consider this fact significant. The first clue came from Singapore. A day after WHO issued its global alert on 12 March, Singapore reported three cases, all of whom had stayed at the Metropole. This information was shared—as part of another conversation—between a doctor in Singapore's Ministry of Health and a doctor in the Hong Kong Department of Health on 8 March.

On 13 March, the Department of Health learned of a 72-year-old Canadian tourist (Mr AC) with atypical pneumonia who had stayed at the Metropole. Then on 18 March, Health Canada, the federal health authority, notified Hong Kong by facsimile that the index case for the Toronto outbreak, Ms KSC, had stayed at the Metropole. Only then did the Department of Health start reviewing all its files on reported cases of severe community-acquired pneumonia.

By 19 March, the Hong Kong Department of Health knew of seven SARS cases who were linked to the 9th floor of the Metropole Hotel. Professor LJL was identified as the index case, as he had fallen ill before all the others. All had been at the hotel, either staying or visiting on the 9th floor, around the same time as Professor LJL. And yet there was no evidence that any of them had been in close contact with him. Certainly, none of those infected could recall meeting him.

How did the virus spread?

"We do not know how the infection took place," Hong Kong Health Director Dr Margaret Chan told reporters. "Perhaps they all stood outside the elevator at the same time and someone sneezed or coughed."[2]

Speculation was rife about how Professor LJL could have infected so many people in the hotel but left others unaffected during his brief stay. The infection, some said, could have been passed on through an elevator button he had touched or while walking through the same corridor. Even more frightening, it could have gone under hotel-room doors to infect occupants inside [see Figure 14.1].

But if the disease was so infectious, why had it infected fewer than 20 guests in the nearly 500-room hotel? And why weren't any members of the hotel staff affected? Of the 285 in the staff, 170 had regular contact with guests. And what about those who had cleaned Professor LJL's room? "A miracle!" was how one hotel employee explained it. A miracle? Or was there a logical explanation? And what was the link to the 9th floor?

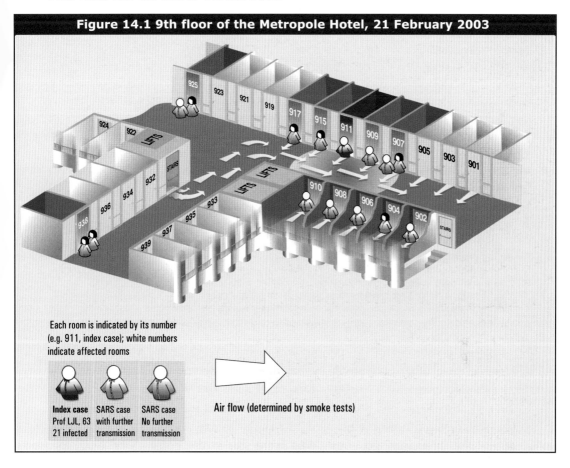

Figure 14.1 9th floor of the Metropole Hotel, 21 February 2003

Each room is indicated by its number (e.g. 911, index case); white numbers indicate affected rooms

Index case — Prof LJL, 63 — 21 infected

SARS case — with further transmission

SARS case — No further transmission

Air flow (determined by smoke tests)

THE INFECTED GUESTS AND VISITOR

While the cause of the disease was being identified, investigators were tracing the viral transmission chains that started at the Metropole Hotel. Fourteen guests and one visitor with SARS who were at the hotel on the night of 21 February were identified [see Table 14.1]. Two of those infected died: the index cases for Hanoi (Mr JC) and Toronto (Ms KSC).

All those infected, except Mr CKL, were on the 9th floor. The hotel staff told the WHO team that the guests in 909 had complained about the coughing in room 911 and had been transferred to room 1409 on the night of 21 February. But there was no record of this move at the hotel and Mr CKL does not recall the incident.

Table 14.1 People infected at the Metropole Hotel and consequences of their infection[a]

Personal details			Hotel stay		Disease event dates			Number directly
	Age	From	Room	Dates	Onset	Admit	Place	infected
Mr JC	47	USA	910	21-23 Feb	23 Feb	26 Feb	Hanoi	>20
Mr CT	26	Hong Kong	906[b]	18-23 Feb	24 Feb	4 Mar	Hong Kong	143
Mr CKW	51	USA	908	19-23 Feb	24 Feb	NA	Hong Kong	0
Ms CHC	42	Canada	907	19-22 Feb	24 Feb	6 Mar	Guangzhou	ND
Ms CJP	36	USA	917	19-22 Feb	24 Feb	2 Mar	USA	0
Ms LYC	33	Singapore	915	20-25 Feb	25 Feb	3 Mar	Singapore	0
Ms EM	22	Singapore	938	21-25 Feb	25 Feb	1 Mar	Singapore	22
Ms KSC	78	Canada	904	18-23 Feb	25 Feb	NA	Toronto	4
Mr TJH	37	UK	925	18-23 Feb	25 Feb	5 Mar	Philippines	0
Mr CHC	40	Canada	907	19-22 Feb	26 Feb	6 Mar	Guangzhou	ND
Mr CKL	55	Canada	1409	20-24 Feb	26 Feb	7 Mar	Vancouver	0
Ms CA[c]	26	Germany	ND	21-22 Feb	26 Feb	NA	Australia	0
Mr AC	72	Canada	902	20 Feb-2 Mar	27 Feb	2 Mar	Hong Kong	9
Ms EMH	33	UK	925	18-23 Feb	27 Feb	6 Mar	Philippines	0
Ms CJE	22	Singapore	938	21-25 Feb	28 Feb	2 Mar	Singapore	0

ND, not determined; NA, not applicable

[a] Two additional guests who were infected on 21 February are not included as details are not available. One hotel guest infected in March is also not included, but detailed in the text.

[b] Mr CT visited a friend in room 906 for those dates; he did not stay there.

[c] Ms CA recalls staying on the ninth floor, but her room number has not been determined.

Follow-up studies of the people who were staying at the Metropole later identified two other people who were infected,[3] bringing the total infected on 21 February to at least 17 people. One other guest (Mr VCC) who stayed on the 9th floor also developed SARS. But since he arrived at the hotel on 1 March and his symptoms did not develop until 13 March, he may have got the virus from one of the three infected guests who were still in the hotel at the time; the source of his infection is not clear. Mr VCC's wife was also infected, most likely by Mr VCC, as her symptoms started six days later than his.

Most of those infected at the hotel did not pass on the virus. But the impact of four infections was dramatic—starting SARS outbreaks outside mainland China, in Hanoi, Hong Kong, Singapore, and Toronto.

Professor LJL had also passed on the virus to his wife, daughter, brother-in-law, and one nurse at the Kwong Wah Hospital. The nurse was in the cubicle next to him during his admission, and had no direct contact with him. The other hospital workers complied fully with infection-control measures during his stay. No one was infected.

The next generation of spread

Mr JC from room 908 would take the virus to Hanoi and trigger the outbreak of 63 cases there, leading to the first alert about the new disease [see Figure 14.2].

Ms KSC, the 78-year-old Canadian, would return to Toronto and pass the virus on to four other members of her family before she died, without going to hospital. Through her family, Ms KSC would be the index case for the first Canadian cluster of 136 cases.

Three Singapore women were infected at the Metropole (they had stayed in rooms 915 and 938). All three were hospitalized within a day of one another, two in the same hospital, and yet only one (Ms EM) transmitted the virus, sparking the Singapore outbreak. Of 238 cases in Singapore, 195 had a contact history leading back to this one index case.

Mr AC, a 72-year-old Canadian in room 902, was admitted to St Paul's Hospital in Hong Kong, where nine of his contacts developed SARS.

But of all those infected at the Metropole, it was a local who passed on the virus to the most number of people. Mr CT, a 26-year-old airport worker, was not a guest at the hotel. However, he had to walk past room 911 to visit his friend in room 906. He thought little of this incident and did not mention it to investigators until 19 March. In all, 143 of his contacts had been infected, all of them at the Prince of Wales Hospital, where he was admitted on 4 March.

Outbreaks that could have been

A British-Filipino couple (Mr TJH and Ms EMH) were infected during their stay in room 925. They developed symptoms later, while travelling in the Philippines, and were hospitalized there on 5 and 6 March. Tests on their return to the United Kingdom were positive, but none of those they had come in contact with showed symptoms.

A German woman (Ms CA) who stayed at the Metropole on the night of 21 February travelled on to Australia, where she developed fever and respiratory symptoms. She was seen by a general practitioner, but was not admitted. On her return home, she tested positive for SARS.[4] But her travelling companion showed no sign of infection. Nor were there any other transmissions among all her contacts, including the doctor who treated her.

These three people could have set off outbreaks in Australia and the Philippines, but they didn't. Was it because their infection was milder and they had fewer close contacts? But the Filipino woman in particular had many contacts while she had symptoms. She had also received nebulizer treatment in the hospital, and that would have spread any droplets widely. Perhaps some people, even though infected, are not infectious.

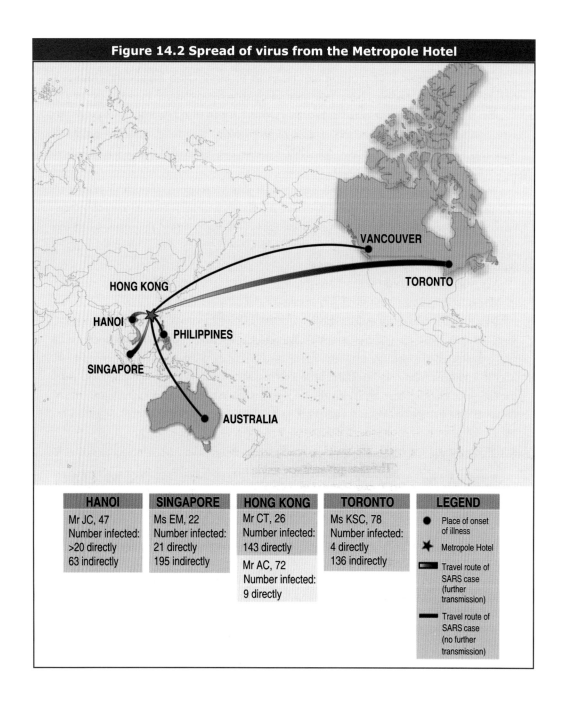

Figure 14.2 Spread of virus from the Metropole Hotel

VANCOUVER

TORONTO

HONG KONG

HANOI

PHILIPPINES

SINGAPORE

AUSTRALIA

HANOI	SINGAPORE	HONG KONG	TORONTO	LEGEND
Mr JC, 47	Ms EM, 22	Mr CT, 26	Ms KSC, 78	● Place of onset of illness
Number infected:	Number infected:	Number infected:	Number infected:	✷ Metropole Hotel
>20 directly	21 directly	143 directly	4 directly	▭ Travel route of SARS case (further transmission)
63 indirectly	195 indirectly	Mr AC, 72	136 indirectly	
		Number infected:		▬ Travel route of SARS case (no further transmission)
		9 directly		

In the case of 55-year-old Mr CKL, he may have been hospitalized early enough and immediately and effectively isolated in Vancouver so he could not infect others. Or he may simply have been one of the many people who did not transmit the virus for reasons that are still unknown.

WHO ENVIRONMENTAL HEALTH TEAM INVESTIGATES

The WHO team of environmental health experts from Health Canada that arrived in late April to investigate the environmental spread at Amoy Gardens [see Chapter 16] also investigated the outbreak at the Metropole. The Hong Kong Department of Health had started an environmental investigation of the hotel right after identifying the link on 19 March. No potential sources had been found in the building's plumbing, as well as its heating, air-conditioning, and ventilation systems.

The WHO team reported their findings on 16 May, at the same press conference where they released their report on the outbreak in Amoy Gardens. They had found traces of genetic material of the SARS virus in eight of 154 samples taken mostly on the 9th floor. Four of the eight positive samples were from the air inlet of the recirculating elevator lobby fan on the 9th floor. The samples taken outside guest rooms 908, 909, 910, and 911 (carpet, door sills, etc.) were also positive. Other sites tested, including the interior of room 911, where Professor LJL had stayed, yielded no traces of the virus. No live virus was found anywhere.

Professor LJL had returned to the hotel in the evening of 21 February after having dinner. The WHO team speculated that he might have contaminated the area of the corridor near his room by vomiting, spitting, or coughing heavily. As there was no record of hotel staff having been called to clean up vomit, his wife, the team said, could have cleaned it up herself, using water and a damp rag but no sanitizer. "The infectious agent would now reside in the damp carpet," the team went on to conjecture, "protected for quite some time by the high level of humidity of the hotel environment (over 80% relative humidity)."

Professor LJL's infected body fluids must have been aerosolized, as indicated by the traces on the inlet of the elevator lobby fan. Anyone who stepped out of the 9th floor lift shortly after the event would have been exposed, while those who walked past room 911 may have been at risk for a longer period. Presumably, by the morning there was no longer any viable virus, or else the staff had quickly disinfected the area without becoming exposed. It certainly appears that only those who were on the 9th floor that night were at risk. Thus, the "miracle" of none of the hotel staff getting SARS could simply have been due to their not having been exposed to the virus.

The rooms in the hotel, atypically, were pressurized; so infected aerosols could not have entered from the corridor. The WHO team dismissed theories that the virus was transmitted through elevators, door handles, or handrails. "In this hotel, these are unlikely scenarios," the report said, "because other guests would have made similar contacts, and indeed, staff would have had intense exposure risk. Staff who served the subject floor did not get infected."[5]

The contamination occurred in the corridor of one wing of one floor, and never moved up or down the building or endangered people inside their rooms.

References

[1] Update: Outbreak of severe acute respiratory syndrome – worldwide, 2003. *Morbidity and Mortality Weekly Report*, 2003, 52(11):226–228.

[2] Crampton T. Killer flu is traced to a hotel in Hong Kong. *International Herald Tribune*, 20 March 2003.

[3] Jones JD et al and the International Hotel M Study Group. *A Cohort Study of SARS Coronavirus Transmission in a Hong Kong Hotel, 2003*. [submitted for publication, 2005]

[4] Radun D et al. SARS: retrospective cohort study among German guests of the Hotel "M", Hong Kong. Euro Surveillance, 2003, 8(12):228–230.

[5] Tilgner I et al. *Final report: Metropole Hotel, WHO Environmental Investigation*. Geneva, World Health Organization, July 2003 (http://www.iapmo.org/common/pdf/ISS-Rome/SARS_Metropole_Hotel_HK.pdf, accessed 1 April 2005).

15 FLIGHT CA112: FACING THE SPECTRE OF IN-FLIGHT ___TRANSMISSION___

INDEX CASE

Mr LSK, a 72-year-old from Beijing, looked pale and sick. He asked a flight attendant for water to take some pills. But nothing appeared out of the ordinary on China Airlines flight 112 from Hong Kong to Beijing on 15 March 2003. No one on the apparently routine three-hour flight knew it yet, as the meal was served and a movie shown, but the SARS virus was in the plane ... and spreading.

Mr LSK had been in Hong Kong (China) from 26 December 2002. His elder brother was in Ward 8A of the Prince of Wales Hospital with *Salmonella* infection from 4 March and died on 9 March. Mr LSK regularly visited him at the hospital. The index case of the Prince of Wales Hospital outbreak was in Ward 8A at the same time; at least 143 of his contacts developed SARS. One of these contacts was Mr LSK; another was Mr LSK's niece, who also visited the ward. Mr LSK developed fever on 11 March and saw a doctor on 14 March, with fever, chills, rigor, cough, and shortness of breath. The doctor advised him to go to hospital, but Mr LSK wanted to return to Beijing on his previously booked flight the next day, 15 March.

On arrival in Beijing he went to a hospital but was not admitted. The next day he was taken to another hospital, where he was resuscitated in the emergency department and admitted. He died there on 20 March, having passed the virus to at least 59 other people in Beijing (three family members, seven or eight members of the hospital staff, other patients and their visitors).[1]

THE FLIGHT

Flight CA112 on 15 March was a Boeing 737-300 aircraft, which can typically carry up to 126 passengers.[2] On this flight there were 112 passengers and eight

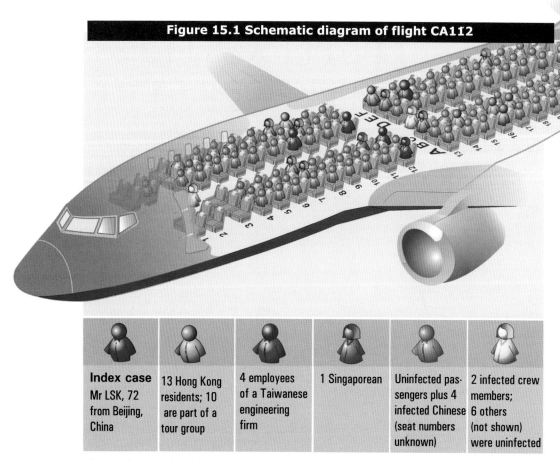

Figure 15.1 Schematic diagram of flight CA112

| Index case Mr LSK, 72 from Beijing, China | 13 Hong Kong residents; 10 are part of a tour group | 4 employees of a Taiwanese engineering firm | 1 Singaporean | Uninfected passengers plus 4 infected Chinese (seat numbers unknown) | 2 infected crew members; 6 others (not shown) were uninfected |

Adapted, by permission of the publisher, from Olsen SJ et al[2]

crew members. At least 22 passengers and two crew members developed SARS, raising the spectre of international spread through air travel [see Figure 15.1].

First detection and alert

On 23 March, a Hong Kong hospital (Tuen Mun) notified the Department of Health that a couple had been admitted the day before with fever that started on 18 March. This couple had been part of a 36-person group (including one guide) that had gone to Beijing on a five-day tour. As other cases came to light, the Department of Health issued a press release on 25 March calling on passengers on flight CA112 of 15 March and the tour group's return flight, CA115 of 19 March, to contact the Department.[3] None of the passengers on CA115 had been infected. But 10 people in the tour group and three other Hong Kong travellers on flight CA112 developed SARS. Eleven of them started showing symptoms between 17 and 20 March, and the two others on 23 March, suggesting a common source of exposure [see Table 15.1].

Table 15.1 Passengers infected during flight CA112

	Sex	Age	Seat	Onset	Admit	Death
Hong Kong tour group 1	F	51	13C	17 Mar	24 Mar	
Chinese official 1	M	41		18 Mar	21 Mar[a]	
Crew member 1 (Ms MCY)	F			18 Mar		
Hong Kong resident 1	M	41	10F	18 Mar	21 Mar	16 Apr
Hong Kong tour group 2	M	44	13F	18 Mar	22 Mar	
Hong Kong tour group 3	F	44	13E	18 Mar	22 Mar	3 May
Hong Kong tour group 4	F	32	9F	18 Mar	23 Mar	
Hong Kong tour group 5	M	33	16A	18 Mar	23 Mar	13 Jun
Hong Kong tour group 6	F	27	7C	18 Mar	23 Mar	
Hong Kong tour group 7	M	48	14B	18 Mar	23 Mar	
Taiwan resident 1	M	43	9D	18 Mar	26 Mar	
Hong Kong tour group 8	M	61	17B	19 Mar	24 Mar	25 Apr
Chinese official 2	M			19 Mar		
China resident 1	M	29		19 Mar		
China resident 2	M	50		19 Mar		
Crew member 2	F			19 Mar		
Singapore resident	F	29	11C	19 Mar	26 Mar	4 Apr
Taiwan resident 2	F	29	12A	19 Mar	26 Mar	
Taiwan resident 3	M	37	12C	19 Mar	26 Mar	
Hong Kong resident 2	F	29	19F	20 Mar	27 Mar	
Hong Kong resident 3	M	36	16B	20 Mar	23 Mar	
Taiwan resident 4	M	47	12D	21 Mar	26 Mar	
Hong Kong tour group 9	F	50	7B	23 Mar	23 Mar	
Hong Kong tour group 10	F	31	10E	23 Mar	27 Mar	

[a] Passenger was hospitalized in Bangkok on 21 March, but discharged himself and was hospitalized again in Beijing.
Source: Olsen SJ et al[2]

SPREAD OF VIRUS

TAIPEI

Seven employees of a Taiwanese engineering firm had been on flight CA112, before returning to Taipei on 21 March. As their laboratory results confirmed, four of them developed SARS, first showing symptoms between 18 and 21 March. But they were admitted only on 26 March after Hong Kong authorities had issued the advisory about flight CA112. Taiwan health authorities scrambled to trace their contacts, including the other passengers on their return flight to Taipei, but none had caught the virus.

SINGAPORE

Ms CPL, a 29-year-old woman from Singapore who was on flight CA112, became the fourth person to import SARS to Singapore (the first three had been infected at the Metropole Hotel). She developed symptoms on 19 March while in Beijing. By the time she returned home on flight CZ355 from Beijing on 26 March she was very ill. From the airport she went straight to Tan Tock Seng Hospital, the SARS-designated hospital. She died on 4 April. The Singapore authorities faced a huge challenge in tracking all the other passengers on that flight, armed only with their names and nationalities. But none of those became ill, nor did the taxi driver who took her from the airport to the hospital.

Beijing via Bangkok; ILO official dies

Two Chinese officials who had been on flight CA112 flew on to Bangkok on 17 March. One of them became ill on 18 March and was admitted to hospital on 21 March, but discharged himself. On 23 March, both officials boarded flight TG614 to Beijing, where they would later be reported as SARS cases. Sitting next to them on that flight was Mr PA, a 52-year-old Finnish official of the International Labour Organisation (ILO). Mr PA developed symptoms on 28 March and died on 5 April.

Mr PA was the first foreigner to develop SARS in China. He had gone from perfect health to death in a matter of days, and had no obvious contact history. He had been in Bangkok since 18 March, and Europe before that. In neither place was there any transmission of SARS. But he recalled the fact that his neighbour on the flight was ill, shivery, and covered by blankets. Mr PA's death greatly affected the international community in Beijing. It may also have contributed to China's perception of SARS as a global concern that needed intense control efforts.

Two other Chinese people who developed SARS were later identified as passengers on flight CA112. Both developed symptoms on 19 March and were hospitalized in Beijing.

Inner Mongolia Autonomous Region, China

In China, Ms MCY, a flight attendant on CA112, began feeling sick on the morning of 18 March. But she kept working and a few days later, still feeling ill, returned to her home in Hohhot, the capital of the Chinese autonomous region of Inner Mongolia.

From Ms MCY, the virus passed to three family members and her doctor in Hohhot, as well as to a close friend, who later became one of the first in Inner Mongolia to die of SARS. "We were told atypical pneumonia was finished in February," Ms MCY said when interviewed by *The New York Times*. "I never imagined that this kind of tragedy would fall on me and my family and take away the person dearest to me."[4]

Health authorities later traced most of Inner Mongolia's 290 SARS cases to Ms MCY and the other flight attendant who had been infected on flight CA112. And from Inner Mongolia, the virus spread to Mongolia [see Chapter 11].

IMPACT OF EVENT: EXIT SCREENING

On 27 March 2003, WHO recommended new measures to reduce the risk of further international spread of SARS. In areas with local transmission of the virus, passengers taking international flights should be asked whether they had fever or respiratory symptoms and contacts with possible SARS cases. Their temperature should also be checked. National authorities in those areas were encouraged to advise travellers with fever to postpone travel until they felt better.[5]

In contrast to entry screening, which many countries introduced at considerable cost and with little apparent benefit, exit screening may have helped prevent the spread of SARS.[6]

TRANSMISSION ON OTHER FLIGHTS

By 22 May, WHO had analysed the outcome of 35 flights with probable SARS cases on board. Virus spread occurred on only four of these flights.[7] Of the 29 people who were infected on these flights, 24 were on CA112.

The first flight with SARS transmission was flight SQ25 [see 15 March in Chapter 1]. A 33-year-old physician who had treated the Singapore index case developed symptoms on 9 March, while attending a medical conference in New York. His 31-year-old wife and 62-year-old mother-in-law were with him. His wife had started showing symptoms on the flight; his mother-in-law, on the day of departure. Therefore, they could not have

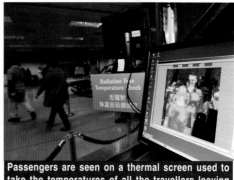

Passengers are seen on a thermal screen used to take the temperatures of all the travellers leaving Changi International Airport in Singapore.

been infected on the flight. Only one person was infected in-flight: a 22-year-old female flight attendant (her symptoms began on 18 March). None of the other passengers (82 in Frankfurt and 28 in Singapore) or the attendants at the medical conference in New York developed SARS.[8] The second flight with SARS transmission was flight CA112. The third was flight AF171 of 22 March, from Hanoi to Paris (via Bangkok). Here the source case was a French physician at the French-Hanoi Hospital who had examined a colleague with SARS on 16 and 17 March without any respiratory protection. He was hospitalized on the day of arrival in Paris. Of the three people infected on that flight, the only one who had clearly come in contact with the source case was the 40-year-old female flight attendant (onset 30 March) who served him on the Hanoi-to-Bangkok leg. The other two were a 55-year old male passenger (onset 26 March) sitting one row ahead and to the right, and a 26-year-old male passenger (onset 29 March) sitting four rows behind the source case.[8]

The fourth and last flight with SARS transmission was flight TG614, where the ILO's Mr PA became infected after sitting next to a person who was infected on CA112 [see above]. Except possibly for flight AF171, and flight CA112, where the mode of transmission is still unclear, all in-flight transmissions were limited to people who had direct contact with the source case.

After the 27 March travel advisory, there were no transmissions of SARS on flights despite at least 21 flights with probable SARS cases on board.[9] The advice from national authorities and exit screening had kept people with SARS symptoms from travelling. But more than this, it appears that what happened on CA112 was unique. Why was this flight the only one where a person with SARS symptoms infected so many others? Was it simply because the virus replicated with high efficiency in Mr LSK? But how was the virus transmitted on this flight? No one knows.

References

[1] Liang W et al. Severe acute respiratory syndrome, Beijing, 2003. *Emerging Infectious Diseases*, 2004, 10(1): 25–31.

[2] Olsen SJ et al. Transmission of the severe acute respiratory syndrome on aircraft. *New England Journal of Medicine*, 2003, 349(25):2416–2422.

[3] *Health surveillance for airline passengers.* Hong Kong Special Administrative Region of the People's Republic of China, Government Information Centre, 25 March 2003 (http://www.info.gov.hk/gia/general/200303/25/0325228.htm, accessed 1 April 2005).

[4] Kahn J. Even in remote China, SARS arrives in force. *The New York Times*, 22 April 2003.

[5] *WHO recommends new measures to prevent travel-related spread of SARS.* Geneva, World Health Organization, 27 March 2003 (http://www.who.int/ csr/don/2003_03_27/en/, accessed 1 April 2005).

[6] Bell DM, World Health Organization Working Group on Prevention of International and Community Transmission of SARS. Public health interventions and SARS spread, 2003. *Emerging Infectious Diseases*, 2004, 10 (11): 1900–1906.

[7] *More than 8000 cases reported globally, situation in Taiwan, data on in-flight transmission, report on Henan Province, China.* Geneva, World Health Organization, 22 May 2003 (http://www.who.int/csr/don/2003_05_22/en/, accessed 1 April 2005).

[8] Desenclos JC et al. Introduction of SARS in France, March–April, 2003. *Emerging Infectious Diseases*, 2004, 10(2):195–200.

[9] *Consensus document on the epidemiology of severe acute respiratory syndrome (SARS).* Geneva, World Health Organization, 2003 (WHO/CDS/CSR/GAR/ 2003.11).

16 LOCKDOWN AT AMOY GARDENS

Police in surgical masks surrounded the block in the dead of night. While the officers secured the area with metal barricades and tape, health workers in full protective gear guarded the door to the high-rise. No one was allowed to go in or come out. Other officials began piling food and supplies near the entrance for those locked inside.

Like a scene out of a movie, this building in the Amoy Gardens apartment complex in Hong Kong (China) was quarantined on 31 March 2003. The eerie news footage of the masked government officials surrounding the buildings sent shock waves around the world and brought home to people everywhere the deadly impact of SARS.

Hong Kong, one of Asia's most prosperous and progressive cities, was forced to use drastic measures to control the outbreak. "We are imposing restrictions on personal freedoms," said Secretary for Health, Welfare and Food Dr Yeoh Eng-kiong. "This is something we have never done before and hope never to do again in the future."[1]

SARS seemed to be entering a new, more frightening phase. Until then, infections had been largely limited to close contacts, mostly in hospital. Now, it appeared that an environmental source was leading to an explosive outbreak. Could Hong Kong control its spread? First, the nature of this unusual outbreak had to be understood.

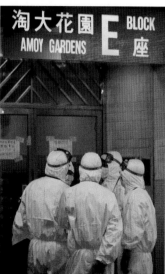

Health workers stand outside Block E of Amoy Gardens. Over 100 residents were infected with the virus and over 200 others quarantined in isolated holiday camps.

INDEX CASE

The index case was identified as Mr LTC, a 33-year-old with autoimmune kidney disease. He lived and worked in Shenzhen, Guangdong Province, but visited Hong Kong twice a week for dialysis at the Prince of Wales Hospital. Each time he would stay with his brother who lived in Block E, one of 14 apartment blocks in the Amoy Gardens complex, which was built in 1981. The complex has about 19,000 residents.

Mr LTC had fever and diarrhoea when he stayed with his brother on the night of 14 March 2003. During his dialysis the next day, his condition worsened and he was transferred to Ward 8A, which had been used since 13 March for cases of suspected atypical pneumonia.

He responded to medical treatment (including an anti-influenza drug) and was discharged on 19 March. None of the control and follow-up measures for SARS cases was implemented, as the diagnosis, based on the isolated virus, was influenza. He returned to Prince of Wales Hospital on 22 March for his scheduled dialysis. On admission, his condition deteriorated rapidly, and he was diagnosed with SARS on 27 March.

Mr LTC had stayed overnight in his brother's unit in Amoy Gardens after being discharged from hospital on 19 March, just as he had on 14 March. He may have transmitted the virus at either or both visits, but the onset dates of the other cases makes it more likely that the virus spread on 19 March. He may have been infected with SARS in Prince of Wales Hospital or in Shenzhen; the source of his infection is not known.

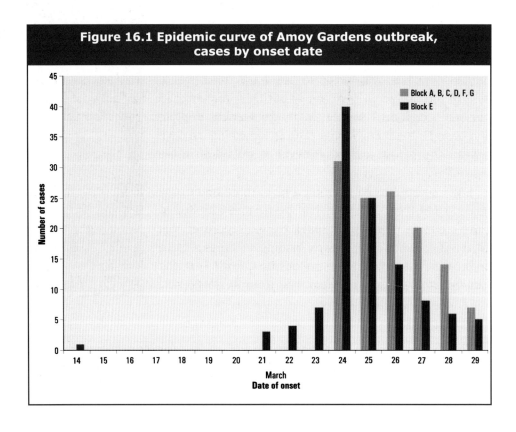

Figure 16.1 Epidemic curve of Amoy Gardens outbreak, cases by onset date

Mr LTC's brother and his brother's wife developed SARS, with the brother first showing symptoms on 23 March and his wife on 28 March. Two nurses who attended Mr LTC at the dialysis session on 22 March were also infected, and both developed symptoms on 26 March [see Figure 16.1]. These cases of infection following close contact were to be expected, but the Amoy Gardens outbreak was to involve a total of 329 residents, 42 of whom died. And they had got the virus in an entirely unprecedented way.

THE OUTBREAK STARTS—AND IS CONFINED

The first alert was raised on 26 March 2003, when 15 residents of Amoy Gardens were reportedly admitted to the United Christian Hospital with suspected SARS. Immediately, the Hong Kong Department of Health sent a team to investigate the common exposure for these cases. None was found. All residents of the complex were warned of the outbreak so that they could be on the alert for symptoms and, once these appeared, they could be isolated and treated early. Daily inspections at Amoy Gardens continued. Still the number of cases continued to rise, mostly in Block E.

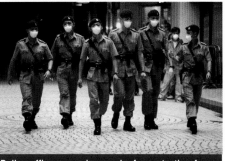

Police officers wearing masks for protection from SARS patrol the grounds of Amoy Gardens. Block E residents were quarantined for 10 days in isolated holiday camps.

On 29 March, a multidisciplinary team from the Department of Health and the Environment, Transport and Works Bureau looked into possible environmental factors. The next day, the Hong Kong SARS Task Force discussed the outbreak and recommended isolating Block E residents. The 1936 Quarantine and Prevention of Disease Ordinance, revised on 27 March to include SARS, empowered the Department of Health to do just that.

In the early morning of 31 March, an isolation order was issued to Block E. Over 240 residents were told that they could not leave the building for 10 days and that they would be hospitalized if they showed symptoms of SARS. Failure to comply could mean prosecution. Many residents fled the building before the area could be sealed off. "Those who have left must contact us," appealed Dr Yeoh Eng-kiong. "Every infected person has the potential to cause another big outbreak like the one at Amoy Gardens."[2]

Locking down Block E was a massive, swift operation involving more than 100 officers from the Departments of Health, Police, Home Affairs, and Social Welfare. Officers went from door to door to serve the notices, explain the need for isolation, and serve meals. The aim, they said, was to protect public health, as well as the health of the residents.

IS THE VIRUS SPREADING THROUGH THE ENVIRONMENT?

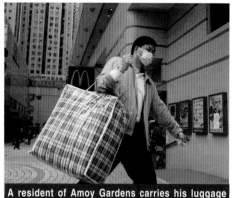

A resident of Amoy Gardens carries his luggage as he leaves the estate. The Government quarantined the housing block in early April.

By the end of the day on 31 March, 213 residents of Amoy Gardens had been admitted to hospital, 107 of them from Block E. Each housing block in Amoy Gardens typically has 33 floors. Each floor has eight units, arranged in pairs [see Figure 16.2]. Most of the cases from Block E were from units 7 and 8, which were next to each other, suggesting vertical spread. But how had it occurred?

On 1 April, new information from field investigations pointed to the building's sewage system as a potential source of the outbreak. It was then decided that the residents should be immediately evacuated to prevent further exposure. By early evening the evacuation had started.

All the Block E residents were to be moved to two holiday camps (Lady MacLehose Holiday Village and Lei Yue Mun Park and Holiday Village) that the Government had turned into quarantine centres. Evacuation was made more challenging by the need to maintain quarantine. But with help from the residents themselves, everyone—all 247 residents from 115 households in Block E—was moved to the centres by the early hours of 2 April.

The evacuation strategy succeeded in ending the outbreak. After 1 April there were only five new cases among Block E residents. Three were household contacts of previous cases, one was exposed to the virus in hospital, and the fifth may have been exposed in travel to Shenzhen.

TWO TEAMS INVESTIGATE THE OUTBREAK

Dr Thomas Tsang Ho-fai, the Department of Health consultant who had helped investigate the outbreak, described the investigations as "fishing expeditions" after the team had established a common source for the outbreak. He said, "We looked at water tanks; we were looking at cockroaches and rodents."[3]

Director of Health Dr Margaret Chan explained that preliminary findings had ruled out a common exposure (through travel or at a banquet or meeting), bioterrorism, and contaminated water or refuse. But positive samples from some rats and cockroach samples made it necessary to look into the sewage system.[4]

On 17 April 2003, the Department of Health investigators concluded that several factors were behind the outbreak. The same conclusions were reached by a WHO team of environmental experts, who arrived on 27 April and submitted their report on 16 May. The team came to assist the Department of Health in investigating the risk factors that made environmental transmission of SARS more likely in several residential buildings including Amoy Gardens and the Metropole Hotel [see Chapter 14].

The WHO team was composed of four experts from Health Canada: Dr Heinz Feldmann, an infectious disease specialist and microbiologist; Immo Tilgner, an engineer specializing in mechanical building systems; Allen Grolla, a laboratory technician with expertise in technical sampling and molecular detection of viruses; and Dr Ramon Flick, a virologist with expertise in mechanical virology sampling and virus isolation from different samples.

Working closely with Hong Kong health officials, the team made an exhaustive examination of the plumbing, heating, ventilation, and air-conditioning systems at Amoy Gardens. In all, they

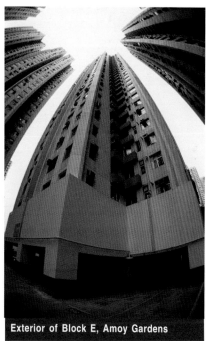

Exterior of Block E, Amoy Gardens

analysed 143 samples from the building. They found no genetic material from the SARS virus.

WHAT CAUSED THE OUTBREAK?

WHO experts concluded that an odd combination of factors had conspired to spread SARS through the building. First, the index case very likely had a high viral load in his faeces because of his medical condition. Second, bathroom drain traps had dried out or been removed, creating an open path for aerosol or droplets to enter the units via drains in the bathroom floor. Third, many residents had bought bathroom exhaust fans that were six to ten times more powerful than needed for use in a small space. These fans, when run with the bathroom door closed, could draw air from the waste pipe through the floor drain. Contaminated exhaust air from nearby bathroom vents could also have carried droplets from adjoining bathrooms via the light well, releasing contaminants through an open window on one floor, and transferring such contaminants into other living units several floors away.

Another factor that may have contributed to the spread of virus was the shutdown of flush water for 16 hours on the evening of 21 March, to allow a broken pipe to be fixed. Many residents were forced to use a bucket to flush their toilets. "Bucket flushing did most likely increase aerosol/droplet formation within the bathroom of the occupants and thus could have contributed to an increased infectious dose," the WHO report concluded. As the virus has been found to survive in stool for at least two days, virus may have survived from the

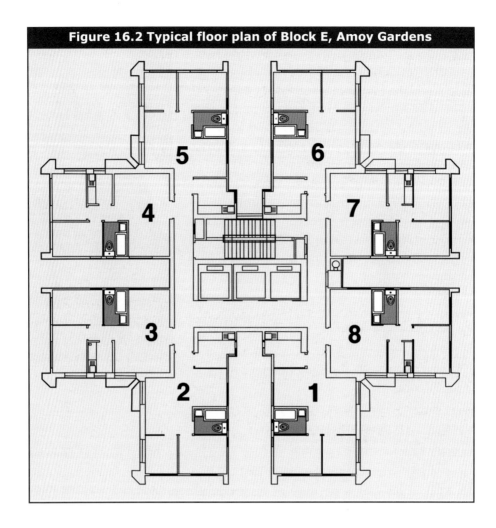

Figure 16.2 Typical floor plan of Block E, Amoy Gardens

overnight stay of the index case on 19 March. The team also found that the virus survived better in fresh water, which was used in bucket flushing, as opposed to seawater, which is generally used for toilet flushing in the building. However, transmission through the sewage system cannot explain the spread to other buildings. Transmission through airflow has been suggested as another possible mechanism [Figure 16.3].[5]

DID RATS OR COCKROACHES PLAY A PART?

The team largely ruled out transmission via pests such as rats or cockroaches. "Rodents and cockroaches are rather passive carriers, meaning that they pick the virus up from contaminated surfaces or from aerosols/droplets," the report noted. "Thus, there is the possibility of transmission of infectious material via these passive carriers. However, the dramatic course of the epidemic does not favour this being the main mechanism of transmission."[6]

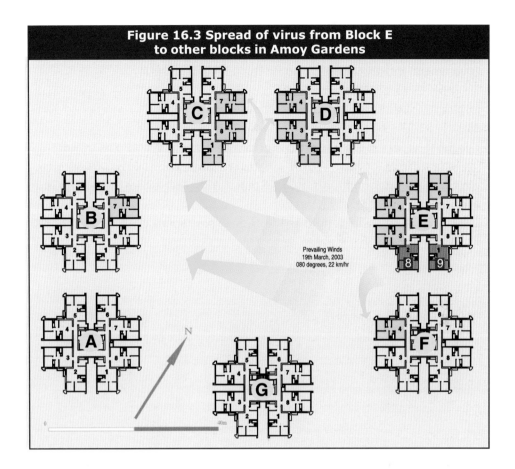

Figure 16.3 Spread of virus from Block E to other blocks in Amoy Gardens

Prevailing Winds
19th March, 2003
080 degrees, 22 km/hr

LIFE AFTER SARS

At Amoy Gardens, life goes on. But for those who have recovered from the disease, life after SARS is anything but normal. "When I visit other people's homes," said one who now suffers from post-traumatic depression, "they always want me to leave as soon as possible."[7]

REFERENCES

[1] Crampton T. 80 new SARS cases bring quarantine in Hong Kong. *International Herald Tribune*, 31 March 2003.

[2] [Anonymous]. Hong Kong seals off apartments when virus cases soar. Reuters, 31 March 2003 (http://yourhealth.stlukesonline.org/HealthNews/reuters/NewsStory0331200315.htm).

[3] Tsang H-F. Testimony before Legislative Council Select Committee to inquire into the handling of the severe acute respiratory syndrome outbreak by the government and the Hospital Authority, 7 February 2004.

[4] Chan M. Testimony before the Legislative Council Select Committee to inquire into the handling of the severe acute respiratory syndrome outbreak by the government and the Hospital Authority, 13 January 2004.

[5] Ignatius TS et al. Evidence of airborne transmission of the severe acute respiratory sysndrome virus. *The New England Journal of Medicine,* 2004, 350: 1731-1739.

[6] Tilgner I et al. Final report : Metropole Hotel, WHO Environmental Investigation. Geneva, World Health Organization, July 2003 (http://www.iapmo.org/common/pdf/ISS-Rome/SARS_Metropole_Hotel_HK.pdf, accessed 1 April 2005).

[7] Lee K. The estate where normal life is a dream. *South China Morning Post,* 11 March 2004 (City):3.

17 Panic in Pasir
__Panjang Market__

Index case

Singapore was in the midst of the SARS crisis when 64-year-old Mr TSC visited his brother (Mr TKC) in Ward 58 at Singapore General Hospital on 31 March 2003. Mr TKC was the index case of the SARS outbreak at that hospital, but because of his atypical symptoms and other medical conditions, his infection had not yet been recognized. On 5 April, Mr TSC began feeling unwell. But still he and his wife took their usual early-morning taxi ride from their suburban home in a high-rise flat on Choa Chu Kang Avenue 4 to the Pasir Panjang Wholesale Market, where he was a vegetable dealer.

On 8 April, feeling too ill to continue his daily routine, Mr TSC went to the emergency department of Singapore's National University Hospital. Twelve hours later he was moved into isolation. By then, he had become the index patient for a SARS outbreak that put more than a thousand people into quarantine and sent government health officials on a frantic mission to trace the chain of contacts.

The virus spreads

On the day that Mr TSC was hospitalized, a 45-year-old colleague at the Pasir Panjang market began feeling ill. Over an eight-day period, he would visit five different clinics seeking treatment before he was isolated at the Tan Tock Seng Hospital, which was specifically designated for SARS patients.

On 10 April, Mr TSC's wife was admitted, and two days later Mr TSC died. Two taxi drivers, colleagues at the market, and several relatives had been infected. Most had no idea they were carrying the virus.

By 20 April, the potential gravity of the situation had become clear. "As time goes on and as each infection wave continues, we will find it more and more difficult to track an infection to a source," Health Minister Lim Hng Kiang told reporters.[1] The Health Ministry put out a notice asking people who had visited the market between 5 and 19 April and felt sick to call a special SARS hotline. The Government also decided to take its strongest action yet to stem the infections originating from the market.

Government closes market, traces contacts, and quarantines more than 1,000

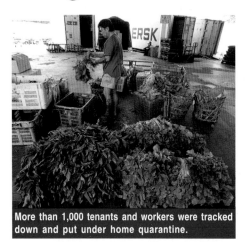

More than 1,000 tenants and workers were tracked down and put under home quarantine.

On the evening of 19 April, dozens of police officers wearing surgical masks cleared the market of people and built barricades to seal off the area. The next day, the Government announced that Singapore's largest wholesale vegetable market would be closed for 10 days and more than 1,000 people would be quarantined at home. Those who defied the orders would be fined or imprisoned, the Health Ministry said.

By 23 April, health officials had linked eight probable and 14 suspect SARS cases to the market. They suspected there might be more.

Senior government officials made it clear that the public had to take an active part in stemming the tide of new infections.

Fighting sars together

During a press conference, Prime Minister Goh Chok Tong pointed out the case of a 72-year-old man who worked at the market and was admitted to Tan Tock Seng Hospital on 19 April. Eight of the man's relatives went to see a general practitioner when they came down with fever. The doctor suspected that they could be SARS cases so he called for an ambulance designated for suspected SARS cases, asked the family to wait for the ambulance, and gave them masks to wear. Instead, they wandered off without their masks to a nearby food centre and a Chinese medical hall.

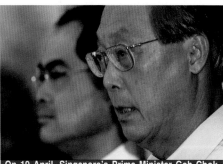

On 19 April, Singapore's Prime Minister Goh Chok Tong (right) spoke to reporters about SARS with Minister for Health Lim Hng Kiang. Prime Minister Goh said that SARS could be the worst crisis that Singapore has faced and announced strict new measures for quarantined carriers.

The Prime Minister also told the story of the 45-year-old colleague of the index patient, who visited a general practitioner, a polyclinic, and two *sinsehs* (practitioners of traditional medicine) before going to Changi General Hospital, which transferred him to Tan Tock Seng Hospital.

Irresponsible actions like these, Mr Goh said, put the health and safety of many others at risk. They were part of the problem, he added.[2]

"If you are unwell, see a doctor immediately," he advised. "If you continue to be unwell, go back to the same doctor. A new doctor would not know how your illness has progressed and would not give you the best treatment. Along the way, you may infect many other people, including your family and friends."

While Singaporeans grappled with the spread of the virus, the Government and the public also had to find a way to supply fresh vegetables with the country's largest produce market closed.

On 24 April, the Government responded to reports of panic buying and hoarding of vegetables with reassurances that there were enough vegetables in the country. Over a 24-hour period 772 tons of fresh vegetables, or more than one-and-a-half times the normal level of imports, were brought in from Malaysia. Yet shoppers at FairPrice, one of Singapore's largest supermarket chains, were allowed to buy no more than S$10 (~US$ 7) worth of vegetables per visit.

Meanwhile, the Government offered daily temperature checks to about 17,000 stall workers at 132 markets throughout Singapore to reassure the public that it was safe to shop again. Many vendors accepted the procedure, hoping that it would improve business. "Having my temperature taken is no problem at all," said Dallar Beebi, a 40-year-old stall operator at Geylang Serai market. "We are in contact with different people every day, so it's good to know we are well."[3]

When the 10-day period of closure of the Pasir Panjang market ended, the Government took the extra step of keeping the market closed for five more days and dispatching a team of 60 nurses to check on the health of those quarantined before allowing them back to work.

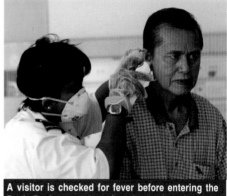

"We thought it would be better for us to reassure ourselves that these people are indeed well," said Health Minister Lim Hng Kiang, when announcing the measure.[4]

A visitor is checked for fever before entering the Pasir Panjang market after the 15-day closure.

Pasir Panjang finally reopened on 5 May, but vendors complained that SARS prevention measures such as temperature checks and registrations for contact tracing were keeping away many shoppers. Even a promotional offer of 1,000 free bags of fruits and vegetables drew only about 100 people. "They have the impression that Pasir Panjang is still not SARS-free," one wholesaler told the media.[5]

But the difficult measures had paid off in one important respect. Swift action by the Government—closing the market, tracing contacts, and placing more than 1,000 persons in quarantine—limited the spread of infection to only 14 other persons, nine of whom were family members.

References

1. Olesen A. Singapore quarantines 2,400 workers, closes vegetable market after SARS outbreak. *The Associated Press*, 20 April 2003.
2. Goh CT. Fighting SARS together. Singapore, Media Relations Division, Ministry of Information, Communications and the Arts, 22 April 2003 (http://app.sprinter.gov.sg/data/pr/2003042204.htm).
3. Arshad A. Enough greens, no need for panic buying. *The Straits Times*, 24 April 2003.
4. Goh Chin Lian. Wholesale centre shut for another five days. *The Straits Times* 29 April 2003.
5. Pasir Panjang Wholesale Centre business yet to recover from SARS impact. *Channel NewsAsia*, 15 July 2003.

18 THE HANOI-FRENCH HOSPITAL: _DR URBANI'S ALERT_

Dr Carlo Urbani had good instincts. As soon as the outbreak in Viet Nam became apparent, he saw the need for immediate action. He had already felt there was something odd about the index case. He was the first person in the world to recognize the significance of the events as they unfolded. His insistence, based on his astute observations, pushed the Viet Nam authorities to rapidly control the outbreak.

FIRST ALERT

Mr JC had been admitted to the Hanoi-French Hospital on 26 February, under the care of the night-duty doctor. In the morning, general physicians Dr Vu Hoang Thu and Dr Olivier Cattin (medical coordinator) took over his care. Mr JC's laboratory results and chest X-ray worried them. Dr Thu remembers, "Mr JC had just arrived from Hong Kong. Through the Internet we had heard about this fatal pneumonia from Guangdong as well as the avian influenza reported by Hong Kong. We discussed a possible connection. So, after the ward round on the morning of 27 February, I called WHO [in Hanoi] to advise them of the case and to get some advice on Mr JC's treatment. They put me through to Dr Urbani."

Dr Thu told Dr Urbani the next afternoon (Friday, 28 March) that the laboratory test for influenza B had turned up positive (a false-positive result). There were no serious concerns yet about Mr JC. He, in fact, seemed to improve the next day, but started getting worse again in the evening. By Sunday he was being intubated and ventilated. On Monday, Drs Thu and Cattin, desperate for help, called in some professors from the Hanoi medical school. They tried but failed to reach Dr Urbani, and left a message for him. After receiving the message, Dr Urbani went to the French-Hanoi Hospital to review Mr JC and see how he could help. "Carlo came without warning and it was a pleasure to see him," recalls Dr Cattin.

Taking action

After his visit, Dr Urbani sent a full clinical report to the WHO Regional Office in Manila. On first hearing about Mr JC, he had discussed the case with Dr Hitoshi Oshitani, Regional Adviser for Communicable Disease Surveillance and Response, including what samples to take and which laboratories to use to reach a diagnosis.

By 5 March, as the cases among the hospital staff started presenting [see Chapter 5], it was clear that Mr JC had indeed brought an infectious disease into Viet Nam. As Drs Thu and Cattin and the hospital staff laboured tirelessly to battle the virus, Dr Urbani was in the hospital every day, organizing samples for laboratory testing, talking to the staff, and strengthening infection-control procedures.

Over the next few days, the situation became alarming. On Thursday morning seven nurses were hospitalized. Dr Urbani spent all morning with the nurses. "He was extremely patient and kind with the staff, [collecting] any piece of information to make sense of what was going on and how the infection might be transmitted," recalled Dr Cattin. "The next day, with 12 nurses hospitalized and other staff getting ill, Carlo helped us a lot. He [isolated] the nurses, initiated contact tracing, and above all [helped with his] positive thinking and fantastic rational approach."

At the end of the day, all the sick nurses were isolated in the middle part of the general ward, personal protective equipment was finally in strict use, and security guards were posted at the only door that was not blocked and nailed shut.

Dr Urbani knew he was dealing with a new and dangerous disease. When his wife, Giuliana Chiorrini, warned him about the danger he was facing, he responded: "If I cannot work in such situations, what am I here for, to answer e-mail and push paper?"

Although more and more people were being hospitalized, Dr Urbani and WHO Representative Pascale Brudon found it difficult at first to convince the local health authorities that they had to do something right away. On 8 March, Dr Urbani emailed his colleagues, "I had a very disappointing discussion with … the Ministry of Health. … All decisions are postponed to next week, as now it's the weekend and he doesn't see any reason to hurry up. … [He] said what we (WHO) are doing is enough and he is very grateful for that support. … To my experience, when they say next week it doesn't necessarily mean Monday morning."

Fortunately, in a long meeting on Sunday, 9 March, Dr Urbani and Ms Brudon were able to persuade Vice-Minister of Health Nguyen Van Thuong that more urgent action was needed [see Chapter 5]. Critical at this stage were Dr Urbani's temperament and sharp intuition and the trust he had built with the authorities.[1] So was the relationship that Ms Brudon had nurtured between WHO and Viet Nam, as well as the leadership and decisiveness shown by Professor Thuong.

As a result, SARS infections in Viet Nam were largely limited to the first wave of infection. Infections took place mostly at the Hanoi-French Hospital, with a small cluster of six cases in Ninh Binh Province.

CONTRIBUTING TO THE GLOBAL RESPONSE

Dr Urbani's early alert was crucial in leading WHO to issue its global alert on 12 March. In an email message to WHO Headquarters on Sunday, 9 March, he provided a detailed clinical description for the global alert.

"High fever, severe myalgia, and mild respiratory symptoms characterize the onset," he wrote. "In some cases, headache, [neck] pain, without meningeal signs. Chills and malaise are also common. Cough increases the following days, and pneumonia is usually diagnosed ... 2–4 days from the onset. The lab [tests show] in some of [the cases] leuco-thrombocytopenia. Then, when pneumonia develops it has usually the X-ray finding of interstitial infiltrate, sometime diffuse and bilateral. The dissociation between auscultation and X-ray [is] similar to common viral/atypical pneumonia. In some cases there is, probably, an alveolar component, with the corresponding auscultatory finding of moist crepitations."

TENSIONS SUBSIDE

By 9 March 2003, Dr Urbani was feeling he could afford to relax somewhat. Not only had he persuaded the Viet Nam authorities to treat the outbreak as something out of the ordinary, but WHO had also received invitations for Dr Oshitani and Dr Tim Uyeki, an influenza expert from the Centers for Disease Control and Prevention, United States of America, to come to Viet Nam. In an email message on 9 March Dr Urbani wrote, "[The Ministry of Health] has agreed this WHO office can receive technical support on the subject of outbreak management. ... It is my impression now that the Ministry of Health is taking the necessary steps." And on 10 March, he wrote, "I [feel] more relaxed today. Things are moving, our recommendations are taken in full consideration, and our 'pressing' action with the Ministry of Health has been effective."

So on 11 March Dr Urbani was able to fly to Bangkok to attend a conference. But he had developed a fever. He was isolated and admitted to hospital on arrival. It was his last journey.

THE WORLD LOSES A HERO

On 29 March 2003, the public-health expert credited with helping contain SARS died of the ailment. He would be remembered not only as a doctor but also as an avid hang glider, motorcycle rider, and musician, who often took sheet music on his field trips in the hope that he might get a chance to play the

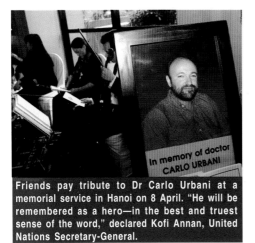

Friends pay tribute to Dr Carlo Urbani at a memorial service in Hanoi on 8 April. "He will be remembered as a hero—in the best and truest sense of the word," declared Kofi Annan, United Nations Secretary-General.

organ in some local church. He left behind his wife, two sons (Tommaso and Luca), and a daughter (Maddalena).

The loss was incalculable. To help himself deal with it, 16-year-old Tommaso leaned on advice from his father. In an email message read to his classmates at the French School in Hanoi on 7 April, Tommaso wrote: "He taught me never to be too fixed on some situations in life but to be ready always to start anew."[2]

Dr Urbani's important work was recognized far and wide. In Hanoi, his death was a blow to many. "Viet Nam has paid a very high price, and WHO also paid a high price in Viet Nam," said Ms Brudon. United Nations Secretary-General Kofi Annan said in a statement delivered at an 8 April Memorial Service in Hanoi, "Had it not been for his recognition that the outbreak of the virus was something out of the ordinary, many more would have fallen victim to SARS. It was the cruellest of ironies that he lost his own life to SARS while seeking to safeguard others from the disease. ... He will be remembered as a hero—in the best and truest sense of the word."[3]

On 16 April 2003, the WHO network of laboratories that detected and characterized the SARS virus dedicated their work to Urbani.[4] On 21 May, in a speech to the Fifty-sixth World Health Assembly, WHO Director-General-elect Dr Lee Jong-wook spoke about how Dr Urbani had told his wife he was needed in the field. "Carlo Urbani has given us WHO at its best," Dr Lee said, "not pushing paper, but pushing back the assault of poverty and disease."[5]

DR URBANI'S EARLIER WORK

Dr Urbani's pioneering work against SARS in its earliest days in Viet Nam was not unusual for him. He had spent his life on the front lines of the fight against infectious disease around the world.

Carlo Urbani was born on 19 October 1956 in Castelplanio, Italy, to a middle-class Catholic family. Both his parents were educators. His mother was headmistress of the local primary school and his father taught at the Ancona Commercial Navy Institute. His mother also served a term as town mayor.

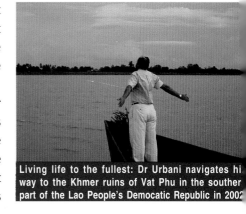

Living life to the fullest: Dr Urbani navigates hi way to the Khmer ruins of Vat Phu in the souther part of the Lao People's Democatic Republic in 2002

Dr Urbani finished medicine at the University of Ancona in 1981 and took a higher degree in infectious diseases three years later. In 1990, he joined the staff of the general hospital in Macerata, Italy. Always interested in international health issues, Dr Urbani approached the World Health Organization and was given assignments in Maldives, Mauritania, and Guinea in the early 1990s.

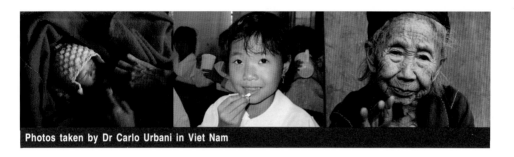
Photos taken by Dr Carlo Urbani in Viet Nam

In Mauritania, Dr Urbani was the first to document the transmission of *Schistosoma mansoni,* an infection affecting over 200 million people worldwide. In 1997, Dr Urbani joined Médecins Sans Frontières (Doctors Without Borders) and did landmark work on the prevention and treatment of a parasitic flatworm often affecting children along the Mekong River. In 1999, he was invited to receive the Nobel Peace Prize on behalf of the organization. He saw the award as recognition "that health and dignity are indissociable in human beings, and that it is a duty to stay close to victims and guarantee their rights".

Dr Urbani began working full time for the World Health Organization in 1998 and was posted to the Viet Nam office in May 2000.

A KIND AND SELFLESS MAN

Several months after the SARS outbreak was contained, Dr Shigeru Omi, Regional Director for WHO's Western Pacific Region, visited Italy to pay respects to Dr Urbani's family. Dr Omi recalled, "I had an opportunity to visit his hometown. I met his wife, his children, and his mother. I now understood why this kind man was so selfless. The life there is simple, and the community is very close-knit. Everyone respects each other. And everyone seemed genuinely solid and warm-hearted. It's not a coincidence that Dr Urbani, who was born and raised in this close-knit community, made such a great contribution to the battle against disease."

REFERENCES

[1] Reilley B et al. SARS and Carlo Urbani. *New England Journal of Medicine*, 2003, 348:1951–1952.

[2] French School in Hanoi reopens as two pupils mourn death of heroic father. *Agence France-Presse*, 8 April 2003.

[3] *Dr Carlo Urbani: A hero—in the best and truest sense of the word.* New York, NY, United Nations, 8 April 2003 (http://www.un.org/News/Press/docs/2003/sgsm8661.doc.htm, accessed 1 April 2005).

[4] *Coronavirus never before seen in humans is the cause of SARS.* Geneva, World Health Organization, 16 April 2003 (http://www.who.int/mediacentre/releases/2003/pr31/en/, accessed 1 April 2005).

[5] Lee J-W. Speech to the Fifty-sixth World Health Assembly. Geneva, World Health Organization, 21 May 2003 (http://www.who.int/dg/lee/speeches/2003/21_05/en/print.html, accessed 1 April 2005).

PART IV: THE SCIENCE OF SARS

19 CLINICAL
FEATURES

Before accurate and rapid diagnostic tests were available, clinical features and radiological findings were the only clues for the diagnosis of SARS. As diagnostic tests are not reliable early in the course of the illness, diagnosis based on clinical findings remains important, so that early public-health control actions can be initiated.

Most of the initial descriptions of SARS came from large cohort studies in Hong Kong (China), Toronto, Singapore, and China.[1,2,3,4,5] These initial descriptions had two limitations. First, not all the cases were confirmed by serology to have SARS coronavirus (SARS-CoV) infection. Some cases of atypical pneumonia with other causes may have been included. Second, many patients received treatments (such as corticosteroid and immunoglobulin) that might modulate the body's response to the infection, and hence the course of the illness.

Like other illnesses, SARS varies in severity. Some of those infected had no symptoms or only very mild influenza-like symptoms that were diagnosed as SARS only by laboratory tests. At the other extreme was the sudden and severe respiratory infections leading to respiratory failure and death. After recovery, some patients were left with pulmonary damage. Variations in SARS-CoV are unlikely to be responsible for the variable manifestations. Host factors such as the major histocompatibility complex (MHC) may explain some of the variability.[6] Age is an important factor, with children generally having milder disease and older people a higher mortality.

The clinical descriptions in this chapter are based on a cohort of 102 serologically confirmed SARS cases from Hong Kong who did not receive corticosteroids, and are supplemented by published reports.

PHASES OF SARS

The typical clinical course of SARS generally follows three phases [Figure 19.1].[7] Phase 1, which is the viral replication phase, usually lasts for about a week after symptom onset. The viral load is noted to increase progressively in respiratory secretions, stool, and urine.[8] Chest X-rays and computed tomography

(CT) scans show only slowly progressing lung damage at this stage.[8] In about a quarter of cases, a transient period of clinical improvement marks the end of phase 1. Phase 2 is the immune hyper-reactive phase, with damage caused by the body's immune system. There is recurrence of fever, oxygen desaturation, and radiological progression of pneumonia or development of adult respiratory distress syndrome (ARDS). This phase is associated with a fall in viral load. Phase 3 is the pulmonary destruction phase. There is usually no fever (unless there are secondary infections) or only a low-grade one. The pulmonary damage, however, persists or even progresses, giving the lungs a honeycomb-like appearance on CT scan. As the pulmonary disease progresses, oxygenation of blood cannot be sustained and the patient may require breathing support. Permanent injury and fibrosis of the lung will set in and the patient may succumb as a result of respiratory failure or may recover with residual impairment of pulmonary functions. Not all patients go through all three phases, especially people who are older or have impaired immune systems.

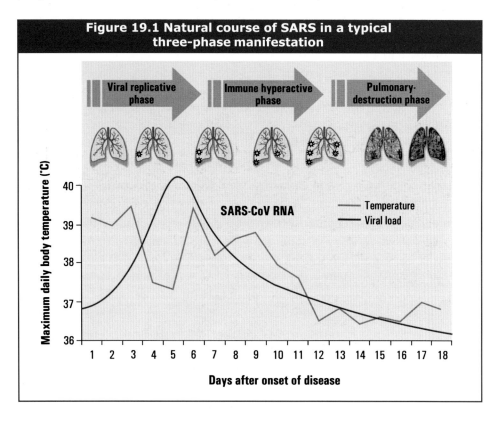

Figure 19.1 Natural course of SARS in a typical three-phase manifestation

Prodromal symptoms

The initial symptoms are fever, chills and rigor, muscle pain, dry cough, headache, and dizziness.[6,7,8,9,10] Fever, chills, and malaise are the three most common symptoms at the time of presentation. These symptoms are non-specific, making early diagnosis extremely difficult, unless there is a known exposure to a known SARS case. Productive cough and sore throat are so uncommon in SARS that they have been suggested as negative diagnostic features.

Pulmonary manifestations

Pulmonary illness is the primary manifestation of SARS. Dry cough is common in the early phase of the disease. If the disease gets worse, patients usually find themselves short of breath while coughing. Inspiratory crackles at the lung bases are often heard but wheezing is usually absent. Towards the end of the first week or at the start of the second week, the pulmonary disease begins to worsen. Shortness of breath increases and limits physical activity. Airspace consolidation, from being unilateral and focal in the early phase of the disease, soon becomes multifocal and more extensive in the second week of the illness [Figure 19.2].

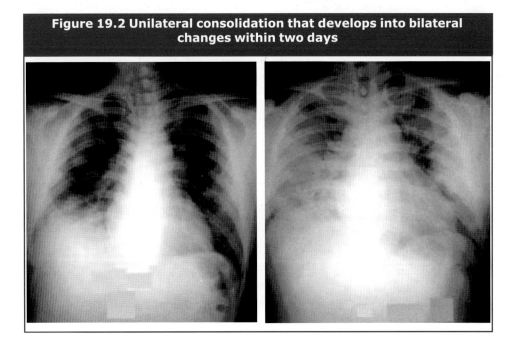

Figure 19.2 Unilateral consolidation that develops into bilateral changes within two days

Although all lung segments can be involved, it is mostly the lower lobes that are affected.[13] In a few cases, pulmonary infiltrates could be detected shifting from one area to another within one or two days. The shifting radiographic shadows coincide with reduction in viral load,[8] suggesting an immune-related damage instead of direct cytolysis by the virus. A high-resolution CT scan of the thorax shows features consistent with, but not specific for, bronchiolitis obliterans organizing pneumonia (BOOP),[9] an immune-mediated disease that responds to corticosteroid therapy [see Figure 19.3]. Other findings include thickening of interlobular septa and intralobular interstitium.

Figure 19.3 Computer tomography showing a mixed ground glass and consolidation opacification resembling bronchiolitis obliterans organizing pneumonia (BOOP)

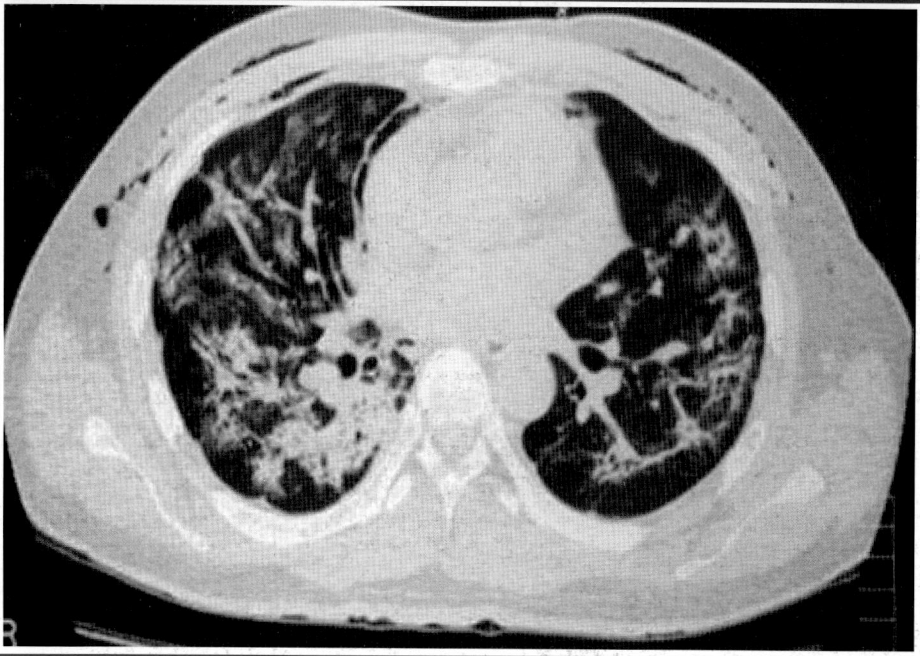

Around 20% to 25% of patients eventually run into severe respiratory failure and ARDS, and thus need care in the intensive care unit (ICU).[10] They will require mechanical ventilation when their oxygen saturation cannot be maintained with high-flow supplementary oxygen. During the epidemic, around 25% of SARS patients who were admitted to the ICU died, mostly from multiple organ failure and secondary nosocomial infections. The mortality rate was higher among those who required mechanical ventilation.

Pneumothorax and pneumomediastinum (air in the chest) were often reported in those severely ill with SARS. These can develop either spontaneously or in association with the use of mechanical ventilation. In one report, 12% of seriously

ill SARS patients developed spontaneous pneumomediastinum.[13] Among patients nursed in the ICU, 25% developed one or the other condition.[14] The incidence of barotraumas (damage from pressure of ventilation) was unusually high despite low-volume, low-pressure mechanical ventilation. The reason is unclear, but reduced lung compliance could be partly responsible, given the pulmonary oedema with hyaline membrane formation and cellular fibromyxoid-organizing exudates in airspaces seen by microscope.

INTESTINAL MANIFESTATIONS

Diarrhoea is the second most common manifestation of SARS. Up to 20% of patients had diarrhoea on presentation,[6] and up to 70% of patients had diarrhoea during the course of illness.[8] The stool is usually watery and high-volume, with no mucus or blood. The profound water and electrolyte loss can lead to volume depletion and electrolyte disturbance in severe cases. In some patients, diarrhoea and fever are the only initial manifestation of SARS in the absence of pneumonia on X-ray. In others, diarrhoea starts in the second week of the illness as fever recurs and pulmonary disease progresses. In a Hong Kong cohort of 1,755 patients, diarrhoea was found to be most common in the second week of the illness, when the fever started to decline. Diarrhoea is associated with more severe pulmonary diseases.[16] Fortunately, it is usually self-limiting and no deaths due to diarrhoea were reported in SARS cases.

Intestinal biopsies obtained by colonoscopy or during autopsy showed minimal inflammation or architectural disruption.[11] However, ultrastructural studies showed the presence of viral particles (60–90nm in size) within both small and large intestinal cells. Viral particles are confined to the epithelial cells, primarily in the apical surface enterocytes and rarely in the glandular epithelial cells. Intracellularly, viral particles are contained within dilated cytoplasmic vesicles consistent with dilated endoplasmic reticulum.[16] During the second week of the illness, the virus can be found by polymerase chain reaction (PCR) in the stool of almost all patients.[8] In vitro studies show that SARS-CoV persists in human colonic cells without causing cell damage.[12]

HEPATIC MANIFESTATIONS

Liver enzyme derangement is common, usually in the second week of the illness. In a cohort of 294 patients, around one quarter had elevated alanine transaminase (ALT) levels on admission.[13] In the rest, two thirds developed elevated ALT after admission. In the few cases where liver biopsy was done, features of acute hepatitis could be seen but no viral particle was identified. Electron microscopy did not reveal viral particles, but PCR suggests that viral protein could be found in some cases.[14] It is likely that in most of these cases, liver dysfunction resulted from acute inflammatory response and cytokine reaction. There is little evidence to show that SARS-CoV directly invaded the liver tissue. Although initial data suggested that co-infection of hepatitis B virus and SARS-CoV led to worse clinical outcome,[8] with larger cohort analysis, this co-infection did not appear to jeopardize the survival of the patients.[18]

HAEMATOLOGICAL MANIFESTATIONS

The haematological features of SARS help to diagnose the disease. Initial and progressive lymphopaenia (absolute lymphocyte count <1000/mm³) is common.[15] The lymphocyte count continues to drop as the disease progresses and in most cases reaches its lowest point in the second week. Lymphopaenia is so common, in fact, that without a progressive drop in lymphocyte count, a diagnosis of SARS would be open to doubt. All T-cell lineages appear to be affected, with the number of CD4 and CD8 cells dropping in parallel; on the other hand, B lymphocytes are relatively unaffected.[20]

The cytokine profile of SARS patients shows a marked elevation of Th1 response (Interferon-gamma, IL-1, IL-6, and IL-12) for at least two weeks after the onset of the disease but little elevation of TNF-alpha and anti-inflammatory cytokinese (IL-10).[16] The chemokine profile demonstrates a significant elevation of neutrophil chemokine IL-8, monocyte chemoattractant protein-1 (MCP-1).[21]

In most cases, the lymphocyte count starts to recover in the third week of illness, coinciding with clinical improvement. However, 30% of patients are still lymphopaenic in the fifth week of SARS.[20] Lower counts of CD4 and CD8 cells are associated with adverse clinical outcomes of ICU admission or death.[20] Moreover, thrombocytopaenia, reactive thrombocytosis, and isolated prolonged activated thromboplastin time are commonly observed.[20] Disseminated intravascular coagulopathy, however, rarely occurs.

RENAL MANIFESTATIONS

Although the virus has been identified in the renal tubules, there is little evidence to suggest that SARS-CoV causes direct injury to the kidney. However, patients with end-stage renal failure and on renal replacement therapy such as hemodialysis may have a more aggressive and yet different presentation of the illness.[17] In a small series of four dialysis patients who contracted SARS-CoV, all four developed respiratory failure requiring mechanical ventilation and eventually died.[18]

CARDIAC MANIFESTATIONS

About half of patients experienced hypotension (systolic blood pressure <100mmHg ± diastolic blood pressure <50mmHg) during hospitalization.[19] The low blood pressure may account for the dizziness felt by many patients. Persistent tachycardia (increased heart rate) was reported in 40% of patients, even in the absence of fever.[24] These abnormal cardiac rhythms were transient and did not warrant therapy. Patients were mostly asymptomatic. Prospective studies using transthoracic echocardiography, in a cohort of 46 patients confirmed to have SARS,[24] disclosed a significantly higher left ventricular index of myocardial performance (IMP) in the acute phase of the infection. Those who required mechanical ventilation had a lower mean left ventricular ejection fraction and a higher mean IMP. These parameters point to a subclinical diastolic impairment without systolic involvement of the heart in SARS. Microscope examination of the heart, however, reveals no interstitial lymphocytic infiltrate or myocyte necrosis.[24] Whether myocardial performance is impaired by cytokine-induced injury, hypoxic damage or drug- (ribavirin) induced alteration is not yet known.

NEUROLOGICAL MANIFESTATIONS

Neurological symptoms of SARS appear to be rare, with only isolated reports of epileptic fits, mental confusion, and disorientation.[20] No focal neurological deficit or structural abnormality on CT and magnetic resonance (MR) scans was found. Lumbar puncture and analysis of spinal fluid were normal in most cases. SARS-CoV RNA were detected in the cerebrospinal fluid of a patient with seizure, but the role of the virus in causing the seizure is not known.[25] A number of patients with SARS developed affective psychosis during the acute phase of their illness. A case-control study found the psychosis to be associated with high-dose steroid use, personal vulnerability, and psychosocial stress.[21]

THROMBISIS AND PULMONARY EMBOLISM

Despite a low platelet count in most cases, venous thrombosis was reported quite often in some series. In Singapore, around one third of the cases had deep venous thrombosis of the legs.[10] Thrombo-embolism was also found in a substantial proportion of postmortem cases.

ATYPICAL PRESENTATION

Individuals may not develop typical features of SARS. Older people often present with clinical or atypical symptoms and may have no documented fever even with progressive pneumonia.[22] They tend to present with common geriatric syndromes such as falls, confusion, incontinence, and poor feeding. The presenting symptoms may be gastrointestinal (such as diarrhoea, nausea, or vomiting) rather than respiratory. In the frail and elderly, diarrhoea may be thought to be due to faecal incontinence and poor feeding rather than infection.

Diagnosis of SARS can be more difficult in the presence of other diseases and in patients with impaired immune systems (e.g. those with chronic renal failure or on immunosuppressive therapy including corticosteroid), who may present with respiratory illness and pneumonia without fever.[23] Plain chest X-rays are difficult to interpret in patients with pre-existing chronic pulmonary diseases (e.g. pulmonary fibrosis) and in the presence of pulmonary oedema (e.g. congestive heart failure) and the radiological features of SARS may mimic some of these conditions.

SARS patients can present in a variety of ways including with acute pulmonary oedema, exacerbation of chronic obstructive airway disease, influenza, bacteraemia, acute abdomen, and even hip fracture. The judicious use of high-resolution CT scan of thorax (HRCT) may be useful in the early diagnosis of SARS in atypical presentations.

RESPIRATORY FAILURE, MORTALITY AND PROGNOSTIC FACTORS

The crude global mortality was 10%, with several factors associated with higher mortality. These include advanced age, male gender, other illnesses (especially cerebrovascular disease, ischaemic heart disease, diabetes mellitus, chronic renal failure, and chronic liver failure), certain laboratory parameters on admission (high neutrophil counts, C-reactive protein levels, low albumin levels, and high levels of urea and creatinine, CPK and LDH, and glucose), and evidence of respiratory failure on admission (low level of oxygen saturation in the blood).[6,7] The major determinant of mortality thus appears to be respiratory failure and multiple organ failure.[6, 24]

Analysis using a multiple logistic regression model (composite model) shows that advanced age, male sex, high neutrophil count, and high LDH and CPK levels are the important predictors of pulmonary failure that requires mechanical ventilation, and of mortality.[29] These parameters are consistently found to carry important prognostic implications both at presentation and on the seventh day after the onset of symptoms.

SUMMARY

SARS can be a dreadful disease that progresses rapidly and leads to high mortality. Most people who contract the virus develop flu-like symptoms followed by lower respiratory tract infection and gastrointestinal complications. Roughly 25% of patients with SARS will develop respiratory failure and 10% succumb despite intensive therapy. Atypical cases with unusual presentations impose further difficulties in early diagnosis.

Diagnosing SARS requires a high index of suspicion, alertness to any contact history of known SARS case, and an updated knowledge of the current prevalence of SARS in the locality.

REFERENCES

1. Lee N et al. A major outbreak of severe acute respiratory syndrome in Hong Kong. *New England Journal of Medicine*, 2003, 348:1986–1994.
2. Booth CM et al. Clinical features and short-term outcomes of 144 patients with SARS in the greater Toronto area. *Journal of the American Medical Association*, 2003, 289:2801–2809.
3. Peiris JS et al. Clinical progression and viral load in a community outbreak of coronavirus-associated SARS pneumonia: a prospective study. *Lancet*, 2003, 361:1767–1772.
4. Wu W et al. A hospital outbreak of severe acute respiratory syndrome in GuangZhou, China. *Chinese Medicine Journal* (English), 2003, 116:811–818.
5. Hsu LY et al. Severe acute respiratory syndrome (SARS) in Singapore: clinical features of index patient and initial contacts. *Emerging Infectious Diseases*, 2003, 9:713–717.
6. Ng MH et al. Association of human-leukocyte-antigen class I (B*0703) and class II (DRB1*0301) genotypes with susceptibility and resistance to the development of severe acute respiratory syndrome. *Journal of Infectious Diseases*, 2004, 190:515–518.
7. Sung JJ et al. Severe acute respiratory syndrome (SARS): report of treatment and outcome after a major outbreak. *Thorax*, 2004, 59:414–420.
8. Antonio GE et al. Imaging of severe acute respiratory syndrome in Hong Kong. *American Journal of Roentgenology*, 2003, 181:11–17.
9. Wong KT et al. Thin-section CT of severe acute respiratory syndrome: evaluation of patients exposed to or with the disease. *Radiology*, 2003, 228:395–400.
10. Gomersall CD et al. Short-term outcome of critically ill patients with severe acute respiratory syndrome. *Intensive Care Medicine*, 2004, 30:381–387.
11. Leung WK et al. Enteric involvement of severe acute respiratory syndrome–associated coronavirus infection. *Gastroenterology*, 2003, 125:1011–1017.
12. Chan PK et al. Persistent infection of SARS coronavirus in colonic cells *in vitro*. *Journal of Medical Virology*, 2004, 74:1–7.
13. Chan HL et al. Retrospective analysis of liver function derangement in severe acute respiratory syndrome. *American Journal of Medicine*, 2004, 116:566–567.
14. Chau TN, Lee KC, Yao H. SARS-associated viral hepatitis caused by a novel coronavirus: report of three cases. *Hepatology*, 2004, 39:291–294.
15. Wong R et al. Haematological manifestations in patients with severe acute respiratory syndrome: retrospective analysis. *British Medical Journal*, 2003, 326:1358–1362.

[16] Wong CK et al. Plasma inflammatory cytokines and chemokines in severe acute respiratory syndrome. *Clinical and Experimental Immunology*, 2004, 136:95–103.

[17] Kwan BC et al. Severe acute respiratory syndrome in a hemodialysis patient. *American Journal of Kidney Diseases*, 2003, 42:1069–1074.

[18] Wong PN et al. Clinical presentation and outcome of severe acute respiratory syndrome in dialysis patients. *American Journal of Kidney Diseases*, 2003, 42:1075–1081.

[19] Li SS et al. Left ventricular performance in patients with severe acute respirtaory syndrome: a 30-day echocardiographic follow-up study. *Circulation*, 2003, 108:1798–1803.

[20] Hung EC et al. Detection of SARS coronavirus RNA in the cerebrospinal fluid of a patient with severe acute respiratory syndrome. *Clinical Chemistry*, 2003, 49:2108–2109.

[21] Lee DT et al. Factors associated with psychosis among patients with severe acute respiratory syndrome: a case-control study. *Clinical Infectious Diseases*, 2004, 39:1247–1249.

[22] Cheng HM, Kwok T. Mild SARS in elderly patients. *Canadian Medical Association Journal*, 2004, 170:927.

[23] Wong AT et al. Coronavirus in an AIDS patient. *AIDS*, 2004, 18:829–830.

[24] Choi KW et al. Outcomes and prognostic factors in 267 patients with severe acute respiratory syndrome in Hong Kong. *Annals of Internal Medicine*, 2003, 139:715–723.

20 EPIDEMIOLOGY

GLOBAL SURVEILLANCE OF SARS

The global surveillance of SARS started with the first WHO alert of 12 March 2003. By 15 March, WHO had received reports of more than 150 new suspected cases of SARS. In the first month, 2,781 SARS cases and 111 deaths had been reported to WHO from 17 countries on three continents.[1] By 5 July 2003, when WHO declared the outbreak over, it had received reports of 8,439 cases and 812 deaths from 32 countries and areas.

Cases continued to be reclassified (according to the results of late-convalescent serology) after the outbreak. The global data set was closed on 31 December 2003, with the total revised to 8,096 cases (21% among health-care workers) and 774 deaths from 29 countries and areas [Table 20.1].[2] Over 95% (n=7,768) of the cases were reported by 12 countries and areas of the Western Pacific Region. Mainland China had the largest outbreak (5,327 cases), and Beijing the largest single site outbreak (2,521 cases). Beijing had a peak of over 100 probable and suspected SARS cases hospitalized daily, for several days [see Chapter 5].[3] The largest outbreak outside Asia occurred in the Greater Toronto Area, Canada (247 cases during a biphasic outbreak).

The global epidemic curve of the outbreak by date of onset shows several peaks in the daily number of reported cases [Figure 20.1]. The peaks reflect the initial outbreak in Guangdong, China, the exponential rise in cases in March 2003 as SARS spread to several countries, the Amoy Gardens outbreak in late March [see Chapter 16], transmission in hospital in Beijing and Taipei beginning in April [see Chapters 5 and 9], and the second wave of the outbreak in Toronto in May [see Chapter 12].

Table 20.1 Probable SARS cases reported to WHO (from 1 November 2002 to 31 July 2003; based on data reported up to 31 December 2003)

Areas	Female	Male	Total	Median age (range)	Number of deaths[a]	Case fatality ratio (%)	Number of cases imported (%)	Number of HCWs affected (%)	Date of onset: first probable case	Date of onset: last probable case
Australia	4	2	6	15 (1–45)	0	0	6 (100)	0 (0)	26 Feb 03	1 Apr 03
Canada	151	100	251	49 (1–98)	43	17	5 (2)	109 (43)	23 Feb 03	12 Jun 03
China	2674	2607	5327[b]	ND	349	7	NA	1002 (19)	16 Nov 02	3 Jun 03
Hong Kong (China)	977	778	1755	40 (0–100)	299	17	NA	386 (22)	15 Feb 03	31 May 03
Macao (China)	0	1	1	28	0	0	1 (100)	0 (0)	5 May 03	5 May 03
Taiwan, China	218	128	346[c]	42 (0–93)	37	11	21 (6)	68 (20)	25 Feb 03	15 Jun 03
France	1	6	7	49 (26–61)	1	14	7 (100)	2 (29)[d]	21 Mar 03	3 May 03
Germany	4	5	9	4 4 (4–73)	0	0	9 (100)	1 (11)	9 Mar 03	6 May 03
India	0	3	3	25 (25–30)	0	0	3 (100)	0 (0)	25 Apr 03	6 May 03
Indonesia	0	2	2	56 (47–65)	0	0	2 (100)	0 (0)	6 Apr 03	17 Apr 03
Italy	1	3	4	30.5 (25–54)	0	0	4 (100)	0 (0)	12 Mar 03	20 Apr 03
Kuwait	1	0	1	50	0	0	1 (100)	0 (0)	9 Apr 03	9 Apr 03
Malaysia	1	4	5	30 (26–84)	2	40	5 (100)	0 (0)	14 Mar 03	22 Apr 03
Mongolia	8	1	9	32 (17–63)	0	0	8 (89)	0 (0)	31 Mar 03	6 May 03
New Zealand	1	0	1	67	0	0	1 (100)	0 (0)	20 Apr 03	20 Apr 03
Philippines	8	6	14	41 (29–73)	2	14	7 (50)	4 (29)	25 Feb 03	5 May 03
Republic of Ireland	0	1	1	56	0	0	1 (100)	0 (0)	27 Feb 03	27 Feb 03
Republic of Korea	0	3	3	40 (20–80)	0	0	3 (100)	0 (0)	25 Apr 03	10 May 03
Romania	0	1	1	52	0	0	1 (100)	0 (0)	19 Mar 03	19 Mar 03
Russian Federation	0	1	1	25	0	0	ND	0 (0)	5 May 03	5 May 03
Singapore	161	77	238	35 (1–90)	33	14	8 (3)	97 (41)	25 Feb 03	5 May 03
South Africa	0	1	1	62	1	100	1 (100)	0 (0)	3 Apr 03	3 Apr 03
Spain	0	1	1	33	0	0	1 (100)	0 (0)	26 Mar 03	26 Mar 03
Sweden	3	2	5	43 (33–55)	0	0	5 (100)	0 (0)	28 Mar 03	23 Apr 03
Switzerland	0	1	1	35	0	0	1 (100)	0 (0)	9 Mar 03	9 Mar 03
Thailand	5	4	9	42 (2–79)	2	22	9 (100)	1 (11)[d]	11 Mar 03	27 May 03
United Kingdom	2	2	4	59 (28–74)	0	0	4 (100)	0 (0)	1 Mar 03	1 Apr 03
United States	13	14	27	36 (0–83)	0	0	27 (100)	0 (0)	24 Feb 03	13 Jul 03[e]
Viet Nam	39	24	63	43 (20–76)	5	8	1 (2)	36 (57)	23 Feb 03	14 Apr 03
Total			**8096**		**774**	**9.6**	**142**	**1706**		

HCW, health-care worker; NA, not applicable; ND, not determined

[a] Includes only cases whose death is attributed to SARS.

[b] Case classification by sex is unknown for 46 cases.

[c] Since 11 July 2003, 325 cases have been discarded in Taiwan, China. Laboratory information was insufficient or incomplete for 135 discarded cases, of which 101 died.

[d] Includes HCWs who acquired illness in other areas.

[e] Due to differences in case definitions, the United States has reported probable cases of SARS with onsets of illness after 5 July 2003.

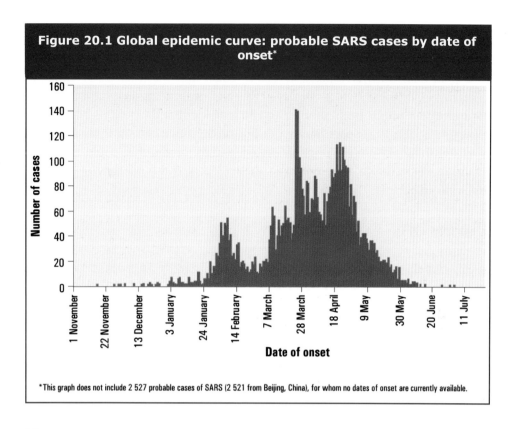

Figure 20.1 Global epidemic curve: probable SARS cases by date of onset*

Number of cases

Date of onset

*This graph does not include 2 527 probable cases of SARS (2 521 from Beijing, China), for whom no dates of onset are currently available.

THE NEED FOR GLOBAL COLLABORATION IN THE EPIDEMIOLOGY OF SARS

WHO established the Ad Hoc Working Group on the Epidemiology of SARS to help reach consensus on the key epidemiological parameters needed for public health control: the incubation period, period of communicability, and modes of transmission of the virus; and identification of risk groups and factors. The group also facilitated information sharing and pooled international data to increase the power of any analysis and ensure that findings were representative.

The Working Group held a weekly teleconference from 28 March 2003. Membership initially included epidemiologists from outbreak sites and from the Global Outbreak Alert and Response Network (GOARN) [see Chapter 2]. Clinical and laboratory experts were later invited to participate in the teleconferences to foster greater collaboration among the disciplines.

To further develop the evidence base for control measures, WHO held a global meeting on the epidemiology of SARS on 16-17 May 2003. This meeting and the ongoing work of the Working Group culminated in the release of the *WHO Consensus Document on the Epidemiology of SARS.*[4] The key epidemiological findings in this document remain valid.

INCUBATION PERIOD

The incubation period is the amount of time it takes for symptoms of a disease to appear after an individual is infected. For SARS, the incubation period is generally reported as two to 10 days,[4,5,6,7] (the mean being five days following exposure), although both shorter and longer incubation periods have been reported.[8,9,10,11,12] It appears likely, but not proven, that the transmission route does not influence the incubation period. Other factors that could affect the incubation period also have not been shown (such as the intensity of exposure and viral load).

PERIOD OF COMMUNICABILITY

The period of communicability of SARS is not as well defined. Evidence from carefully constructed transmission trees supports earlier observations that transmission only occurs when cases are symptomatic. This is consistent with the finding that the amount of virus shed from the respiratory secretions, urine, and faeces of infected patients in the first few days of illness is usually low or undetectable.[13] There have been no reports of the transmission of SARS before the onset of symptoms or in asymptomatic cases. The risk of secondary transmission is low when cases are identified and isolated within three days of symptom onset.[4]

Transmission appears to be most likely from severely ill patients or those experiencing rapid clinical deterioration, usually during the second week of illness, and correlates with peak viral excretion from the respiratory tract.[14] Convalescent patients have limited infectivity and have not been implicated in transmission.[13] There are no reports of transmission beyond 10 days of fever resolution, consistent with the total period of isolation recommended by WHO.[15]

Viral shedding in respiratory secretions beyond the sixth week after the onset of illness is rare,[16] although prolonged shedding of SARS-CoV RNA in stool samples of recovering patients has been reported by several authors.[16,17,18] One respiratory sample in a severely ill patient collected on day 50 was positive by reverse transcriptase-polymerase chain reaction (RT-PCR).[19] The longest period of continuing detection of viral RNA from stool samples of a recovering patient is 73 days.[18] However, no virus was successfully isolated from those patients indicating low, if any, infectivity. There is no evidence of disease recrudescence.

TRANSMISSION OF SARS

Transmission was mostly limited to close contacts—those who had cared for, lived with, or had direct contact with the respiratory secretions or body fluids of a person with SARS. Large, virus-laden respiratory droplets from symptomatic cases of SARS are deposited onto mucous membranes (eyes, nose, and mouth) or by contact with infectious fomites. Saliva, tears, urine, and faeces also contain virus but have not been implicated in hospital-acquired infections when standard infection-control precautions are observed. Transmission from pregnant mothers to their babies has not been reported.[5]

The route(s) of transmission have not been fully determined for some cases and clusters. Faecal aerosolization from faulty plumbing was implicated in the Amoy Gardens outbreak [see Chapter 16].[20] Aerosolization spread is likely to have also been responsible for spread in the Metropole Hotel [see Chapter 14] and in some hospitals,[21,22,23] and may have been responsible for in-flight transmission [see Chapter 15].

Environmental contamination with infectious respiratory secretions or other body fluids may have contributed to transmission. Although diarrhoea is common in SARS and viral shedding in faeces can be prolonged, true faecal-oral transmission did not appear to occur, and there are no reports of food or waterborne transmission.

Experimental evidence on the stability of SARS-CoV supports a role for contact transmission in contaminated environments. SARS-CoV was still infective for up to nine days in suspension and up to six days when dried.[24]

TRANSMISSION SETTINGS

Hospitals were sites of transmission amplification,[25] and the main site for SARS transmission. This was first noted in Guangdong, China, where after mid-January 2003, SARS cases were concentrated in hospitals and household contacts of SARS cases.[26] In all outbreak sites, a large number of health-care workers were infected by the primary case presenting at their facility with atypical pneumonia of unknown aetiology. Later, the management or transfer of unrecognized cases led to continued transmission after control measures had been implemented.[6,27,28] In Singapore, about 76% of SARS cases were infected in hospitals, of which 42% were health-care workers.[29]

The second wave of SARS transmission in Canada was attributed to the inherent difficulties in diagnosing SARS when the clinical presentation is atypical, and prematurely decreasing respiratory precautions in hospitals.[30,31]

Most of the Viet Nam cases were infected in the hospital where the index case was admitted, but transmission did not occur in the other hospital where infectious SARS cases were admitted, in spite of the inconsistent adherence to infection control and use of personal protective equipment.[32]

In health-care settings, medical procedures leading to aerosolization of respiratory secretions (such as intubation,[33] the use of nebulisers,[21,22] suction,[22] or assisted ventilation[23]) resulted on occasion in transmission to health-care workers despite use of personal protective equipment. A Hong Kong study found infection of health-care workers was strongly associated with inconsistent use of personal protection equipment and with inadequate training in and poor understanding of infection-control procedures.[13]

In Hong Kong (China), non-clinical support staff had the highest attack rate of 2.7% (overall rate of 1.2% for all hospital staff), and were 2.3 and 9.8 times more likely to contract SARS than nurses and doctors, respectively.[34] Non-clinical staff also had the highest attack rate in Viet Nam.[32]

Households with at least one probable SARS case were the second most important transmission setting.[35] In Hong Kong, the number of secondary household transmissions for 1,214 SARS cases was studied for two phases of the epidemic.[36] Transmission occurred in 15% of all households (22% and 11% for earlier and later phases, respectively) and to 8% of all household members (12% and 6% for earlier and later phases, respectively). Duration before hospitalization, visiting the SARS patient in hospital (and mask use during the visit), and frequency of close contact were independent predictors of transmission in a multivariate analysis. A Singapore study of 114 households with 417 contacts reported an attack rate of 6%,[37] similar to the 5% reported in Beijing.[38]

Household contacts may have been infected in hospitals, rather than in their homes. An analysis of the onset dates of the contacts of the first Singapore index case suggests that all her household and social contacts were infected when they visited her in hospital.

During the 2002–2003 SARS epidemic, transmission to social and casual contacts was occasionally reported as a result of short but intense exposure to a severely ill case in an enclosed space (e.g. in a hospital,[5,39] market,[29] office,[40] airplane,[41] private transport,[39,29] and train[42]) or from longer exposure to patients who were less severely ill. Community-acquired infection has been associated with religious gatherings.[43] Overall, the risk of acquiring SARS from air travel, even before the second travel advisory, was extremely small.[44] The incidence density of secondary transmission was calculated as 1 per 100 person-hours of travel in one study.[45] Transmission in public buildings, schools, or open-air settings has not been reported.[50,46]

PATIENT CHARACTERISTICS

Most SARS transmissions were from sick people who had been hospitalized. As a result, 21% of all cases were health-care workers, with a range from 19% to 57% in the different outbreak sites [Table 20.2]. It also led to 53% of all cases being women, as they are over-represented among health-care workers. These data do not include cases in other patients and visitors within health-care settings so it underestimates the total risk of SARS in hospitals during the epidemic. In Canada, for example, SARS transmission was almost exclusively health-care associated with only a few cases acquired within affected households or in the broader community.

All age groups were affected (age range 0-100 years, median age 42 years). It is not fully understood why SARS was uncommon in younger children, but it may be partly due to the fact that children were less likely to be exposed to

Table 20.2 SARS in health-care workers at outbreak sites, November 2002–July 2003

Area	Total cases	Health-care worker cases Number	Percentage (%)
Canada	251	109	43
China	5,327	1002	19
Hong Kong (China)	1,755	386	22
Taiwan, China	346	68	20
The Philippines	14	3	21
Singapore	238	97	41
Viet Nam	63	36	57
All outbreak sites	7,994	36	57

Source: Data reported to WHO

SARS as a result of protective behaviours by exposed parents (especially health-care workers) and a lower likelihood of exposure within health-care settings. Most children experienced only mild illness.[47,48] There is no evidence that young children were asymptomatically infected. In Beijing, only 1% of cases were children below 10 years.[3] Age-stratified serosurveys in Guangdong Province, where a higher proportion of cases were acquired in the community, may provide a better understanding of the risk to children before control measures were fully implemented. Children did not appear to be implicated in transmission in schools or to adults. In the only well-documented chain of transmission from a child to household contacts, an 11-year-old child transmitted SARS to four people (three adults and one child) in another household.[49] Adolescents with SARS may develop severe disease requiring oxygen therapy or assisted ventilation.[50,51] SARS acquired during pregnancy was associated with a high incidence of spontaneous miscarriage, preterm delivery, and intrauterine growth retardation.[52] Pregnant women also experienced a higher case fatality rate.[53, 54]

The case fatality rate in adults increased with age in all centres and exceeded 50% in cases aged 55 years and over.[4] Overall, 20%–25% of cases required intensive care during their illness.

ASYMPTOMATIC INFECTION AND CONTRIBUTION TO SARS TRANSMISSION

Serological surveys of populations at risk of SARS in 2003 found that asymptomatic infections were very uncommon.[55,56,57,58,59] In Hong Kong, only two of 1,068 contacts of SARS cases (0.19%) who did not develop symptoms had SARS antibodies.[56] A survey of 12,000 Hong Kong residents found only seven positive results (0.009%).[59] In Taiwan, China, a survey of 623 healthy health-care workers who treated SARS patients found asymptomatic seroconversions in only two hospitals where four out of 433 health-care workers had SARS antibodies (0.92%).[60]

Most laboratory-confirmed SARS cases met the WHO clinical case definition (of severe disease), but mild infections have been reported. Mild cases of infection with SARS-CoV may be difficult to detect, and could theoretically have been important in transmission. However, there is no evidence that they played an important role in transmission during the epidemic. Mild infections have not been implicated in super-spreading events.[19,57,61,62]

Despite close examination of contacts prior to symptoms, there was no observed transmission from asymptomatic infections.[51,63] If asymptomatic transmission does occur, it must be extremely rare.

REPRODUCTION NUMBER IN DIFFERENT TRANSMISSION SETTINGS AND UNDER DIFFERENT CONTROL STRATEGIES

The basic reproduction number (R_0) is the *average* number of secondary cases infected by an infected person, during their entire infectious period, when entering a totally susceptible population and before control measures are instituted. For SARS, R_0 was estimated at about 3,[64] consistent with a condition of relatively low infectivity spread by direct contact or larger virus-laden droplets that travel only a few metres rather than by aerosols.

The serial interval is the *average* number of days between the onset of symptoms in a primary case and the onset of symptoms in secondary cases. For SARS, it was relatively long at 8.4 days (SD 3.8 days),[65] which assisted in the early identification of contacts and rapid application of control measures.

Data from Singapore where contact tracing was complete indicate that the majority of SARS cases did not transmit the infection to others.[65] Of the remaining cases, most transmitted infection to only a few others, but five cases transmitted infection to about 20 or more. These events with large numbers (variably defined) of transmissions were called "super-spreading" events and are discussed in Chapter 13.

Super-spreading events played a major role in transmission of SARS in all sites.[21,66,67,68,69,70,71] They accounted for 71% and 75% of SARS cases in Hong Kong and Singapore, respectively.[72] A meta-analysis of super-spreading events is still needed to better understand the underlying behavioural, biological, and environmental factors.

MODELLING CONTROL MEASURES

Modelling the Hong Kong data supports the findings from Singapore that the daily rate of infection was correlated with the number of symptomatic cases who were not isolated within four days of symptom onset.[72]

A modelling study found that hospital-based case management with precautions to prevent transmission had the greatest impact on the reproduction number.[64] Their model showed that for an R_0 of 3, case isolation as a single measure can control a SARS outbreak if isolation reduces transmission four-fold and the mean time to isolation is within three days of symptom onset. Even small delays in case isolation substantially reduced the effectiveness of case isolation. These results are consistent with the finding that reducing the mean time from symptom onset to isolation from 4.8 days to 3.7 days was insufficient to control the outbreak in Hong Kong.[73] Additional analysis of 1,709 cases in Hong Kong showed that laboratory-confirmed SARS cases were highly clustered geographically.[74] Using cartographic and geostatistical methods epidemiological investigations can provide real-time quantitative data for identifying and tracking the geospatial spread of infectious diseases.

Summary

The key epidemiological features of SARS, which were defined early on with limited information, remain valid. The most critical finding was that SARS transmission did not occur until after symptom onset, allowing early isolation of cases to terminate the outbreak. The main mode of transmission is through respiratory droplets that require close contact or transfer through fomites. However, under special circumstances, aerosolization can occur, leading to airborne spread.

References

[1] *Severe acute respiratory syndrome (SARS): multicountry outbreak – Update 27*. One month into the global SARS outbreak: Status of the outbreak and lessons for the immediate future. Geneva, World Health Organization, 2003 (http://www.who.int/csr/don/2003_04_11/en/).

[2] *Summary of probable SARS cases with onset of illness from 1 November 2002 to 31 July 2003* (based on data as of 31 December 2003). Geneva, World Health Organization, 2004 (http://www.who.int/csr/sars/country/table2004_04_21/en/).

[3] Liang W et al. Severe acute respiratory syndrome, Beijing, 2003. *Emerging Infectious Diseases*, 2004, 10:25–30.

[4] *Consensus document on the epidemiology of acute severe respiratory syndrome (SARS)*. Geneva, World Health Organization, 2003 (WHO/CDS/CSR/GAR/2003.11).

[5] Varia M et al. (for the Hospital Outbreak Investigation Team). *Investigation of a nosocomial outbreak of severe acute respiratory syndrome (SARS) in Toronto, Canada*. Canadian Medical Association Journal, 2003, 169:285–292.

[6] Chow KY et al. Outbreak of severe acute respiratory syndrome in a tertiary hospital in Singapore, linked to an primary patient with atypical presentation: epidemiological study. *British Medical Journal*, 2004,328:195.

[7] Donnelly CA et al. Epidemiological determinants of spread of causal agent of severe acute respiratory syndrome in Hong Kong. *Lancet*, 2003, 361:1761–1766.

[8] Zhao CH et al. Clinical manifestation, treatment, and outcome of severe acute respiratory syndrome: analysis of 108 cases in Beijing. *Zhonghua Yi Xue Za Zhi*, 2003, 83:897–901. [Abstract. Article in Chinese]

[9] Wu W et al. A hospital outbreak of severe acute respiratory syndrome in Guangzhou, China. *Chinese Medical Journal* (English), 2003, 116:811–818.

[10] Chan-Yeung M et al. Severe acute respiratory syndrome. *International Journal of Tuberculosis and Lung Disease*, 2003, 7:1117–1130.

[11] Tsang KW et al. A cluster of cases of severe acute respiratory syndrome in Hong Kong. *New England Journal of Medicine*, 2003, 348:1977–1985.

[12] Chan W et al. Epidemiologic linkage and public health implications of a cluster of severe acute respiratory syndrome in an extended family. *Paediatric Infectious Disease Journal*, 2004, in press.

[13] Lau JT et al. SARS transmission among hospital workers in Hong Kong. *Emerging Infectious Diseases*, 2004, 10:280–286.

[14] Peiris JSM et al. Clinical progression and viral load in a community outbreak of coronavirus-associated SARS pneumonia: a prospective clinical trial. *Lancet*, 2003, 361:1767–1772.

[15] Management of severe acute respiratory syndrome (SARS). Revised 11 April 2003. Geneva, World Health Organization, 2003 (http://www.who.int/csr/sars/management/en/).

[16] Chan PKS et al. Laboratory diagnosis of SARS. *Emerging Infectious Diseases*, 2004, 10:825–831.

[17] Liu W et al. Long-term SARS coronavirus excretion from patient cohort, China. *Emerging Infectious Diseases*, 2004, 10:1841–1843.

[18] Leung WK et al. Enteric involvement of severe acute respiratory syndrome-associated coronavirus infection. *Gastroenterology*, 2003, 125:1011–1017.

[19] Chang W-T et al. SARS exposure and emergency department workers. *Emerging Infectious Diseases*, 2004, 10:1117–1119.

[20] Yu IT et al. Evidence of airborne transmission of the severe acute respiratory syndrome virus. *New England Journal of Medicine*, 2004, 351:609–611.

[21] Wong T-W et al. Cluster of SARS among medical students exposed to single patient, Hong Kong. *Emerging Infectious Diseases*, 2004, 10:269–276.

[22] Loeb M et al. SARS among critical care nurses, Toronto. *Emerging Infectious Diseases*, 2004, 10:251–255.

[23] Lee N et al. A major outbreak of severe acute respiratory syndrome in Hong Kong. *New England Journal of Medicine*, 2003, 348:1986–1994.

[24] Rebenau HF et al. Stability and inactivation of SARS coronavirus. *Medical Microbiology and Immunology* (Berlin), 2005, 194:1–6.

[25] Drazen JM. Case clusters of the severe acute respiratory syndrome. *New England Journal of Medicine*, 2003, 348:e6–7.

[26] He J-F et al. An epidemiological study on the primary cases of severe acute respiratory syndrome which occurred in different cities in Guangdong province (English abstract). In Chinese Medical Association Journals. Beijing:Chinese Medical Association, 27 May 2003, p44.

[27] Wong T et al. Late recognition of SARS in a nosocomial outbreak, Toronto, Canada. *Emerging Infectious Diseases* [submitted].

[28] McDonald LC et al. SARS in healthcare facilities, Toronto and Taiwan. *Emerging Infectious Diseases*, 2004, 10:777–781.

[29] Centers for Disease Control and Prevention. Severe acute respiratory syndrome, Singapore, 2003. *Morbidity and Mortality Weekly Report*, 2003, 52:405–411.

[30] Low DE, McGeer A. SARS: one year later. *New England Journal of Medicine*, 2003, 349:2381–2382.

[31] Svoboda T et al. Public health measures to control the spread of severe acute respiratory syndrome during the outbreak in Toronto. *New England Journal of Medicine*, 2004, 350:2352–2361.

[32] Ha LD et al. Lack of SARS transmission among public hospital workers, Viet Nam. Emerging Infectious Diseases, 2004, 10:265–268.

[33] Scales DC et al. Illness in intensive care staff after brief exposure to severe acute respiratory syndrome. Emerging Infectious Diseases, 2004, 10:1205–1210 .

[34] Lau JT et al. SARS in three categories of hospital workers, Hong Kong. *Emerging Infectious Diseases*, 2004, 10:1399–1404.

[35] Tomlinson B, Cockram C. SARS: experience at Prince of Wales Hospital, Hong Kong. *Lancet*, 2003, 361:1486–1487.

[36] Lau JT et al. Probable secondary infections in households of SARS patients in Hong Kong. *Emerging Infectious Diseases*, 2004, 10:235–243.

[37] Goh DL-M et al. Secondary household transmission of SARS, Singapore. *Emerging Infectious Diseases* [serial online] 2004 February [date cited] (http://www.cdc.gov/ncidod/EID/vol10no2/03-0676.htm).

[38] Centers for Disease Control and Prevention. Efficiency of quarantine during an epidemic of severe acute respiratory syndrome, Beijing, China, 2003. *Morbidity and Mortality Weekly Report*, 2003, 52:1037.

[39] World Health Organization. SARS outbreak in the Philippines. *Weekly Epidemiological Record*, 2003, 78:189–192.

[40] Health Canada. Learning from SARS. Renewal of public health in Canada. A report of the National Advisory Committee on SARS and Public Health, October 2003 (http://www.hc-sc.gc.ca/english/pdf/sars/sars-e.pdf).

[41] Olsen SJ et al. Transmission of severe acute respiratory syndrome on aircraft. *New England Journal of Medicine*, 2003:349:2414-20.

[42] Chiu RWK, Chim SSC, Lo YMD. Molecular epidemiology of SARS – from Amoy Gardens to Taiwan. *New England Journal of Medicine*, 2003, 349:1875–1876.

[43] Health Canada. *Summary of Severe Acute Respiratory Syndrome (SARS) Cases: Canada and International*. Ottawa, 16 April 2003 (http://www.hc-sc.gc.ca/pphb-dgspsp/sars-sras/eu-ae/sars20030416_e.html, accessed 1 April 2005).

[44] Wilder-Smith A, Paton NI, Goh KT. Low risk of severe acute respiratory syndrome on airplanes: the Singapore experience. *Tropical Medicine and International Health*, 2003, 8:1035–1037.

[45] Desenclos JC et al. Introduction of SARS in France, March–April 2003. *Emerging Infectious Diseases*, 2004, 10:195–200.

[46] Wang M et al. Study on the epidemiology and measures for control of severe acute respiratory syndrome in Guangzhou City (English abstract). In collection of papers on SARS published in *Chinese Medical Association Journals*. Beijing: Chinese Medical Association, 27 May 2003:50.

[47] Leung TF et al. Severe acute respiratory syndrome (SARS) in children: epidemiology, presentation and management. *Paediatric Respiratory Reviewsm*, 2003, 4:334–339.

[48] Ng PC et al. SARS in newborns and children. *Biology of the Neonate*, 2004, 85:293–298.

[49] Chan WM et al. Epidemiologic linkage and public health implication of a cluster of severe acute respiratory syndrome in an extended family. *The Pediatric Infectious Disease Journal*, 2004, 23(12):1156–1159.

[50] Hon KLE et al. Clinical presentations and outcome of severe acute respiratory syndrome in children. *Lancet*, 2003, 361:1701–1703.

[51] Fong NC et al. Adolescent twin sisters with severe acute respiratory syndrome (SARS). *Paediatrics*, 2004, 113:146–149.

[52] Wong SF et al. Pregnancy and perinatal outcomes of women with severe acute respiratory syndrome. *American Journal of Obstetrics and Gynecology*, 2004, 191:292–297.

[53] Lam CM et al. A case-controlled study comparing clinical course and outcomes of pregnant and non-pregnant women with severe acute respiratory syndrome. *British Journal of Gynaecology*, 2004, 111:771–774.

[54] Shek CC et al. Infants born to mothers with severe acute respiratory syndrome. *Pediatrics*, 2003, 112:e254–e256.

[55] Lee HKK et al. Asymptomatic severe acute respiratory syndrome-associated coronavirus infection. *Emerging Infectious Diseases*, 2003, 9:1491–1492.

[56] Leung GM et al. SARS-CoV antibody prevalence in all Hong Kong patient contacts *Emerging Infectious Diseases*, 2004, 10:1653–1656.

[57] Rainer TH et al. The spectrum of severe acute respiratory syndrome-associated coronavirus infection. *Annals of Internal Medicine*, 2004, 140:614–619.

[58] Yu IT, Sung JJ. The epidemiology of the outbreak of severe acute respiratory syndrome (SARS) in Hong Kong: what we do know and what we don't. *Epidemiology and Infection*, 2004, 132:781–786.

[59] Chinese University of Hong Kong. *Territory-wide SARS seroprevalence study suggests Hong Kong is not a human reservoir for SARS coronavirus.* Hong Kong, 2004 (http://www.cuhk.edu.hk/ipro/pressrelease/040315e.htm, accessed 26 October 2004).

[60] Hsueh P-R et al. SARS antibody test for serosurveillance. *Emerging Infectious Diseases*, 2004, 10:1558–1562.

[61] Li G et al. Mild severe acute respiratory syndrome. *Emerging Infectious Diseases*, 2003, 9:1182–1183.

[62] Lim PL et al. Laboratory-acquired severe acute respiratory syndrome. *New England Journal of Medicine*, 2004, 350:1740–1745.

[63] Vu TH et al. SARS in Northern Viet Nam. *New England Journal of Medicine*, 2003, 348:2035.

[64] Lloyd-Smith JO, Galvani AP, Getz W. Curtailing transmission of severe acute respiratory syndrome within a community and its hospital. *Proceedings of the Royal Society London, B series*, 2003, 270:1979–1989.

[65] Lipsitch M et al. Transmission dynamics and control of severe acute respiratory syndrome. *Science*, 2003, 300:1966–1970.

[66] World Health Organization. Severe Acute Respiratory Syndrome – Singapore. *Weekly Epidemiological Record*, 2003, 78:157–162.

[67] Gopalakrishna G et al. SARS transmission and hospital containment. *Emerging Infectious Diseases*, 2004, 10:395–400.

[68] Peiris JSM et al. The severe acute respiratory syndrome. *New England Journal of Medicine*, 2003, 349:2431–2441.

[69] Shen Z et al. Superspreading SARS events, Beijing, 2003. *Emerging Infectious Diseases*, 2004, 10:256–260.

[70] Xie S et al. Analyses of one case of severe acute respiratory syndrome "super-transmitter" and chain of transmission. Chinese Journal of Epidemiology, 2003, 24:449–453.

[71] Poutanen SM et al. Identification of severe acute respiratory syndrome in Canada. *New England Journal of Medicine*, 2003, 348:1995–2005.

[72] Li Y et al. Predicting super spreading events during the 2003 severe acute respiratory syndrome epidemics in Hong Kong and Singapore. *American Journal of Epidemiology*, 2004, 160:719–728.

[73] Riley S et al. Transmission dynamics of the aetiological agent of severe acute respiratory syndrome (SARS) in Hong Kong: the impact of public health interventions. *Science*, 2003, 1961–1966.

[74] Lai PC et al. Understanding the spatial clustering of severe acute respiratory syndrome (SARS) in Hong Kong. *Environmental Health Perspectives*, 2004, 112:1550–1556.

21 ANIMAL CORONAVIRUSES

CORONAVIRUS FAMILY

The family *Coronaviridae* comprises three genera: *Coronavirus, Torovirus,* and *Arterivirus*—enveloped, positive-strand RNA viruses with nonsegmented genomes that share similarities in genome organization and expression. Historically, the genus *Coronavirus* comprised three antigenically and genetically distinct groups [Table 21.1]. The newly emerged SARS/SARS-like coronaviruses (CoVs) are only distantly related genetically to known CoVs and provisionally compose group IV,[1,2,3] or a subgroup of group II.[4] These CoVs include human,[1,5,6] civet cat, and raccoon dog isolates.[7]

All CoVs contain at least four structural proteins: the nucleocapsid (N) protein, the protruding spike (S) glycoprotein (cleaved or uncleaved depending on the CoV species), the integral membrane glycoprotein (M), and the envelope protein.[8] Several group II CoVs including bovine CoV (BCoV) also contain a surface hemagglutinin-esterase (HE), which has homology with the HE of group C influenza viruses suggesting a prior recombination event between these two viruses.[8] The S (and HE when present) functions in viral attachment and fusion and induction of neutralizing antibodies. Except for a very large RNA polymerase gene with two open reading frames (ORFs), the remaining CoV nonstructural protein ORFs are diverse in number, size, and genome arrangement.[8]

RESPIRATORY AND ENTERIC ANIMAL CORONAVIRUSES

Animal CoVs cause a broad spectrum of diseases in their hosts including enteric, respiratory, reproductive, neurologic, hepatic, nephritic, and generalized systemic disease [Table 21.1]. They infect diverse host species (humans, wild and domestic animals, avian species, rodents), producing both acute and persistent infections of variable severity. Because both pneumonia and diarrhoea occur in SARS cases, this review gives a brief overview of key aspects of respiratory and enteric animal CoV infections with potential analogies to SARS-CoV. A more detailed review of these animal CoVs with comparisons to SARS is available.[9]

Table 21.1 Members of the *Coronavirus* genus, target tissues, and diseases

Genetic group	Virus	Host	Disease/infection site		
			Respiratory	Enteric	Other
I	HCoV-229E	Human	X upper		
	TGEV	Pig	X upper	X SI	
	PRCV	Pig	X upper/lung		Viremia
	PEDV	Pig		X SI, Colon	
	FIPV/FCoV	Cat	X upper	X SI	Systemic
	CCoV	Dog		X SI	
	RaCoV	Rabbit			Systemic
II	HCoV-OC43	Human	X upper	BCoV?[a]	
	MHV	Mouse		X	Hepatitis, CNS, systemic,
	RcoV (sialodocry-adenitis)	Rat	X		eye, salivary glands
	HEV	Pig	X		CNS
	BCoV	Cattle	X upper/lung	X SI, Colon	
III	IBV	Chicken	X upper	X	Kidney, oviduct
	TCoV (TECoV)	Turkey		X SI	
IV?	SARSCoV	Human	X lung	X?	Viremia, kidney?
IIA?	Civet cat	Himalayan palm civet Raccoon dog	X	X	subclinical?
	Raccoon dog CoV		?	X	subclinical?

SI = small intestine; CNS = central nervous system; ? = unknown

[a] Possibly a BCoV-like CoV from a child[10]

EMERGENCE OF NEW CoVs

Like SARS, new CoVs like the group I porcine epidemic diarrhoea virus (PEDV) in pigs have arisen from unknown sources. PEDV caused fatal diarrhoeal disease in naive populations, then diminished in severity and became endemic as the population acquired immunity.[11] PEDV is genetically more closely related to human CoV 229E than to the other animal group I CoVs,[12] and, unlike the other group I CoVs, it grows only in Vero cells like SARS-CoV,[13] raising intriguing, but unanswered, questions about its origin.

New animal CoVs with altered tissue tropisms (the preferred tissue that the virus grows in) and virulence may also arise spontaneously from existing strains. The group I porcine respiratory CoV (PRCV) is a naturally occurring S gene deletion mutant of the highly virulent porcine enteric transmissible gastroenteritis virus (TGEV).[14,15] PRCV strains emerged independently in Europe and the United States of America in the 1980s, as shown by differences in the sizes of the 5' end S gene deletion region (621–681 nucleotides). Deletion of this region presumably accounted for altered tissue tropism (from enteric to respiratory) and reduced virulence of the PRCV strains.[16,17]

SIMILARITIES TO SARS CORONAVIRUS

PRCV has several similarities to SARS-CoV, including clinical signs of fever, dyspnoea, polypnoea, and anorexia and less coughing and rhinitis. It spreads by droplets and replicates in the lung at high levels (10^7–10^8 $TCID_{50}$) producing interstitial pneumonia (affecting 5%–60% of the lung). It infects lung epithelial cells and possibly macrophages, resulting in bronchiolar infiltration of mononuclear cells, lymphohistiocytic exudates, and epithelial cell necrosis.[14,15,18,19] PRCV induces transient viraemia with virus also detected from nasal secretions, tonsil, and trachea. PRCV further replicates in undefined cells in the intestinal lamina propria, but without inducing villous atrophy or diarrhoea and with limited faecal shedding.[15] Recently, however, faecal isolates of PRCV were detected with minor (point mutations) in the S gene compared with the nasal isolates from the same pig.[20] Such observations suggest the presence of CoV quasispecies in the host with some strains more adapted to the intestine, a potential corollary for the faecal shedding of SARS-CoV. The widespread dissemination of PRCV in Europe has displaced the more virulent TGEV, acting as a natural vaccine.[14,15]

Although not yet evident for SARS-CoV, the ability of certain CoVs to persist in their host also provides a longer opportunity for new mutants to be selected with altered tissue tropisms and virulence from among the viral RNA quasispecies (or swarm of viruses). An example is the virulent systemic variant, the group I CoV feline infectious peritonitis virus (FIPV), which very likely arises from persistent infection of cats with the less virulent feline enteric CoV.[21,22]

THE ROLE OF COFACTORS

Respiratory and enteric CoV infections in the natural animal host (swine, cattle, poultry) have provided important information on CoV disease pathogenesis that is potentially applicable to SARS-CoV. Enteric CoV infections (TGEV, BCoV) alone often cause fatal infections in young animals. However, in adults, respiratory CoV infections are more severe or often fatal when combined with other factors including respiratory co-infections (viruses, bacteria) and stress and transport of animals (shipping fever of cattle).[27,28,29,30]

Underlying disease or respiratory co-infections, dose, aerosols, and route of infection and immunosuppression (corticosteroids) are all potential cofactors related to the severity of SARS. These cofactors can also exacerbate the severity of infectious bronchitis virus (IBV), BCoV, TGEV, or PRCV infections

PNEUMOENTERIC CORONAVIRUSES

SARS may be pneumoenteric like group II BCoVs.[9] Besides the respiratory disease complex, shipping fever, BCoV causes two other distinct clinical syndromes in cattle: calf diarrhoea and winter dysentery with hemorrhagic diarrhoea in adults [Table 21.1].[9,23,24,25,26,27,28,29,30,31] On the basis of BCoV antibody seroprevalence, the virus is ubiquitous in cattle worldwide. All BCoV isolates from both enteric and respiratory infections are antigenically similar and are pneumoenteric, inducing both nasal and faecal shedding, often with lung, and invariably with intestinal, lesions in inoculated calves.[9,32,33] Only point mutations, but not deletions have been detected in the S gene between enteric and respiratory BCoV isolates, including ones from the same animal.[34,35] Subclinical nasal and faecal virus shedding were detected in BCoV-experimentally- infected calves challenged with heterologous BCoV strains,[32,33] confirming field studies showing that repeated upper respiratory BCoV infections occur frequently in calves and that subclinically infected animals may be reservoirs for BCoV.[36]

Shipping fever is recognized as a multifactorial, polymicrobial respiratory disease complex in young adult feedlot cattle. BCoV infections are common in feedlot cattle with several factors exacerbating BCoV respiratory disease and the shipping fever disease complex.[27,28,29,30] The shipping of cattle long distances in close confinement to feedlots and the commingling of cattle from several farms create physical stresses that overwhelm the animal's defence mechanisms and provide close contact for exposure to new pathogens or strains not previously encountered.

For shipping fever, various predisposing factors (viruses, stress) allow commensal bacteria of the nasal cavity (*Mannheimia haemolytica, Pasteurella sp, Mycoplasma sp*, etc.) to infect the lungs, leading to fatal fibrinous pneumonia.[23,24,25,30] As with PRCV or SARS infections, antibiotic treatment of such individuals with massive release of bacterial lipopolysaccharides (LPS) could potentially precipitate the induction of proinflammatory cytokines, which may further worsen lung damage. Pigs infected with PRCV followed by a subclinical dose of *E. coli* LPS within 24 hours developed higher fever and more severe respiratory disease than when exposed to each agent alone, with the disease most likely accentuated by proinflammatory cytokines induced by the bacterial LPS in concert with the virus.[37]

Sequential infections of pigs with the arterivirus (family *Coronaviridae*) PRRSV, followed in five days by PRCV, significantly increased lung lesions and reduced weight gain compared with infections with each virus alone.[19] The dual infections also led to more pigs shedding PRCV nasally for a prolonged period and, surprisingly, to increased faecal shedding of PRCV. Pigs inoculated with PRCV followed in two to three days by swine influenza A virus (SIV) had reduced SIV lung titres but more severe lung lesions than the singly infected pigs.[38] The high levels of interferon (INF)-alpha induced by PRCV may have interfered with SIV replication but also may have contributed to the increased lung lesions via immunopathologic mechansims. Such studies are highly relevant to potential dual infections with SARS-CoV and influenza virus and proposed treatments of SARS patients with IFN-alpha.

Experimental inoculation of pigs showed that administration of PRCV by aerosol rather than the oronasal route, or in higher doses, resulted in higher virus titres shed and longer shedding.[39] Also, high PRCV doses induced more severe respiratory disease than lower doses. Pigs given $10^{8.5}$ TCID$_{50}$ of PRCV had more severe pneumonia and deaths than pigs exposed by contact,[40] and higher intranasal doses of another PRCV strain (AR310) induced moderate respiratory disease whereas lower doses produced subclinical infections.[18]

A recrudescence of BCoV faecal shedding was observed in one of four winter dysentery BCoV–infected cows treated with dexamethasone.[30] Similarly, treatment of older pigs with dexamethasone prior to TGEV challenge led to profuse diarrhoea and reduced lymphoproliferative responses in the treated pigs.[41] These data raise issues for corticosteroid treatment of SARS patients related to possible transient immunosuppression leading to worsened respiratory disease or increased and prolonged CoV shedding. Alternatively, corticosteroid treatment may help reduce proinflammatory cytokine levels if they are found to play a major role in lung immunopathology.

AVIAN RESPIRATORY CORONAVIRUS

Unlike SARS, which targets the lung resulting in pneumonia, the avian group III CoV infectious bronchitis virus (IBV) is a highly contagious upper respiratory disease of chickens. It is spread by aerosol or possibly faecal-oral transmission and distributed worldwide.[42,43] Genetically and antigenically closely related CoVs have been isolated from pheasants and turkeys,[44,45] but in young turkeys, they cause only enteritis. Respiratory infections of chickens are characterized by upper respiratory clinical signs including tracheal rales, coughing, and sneezing.[42,43] IBV infection is most severe in chicks. IBV replicates in epithelial cells of the trachea and bronchi, intestinal tract, oviduct, and kidney, causing necrosis and oedema with small areas of pneumonia near large bronchi, decreased egg production, and interstitial nephritis in the kidney.[42,43] Whether SAR-CoV also infects the kidney like IBV or is present in urine as a consequence of the viremia it induces, is unkown. In older birds, severe disease or death ensues from systemic E. coli co-infections after IBV damage to the respiratory tract or Mycoplasma sp co-infections with IBV.[42,43] The IBV is recovered intermittently from the respiratory tract for about 28 days after infection and from the faeces after clinical recovery, with the caecal tonsil being a possible reservoir for IBV persistence, similar to the persistence of FIPV in the intestine of cats.[21] Unlike many group I or II CoVs or SARS-CoV, which have only one serotype, IBV has multiple serotypes, complicating its diagnosis and control.[42,43]

Interspecies transmission of coronavirus

The likelihood that SARS is a zoonosis transmitted from wild animals is not unprecedented for CoVs in view of previously documented interspecies transmission of animal CoVs and wildlife reservoirs for CoV. For example, the antigenically closely related porcine (TGEV), canine, and feline CoV (FIPV) cross-infect pigs, with variable disease expression and cross-protection.[9,15,28] Captive wild ruminants harbour CoVs antigenically like bovine CoV,[46,47] and these CoVs experimentally infect calves.[46] Bovine CoV can naturally infect mammalian species (humans, dogs),[48,49] but they can also experimentally infect and cause disease even in diverse avian hosts.[45] Clearly, CoVs can and have circumvented host species barriers to adapt to new hosts.

Vaccine development

The need to target vaccines to protect mucosal tissues (lung, intestine) to prevent respiratory and enteric CoV infections has been and is still a major challenge for the design of effective animal or SARS-CoV vaccines. Existing CoV vaccines are often only marginally effective in the field. Live vaccines are usually more effective than killed vaccines for TGEV in pigs,[15] and IBV in chickens.[42] Neutralizing IgG antibodies in the serum generally fail to correlate with protection, whereas IgA antibodies in the milk or intestine are a correlate of immunity to the enteric CoV TGEV.[15,50] For the persistent systemic FIPV infection of cats, neutralizing serum IgG antibodies to the S protein not only fail to protect but exacerbate disease by contributing to the immunopathology.[51] For both TGEV and IBV, priming with live virus followed by boosting with killed virus was an effective strategy to raise protective mucosal immunity.[15] Subunit vaccines including the S protein were only partially effective unless delivered via an effective live replicating vector (like adenovirus) that preserved conformationally dependent antigenic sites on the S protein and induced local neutralizing antibody responses.[15] Although highly effective vaccines for many animal CoV infections are still elusive, understanding the basis for their successes and failures provides invaluable lessons for the development of SARS vaccines.

Summary

Studies of animal CoV infections can improve our understanding of the similarities and divergence of CoV disease pathogenesis and targets for control. Many unanswered questions for SARS pathogenesis are highly relevant to strategies for the prevention and control of SARS. What is the initial site of viral replication? Is SARS-CoV pneumoenteric like BCoV with variable degrees of infection of the intestinal and respiratory tracts and disease precipitated by the co-factors discussed or unknown variables? Alternatively, is SARS primarily targeted to the lung like PRCV with faecal shedding of swallowed virus and with undefined sequelae contributing to the diarrhoea cases? Does SARS-CoV infect the lung directly or via viraemia after initial replication in another site (oral cavity, tonsil, upper respiratory tract) and does it productively infect secondary target organs (intestine, kidney) via viraemia after replication in the lung? Finally, the persistent, macrophage-tropic, systemic FIPV infection of cats presents yet another CoV disease model and a dilemma for attempted control strategies because antibodies enhance FIPV disease, making protection by vaccine difficult.

The suspected zoonotic origin of SARS CoV [see Chapter 24], and the recognized propensity of several CoVs to cross species barriers illustrate the need for more animal transmission studies to understand how virus circumvents the host-species barrier and adapts to new host species. The SARS epidemic should generate new investigations of fundamental research questions applicable to SARS-CoV and the other newly emerging or re-emerging zoonotic human diseases, many of which, like SARS-CoV are caused by highly variable RNA viruses.[52]

References

1 Drosten C et al. Identification of a novel coronavirus in patients with severe acute respiratory syndrome. *New England Journal of Medicine*, 2003, 348:1967–1976.
2 Marra MA et al. The genome sequence of the SARS-associated coronavirus. *Science*, 2003, 300:1399–404.
3 Rota PA et al. Characterization of a novel coronavirus associated with severe acute respiratory syndrome. *Science*, 2003, 300:1394–1399.
4 Snijder EJ et al. Unique and conserved features of genome and proteome of SARS-coronavirus, an early split-off from the coronavirus grou: p 2 lineage. *Journal of Molecular Biology*, 2003, 331:991–1004.

[5] Marra MA et al. The genome sequence of the SARS-associated coronavirus. *Science*, 2003, 300:1399–404.

[6] Rota PA et al. Characterization of a novel coronavirus associated with severe acute respiratory syndrome. *Science*, 2003, 300:1394–1399.

[7] Guan Y et al. Isolation and characterization of viruses related to the SARS coronavirus from animals in southern China. *Science*, 2003, 302:276–278.

[8] Lai MMC, Cavenagh D. The molecular biology of coronaviruses. *Advances in Virus Research*, 1997, 48:1–100.

[9] Saif LJ. Comparative biology of coronaviruses: lessons for SARS. In Peiris M, ed. *SARS: The first new plague of the 21st century*, Oxford, UK, Blackwell Publishing, 2005 (in press).

[10] Zhang XM et al. Biologic and genetic characterization of a hemagglutinating coronavirus isolated from a diarrhoeic child. *Journal of Medical Virology*, 1994, 44:152–161.

[11] Pensaert MB. Porcine epidemic diarrhea. In Straw B. et al., eds. *Diseases of Swine*, 8th ed. Ames, Iowa, Iowa State Press, 1999:179–185.

[12] Duarte M et al. Sequence analysis of the porcine epidemic diarrhea virus genome between the nucleocapsid and spike protein genes reveals a polymorphic ORF. *Virology*, 1994, 198:466–476.

[13] Hoffman M, Wyler R. Propagation of the virus of porcine epidemic diarrhea in cell culture. *Journal of Clinical Microbiology*, 1988, 26:2235–2239.

[14] Laude H, Van Reeth K, Pensaert M. Porcine respiratory coronavirus: molecular features and virus-host interactions. *Veterinary Research*, 1993, 24:125–150.

[15] Saif LJ, Wesley R. Transmissible gastroenteritis virus. In Straw B. et al., eds. *Diseases of Swine*, 8th ed. Ames, Iowa, Iowa State Press, 1999:295–325.

[16] Ballesteros ML, Sanchez CM, Enjuanes L. Two amino acid changes at the N-terminal of the transmissible gastroenteritis coronavirus spike protein result in the loss of enteric tropism. *Virology*, 1997, 227:378–388.

[17] Sanchez CM et al. Targeted recombination demonstrates that the spike gene of transmissible gastroenteritis coronavirus is a determinant of its enteric tropism and virulence. *Journal of Virology*, 1999, 73:7607–7618.

[18] Halbur PG et al. Experimental reproduction of pneumonia in gnotobiotic pigs with porcine respiratory coronavirus isolate AR310. *Journal of Veterinary Diagnostic Investigation*, 1993, 5:184–188.

[19] Hayes JR. *Evaluation of dual infection of nursery pigs with US strains of porcine reproductive and respiratory syndrome virus and porcine respiratory coronavirus* [master's thesis]. Columbus, Ohio, The Ohio State University, 2000.

[20] Costantini V et al. Respiratory and enteric shedding of porcine respiratory coronavirus (PRCV) in sentinel weaned pigs and sequence of the partial S gene of the PRCV isolates. *Archives of Virology*, 2004, 149:957-974.

[21] Herrewegh AAPM et al. Persistence and evolution of feline coronavirus in a closed cat-breeding colony. *Virology*, 1997, 234:349–363.

[22] Vennema H et al. A comparison of the genomes of FECVs and FIPVs and what they tell us about the relationships between feline coronaviruses and their evolution. *Feline Practitioner*, 1995, 23:40–44.

[23] Lathrop SL et al. Association between infection of the respiratory tract attributable to bovine coronavirus and health and growth performance of cattle in feedlots. *American Journal of Veterinary Research*, 2000, 61:1062–1066.

[24] Storz J et al. Coronavirus isolation from nasal swab samples in cattle with signs of respiratory tract disease after shipping. *Journal of American Veterinary Medical Association*, 1996, 208:1452–1455.

[25] Storz J et al. Coronavirus and Pasteurella infections in bovine shipping fever pneumonia and Evan's criteria for causation. *Journal of Clinical Microbiology*, 2000, 38:3291–3298.

[26] Hasoksuz M et al. Isolation of bovine respiratory coronaviruses from feedlot cattle and comparison of their biologic and antigenic properties with bovine enteric coronaviruses. *American Journal of Veterinary Research*, 1999, 60:1227–1233.

[27] Cho KO et al. Evaluation of concurrent shedding of bovine coronavirus via the respiratory and enteric route in feedlot cattle. *American Journal of Veterinary Research*, 2001, 62:1436–1441.

[28] Saif LJ, Heckert RA. Enteric coronaviruses. In: Saif LJ, Theil KW, eds. *Viral Diarrheas of Man and Animals*, Boca Raton, Florida, CRC Press, 1990:185–252.

[29] Tsunemitsu H, Saif LJ. Antigenic and biological comparisons of bovine coronaviruses derived from neonatal calf diarrhea and winter dysentery of adult cattle. *Archives of Virology*, 1995, 140:1303–1311.

[30] Tsunemitsu H, Smith DR, Saif LJ. Experimental inoculation of adult dairy cows with bovine coronavirus and detection of coronavirus in feces by RT-PCR. *Archives of Virology*, 1999, 144:167–175.

[31] Traven M et al. Experimental reproduction of winter dysentery in lactating cows using BCV: comparison with BCV infection in milk-fed calves. *Veterinary Microbiology*, 2001, 81:127–151.

[32] Cho KO et al. Cross-protection studies of respiratory, calf diarrhea and winter dysentery coronavirus strains in calves and RT-PCR and nested PCR for their detection. *Archives of Virology*, 2001, 146:2401–2419.

[33] El-Kanawati Z et al. Infection and cross-protection studies of winter dysentery and calf diarrhea bovine coronavirus strains in colostrum-deprived and gnotobiotic calves. *American Journal of Veterinary Research*, 1996, 57:48–53.

[34] Chouljenko VN et al. Comparison of genomic and predicted amino acid sequences of respiratory and enteric bovine coronaviruses isolated from the same animal with fatal shipping pneumonia. *Journal of General Virology*, 2001, 82:2927–2933.

[35] Hasoksuz M et al. Molecular analysis of the S1 subunit of the spike glycoprotein of respiratory and enteric bovine coronavirus isolates. *Virus Research*, 2002, 84:101–109.

[36] Heckert RA, Saif LJ, Agnes AG. A longitudinal study of bovine coronavirus enteric and respiratory infections in dairy calves in two herds in Ohio. *Veterinary Microbiology*, 1990, 22:187.

[37] Van Reeth K, Nauwynck H, Pensaert M. A potential role for tumour necrosis factor-alpha in synergy between porcine respiratory coronavirus and bacterial lipopolysaccharide in the induction of respiratory disease in pigs. *Journal of Medical Microbiology*, 2000, 49:613–620.

[38] Van Reeth K, Pensaert MB. Porcine respiratory coronavirus-mediated interference against influenza virus replication in the respiratory tract of feeder pigs. *American Journal of Veterinary Research*, 1994, 55:1275–1281.

[39] Van Cott JL et al. Antibody-secreting cells to transmissible gastroenteritis virus and porcine respiratory coronavirus in gut- and bronchus-associated lymphoid tissues of neonatal pigs. *Journal of Immunology*, 1993, 150:3990–4000.

[40] Jabrane A, Girard C, Elazhary Y. Pathogenicity of porcine respiratory coronavirus isolated in Quebec. *Canadian Veterinary Journal*, 1994, 35:86–92.

[41] Shimizu M, Shimizu Y. Effects of ambient temperatures on clinical and immune responses of pigs infected with transmissible gastroenteritis virus. *Veterinary Microbiology*, 1979, 4:109–116.

[42] Cavanagh D, Naqi S. Infectious bronchitis. In: Saif YM et al., eds. *Diseases of Swine*, 11th ed. Ames, Iowa, Iowa State Press, 2003:101–119.

[43] Cook J, Mockett APA. Epidemiology of infectious bronchitis virus. In: Siddell SG, ed. *The Coronaviridae*. New York, Plenum Press, 1995:317–335.

[44] Guy JS et al. Antigenic characterization of a turkey coronavirus identified in poult enteritis and mortality syndrome–affected turkeys. *Avian Diseases*, 1997, 41:583–590.

[45] Ismail MM et al. Experimental bovine coronavirus in turkey poults and young chickens. *Avian Diseases*, 2001, 45:157–163.

[46] Tsunemitsu H et al. Isolation of coronaviruses antigenically indistinguishable from bovine coronavirus from a Sambar and white tailed deer and waterbuck with diarrhea. *Journal of Clinical Microbiology*, 1995, 33:3264–3269.

[47] Majhdi F, Minocha HC, Kapil S. Isolation and characterization of a coronavirus from elk calves with diarrhea. *Journal of Clinical Microbiology*, 1997, 35:2937–2942.

[48] Zhang XM et al. Biologic and genetic characterization of a hemagglutinating

coronavirus isolated from a diarrhoeic child. *Journal of Medical Virology*, 1994, 44:152–161.

[49] Erles K et al. Detection of a novel canine coronavirus in dogs with respiratory disease. In: *Proceedings of the 9th International Symposium on Nidoviruses*. The Netherlands, 2003:49.

[50] Van Cott JL, Brim TA, Lunney J. Contribution of antibody secreting cells induced in mucosal lymphoid tissues of pigs inoculated with respiratory or enteric strains of coronavirus to immunity against enteric coronavirus challenge. *Journal of Immunology*, 1994, 152:3980–3990.

[51] Olsen CW. A review of feline infectious peritonitis virus: molecular biology, immunopathogenesis, clinical aspects, and vaccination. *Veterinary Microbiology*, 1993, 36:1–37.

[52] Taylor LH. Risk factors for human disease emergence. *Philosophical Transactions of the Royal Society of London B: Biological Sciences*, 2001, 356:983–990.

22 THE SARS CORONAVIRUS (SARS-COV)

In March 2003, WHO alerted the world to the probability of a new disease, now designated as severe acute respiratory syndrome (SARS). To find its cause, WHO immediately formed a virtual network of laboratories working on clinical specimens from patients with SARS.[1] This network investigated patients from outbreaks in Viet Nam, Hong Kong (China), and Singapore and cases in Germany. Collectively, these laboratories were able to exclude a number of potential pathogens including influenza, as the cause of SARS. Detection of paramyxoviruses by electron microscopy and human metapneumovirus by reverse transcriptase-polymerase chain reaction (RT-PCR) and culture were reported in some patients with SARS,[1] and there were also reports that *Chlamydia* had been observed in lungs of patients at autopsy in Guangdong.[1] However, none of these agents could be detected in all patients at all sites. Between 21 and 24 March, three laboratories in the WHO network reported that they had independently isolated a novel virus on FRhK-4 or Vero E6 cells.[2,3,4] The virus was identified by electron microscopy to be a coronavirus. Similar virus particles were observed by electron microscopy in the lung biopsy of a patient with SARS.[2] Genetic analysis appeared to indicate that this was a novel coronavirus.[2,3,4] This chapter provides an overview of this virus, now called SARS coronavirus (SARS-CoV).

AETIOLOGY

Patients with SARS consistently seroconverted to SARS-CoV while there was little serological evidence of past infection in healthy controls, or in blood donations taken before the outbreak. Experimental inoculation of SARS-CoV into cynomolgous macaques resulted in a disease similar to SARS, satisfying the last of Koch's postulates for establishing the aetiology of an infectious disease.[5,6]

The lack of serological evidence in human samples collected prior to 2002 suggested that SARS-CoV was not a virus that had been previously circulating in humans. As with most novel, previously unrecognized viruses over the past two decades, it was probable that SARS-CoV originated from an animal source [see Chapter 24].

GENETIC CLUES

Within weeks of the initial isolation of SARS-CoV, the viral genome had been completely sequenced.[7,8] These findings confirmed that SARS-CoV was distinct from previously known animal and human coronaviruses across the full extent of its genome. This excluded the possibility that SARS-CoV arose by the natural or artificial recombination of the genomes of previously known coronaviruses. The genome organization and phylogeny suggests that SARS-CoV is probably a group II coronavirus, but only distantly related to other coronaviruses in the group.[9] Its formal taxonomic position within the *Coronaviridae* still has to be established by the International Committee on the Taxonomy of Viruses.

Studies on the molecular evolution of the virus confirmed the epidemiological deduction[10] that the global epidemic was linked to the index patient in the Metropole Hotel [see Chapter 14].[11,12,13,14] However, the earliest cases of SARS in Guangdong Province, China, in late 2002 and January 2003, as well as in Hong Kong in February 2003, were genetically more diverse.[15,16] These early SARS-CoV isolates showed higher rates of nonsynonymous mutation, suggesting that the virus was still adapting to the human host.[14] Some of these early SARS-CoV strains had an additional 29-nucleotide segment in ORF8. In this regard, they were similar to SARS-CoV-like animal strains detected in markets in Guangdong,[16] supporting the contention that SARS had a zoonotic origin.

SPREAD

In comparison with other respiratory viruses, SARS-CoV was unusually stable in the environment. It stayed infective for many days even after it had dried on surfaces or in faeces.[17,18] This property may partly explain its infectivity in a hospital setting through fomite and indirect contact. It is thought to have contributed to the extent of the outbreak in the Amoy Gardens housing estate in Hong Kong.[19] Other factors in hospital spread are procedures related to intubation, ventilation, and oxygen supplementation, contributing to aerosolized SARS droplets.[20]

PATHOGENESIS

Infectious virus was detected in the faeces and urine as well as the respiratory tract, indicating that SARS was a disseminated infection, not one confined to the respiratory tract.[21,22,23] The detection of infectious virus in the urine implies that the virus spreads via a viraemic phase. While infectious virus has not been conclusively documented in the peripheral blood, viral RNA is reproducibly detected in the serum[24] and peripheral white blood cells.[25] Viral RNA in respiratory secretions and faeces can be demonstrated by RT-PCR for three to four weeks or even longer.[22] However, infectious virus is rarely isolated after the third week of illness,[22,23] a finding that is consistent with the lack of evidence for transmission of SARS during convalescence.

Quantitative RT-PCR assays of SARS-CoV in the respiratory tract and the faeces revealed that viral load continues to increase during the first week of illness and peaks around the tenth to eleventh day of disease.[21,26] This explains why, in the first five days of illness, transmission appeared to be less common.[27] Higher viral load in the serum at the time of admission,[24] or in the respiratory tract in the second week of illness,[28] correlates with poor prognosis, suggesting that continued viral replication plays a significant role in pathogenesis and that an effective antiviral agent would help improve the chances of recovery. While the window of opportunity for therapeutic intervention with an antiviral agent is relatively narrow in influenza (36 to 48 hours after the onset of disease), with SARS, the opportunity for clinical benefit may be wider. One aspect of pathogenesis that is not easily explained by direct viral cytolysis is the marked lymphopenia consistently observed in patients with SARS,[29] because so far there is to date no evidence *in vivo* or *in vitro* that SARS-CoV infects lymphocytes or their precursors.

The pathological changes predominant in patients with SARS are diffuse alveolar damage, lung oedema, a mixed alveolar infiltrate with a preponderance of macrophages and hyaline membranes. The later stages of the disease show organizing diffuse alveolar damage with focal squamous metaplasia of the bronchial epithelium and fibrosis of the alveolar walls, as well as multinucleate giant cells of macrophage or epithelial cell origin.[30,31] Electron microscopy, *in situ* hybridization, and immunohistological methods conclusively demonstrated virus infection in pneumocytes and enterocytes (epithelial cells of the lung alveoli and the intestine, respectively).[32,33,34,35,36] There appears to be little cell damage or cell infiltrate in the intestinal mucosa, and the mechanisms leading to diarrhoea are unclear.

Like many other viral infections, SARS-CoV infection triggers a number of cytokine responses.[37,38,39,40] It is not yet clear whether these play a role in pathogenesis.[41] As with other coronaviruses, the spike protein of SARS-CoV is the critical determinant of viral attachment to the cell.[42,43,44] The main functional receptor for SARS-CoV has been identified to be the metallopeptidase angiotensin converting enzyme 2 (ACE-2).[45,46] ACE-2 is expressed on alveolar pneumocytes and enterocytes,[47] within which the virus is known to replicate. However, not all cells that express ACE-2 support viral replication *in vivo* or *in vitro*.[48]

The glycosylated S protein has been shown to bind the C-type lectin DC-specific ICAM-3 grabbing non-integrin (DC-SIGN) expressed on dendritic cells, which then mediate SARS-CoV infection *in trans* of cells that express human ACE-2, but the DC-SIGN does not initiate SARS-CoV into the dendritic cells.[42] Human CD209L (also known as L-SIGN) which is 77% identical to human DC-SIGN, can also bind to S protein and mediate virus entry,[49] but its role in initiating productive virus replication remains unclear.

A full-length infectious clone of SARS-CoV has been developed and will permit a more detailed analysis of the virulence factors of the SARS-CoV through the reverse genetics approach.[50]

The genetics of host susceptibility or resistance are being explored although the findings are still preliminary. HLA-B*4601 has been associated with severe SARS disease in Taiwan, China,[51] but the association has not been confirmed in studies elsewhere.[43] HLA-B*0703 has been associated with disease susceptibility, and HLA-DRB1*0301 with resistance to SARS.[52] The mechanisms underlying these disease associations are still unclear.

SUMMARY

SARS-CoV is a previously undetected coronavirus that has been confirmed through several lines of evidence as the cause of SARS. Its survival in the environment and in aerosols generated during medical procedures such as nebulization promoted the spread of SARS-CoV. The SARS outbreak demonstrated the potential for a novel, emerging viral disease to cause a pandemic with a major global impact. The importance of global surveillance measures to rapidly detect outbreaks of infectious diseases of potential international significance, such as SARS, cannot be over-emphasized.[53,54] The experience gained from SARS also demonstrated the importance of international coordination in responding to a major outbreak,[55,56] and specifically the rapid establishment of international networks of experts, as exemplified by the laboratory network.[1] The success of the laboratory network in rapidly isolating and characterizing SARS-CoV was an important step in the battle to control the spread of SARS, resulting in the development of diagnostic tools and, through our knowledge of the aetiological agent, in being able to better understand the transmission, pathogenesis, and ecology of the disease.

REFERENCES

[1] World Health Organization. A multicentre collaboration to investigate the cause of severe acute respiratory syndrome. *Lancet*, 2003, 361:1730–1733.
[2] Peiris JS et al. Coronavirus as a possible cause of severe acute respiratory syndrome. *Lancet*, 2003, 361:1319–1325.
[3] Ksiazek TG et al. A novel coronavirus associated with severe acute respiratory syndrome. *New England Journal of Medicine*, 2003, 348:1953–1966

[4] Drosten C et al. Identification of a novel coronavirus in patients with severe acute respiratory syndrome. *New England Journal of Medicine*, 2003, 348:1967–1976.

[5] Fouchier RA et al. Aetiology: Koch's postulates fulfilled for SARS virus. *Nature*, 2003, 423:240.

[6] Kuiken T et al. Newly discovered coronavirus as the primary cause of severe acute respiratory syndrome. *Lancet*, 2003, 362:263–270.

[7] Marra MA et al. The genome sequence of the SARS associated coronavirus. *Science*, 2003, 300:1399–1404.

[8] Rota PA et al. Characterization of a novel coronavirus associated with severe acute respiratory syndrome. *Science*, 2003, 300:1394–1399.

[9] Snijder EJ et al. Unique and conserved features of genome and proteome of SARS-coronavirus: an early split-off from the coronavirus group 2 lineage. *Journal of Molecular Biology*, 2003, 331:991–1004.

[10] Centers for Disease Control and Prevention. Update: Outbreak of severe acute respiratory syndrome—worldwide, 2003. *Morbidity and Mortality Weekly Report*, 2003, 52:241–248.

[11] Ruan YJ et al. Comparative full-length genome sequence analysis of 14 SARS coronavirus isolates and common mutations associated with putative origins of infection. *Lancet*, 2003, 361:1779–1785.

[12] Guan Y et al. Molecular epidemiology of the novel coronavirus that causes severe acute respiratory syndrome. *Lancet*, 2004, 363:99–104

[13] Yeh SH et al. Characterization of severe acute respiratory syndrome coronavirus genomes in Taiwan: molecular epidemiology and genome evolution. *Proceedings of the National Academy of Sciences USA*, 2004, 101:2542–2547;

[14] The Chinese SARS Molecular Epidemiology Consortium. Molecular evolution of the SARS coronavirus during the course of the SARS epidemic in China. *Science*, 2004, 303:1666–1669.

[15] Zhong NS et al. Epidemiology and cause of severe acute respiratory syndrome (SARS) in Guangdong, People's Republic of China, in February 2003. *Lancet*, 2003, 362:1353–1358.

[16] Guan Y et al. Isolation and characterization of viruses related to SARS coronavirus from animals in southern China. *Science*, 2003, 302:276–278.

[17] *First data on stability and resistance of SARS coronavirus compiled by members of WHO laboratory network.* Geneva, World Health Orgization, 2003 (http://www.who.int/csr/sars/survival_2003_05_04/en/index.html, accessed 1 April 2005).

[18] Rabenau HF et al. Stability and inactivation of SARS coronavirus. *Medical Microbiology and Immunology*, 2005, 194:1-6.

[19] Yu IT et al. Evidence of airborne transmission of the severe acute respiratory syndrome virus. *New England Journal of Medicine*, 2004, 350:1731–1739.

[20] Somogyi R et al. Dispersal of respiratory droplets with open versus closed oxygen delivery masks. *Chest,* 2004, 125:1155–1157.

[21] Peiris JS et al. Clinical progression and viral load in a community outbreak of coronavirus-associated SARS pneumonia: a prospective study. *Lancet,* 2003, 361:1767–1772.

[22] Chan KH et al. Detection of SARS coronavirus in patients with suspected SARS. *Emerging Infectious Diseases,* 2004, 10:294–299.

[23] Chan PK et al. Laboratory diagnosis of SARS. *Emerging Infectious Diseases,* 2004, 10: 825–831.

[24] Ng EK et al. Serial analysis of the plasma concentration of SARS coronavirus RNA in pediatric patients with severe acute respiratory syndrome. *Clinical Chemistry,* 2003, 49:2085–2088.

[25] Li L et al. SARS-coronavirus replicates in mononuclear cells of peripheral blood (PBMCs) from SARS patients. *Journal of Clinical Virology,* 2003, 28:239–244.

[26] Cheng PKC et al. Viral shedding patterns of coronavirus in patients with probable severe acute respiratory syndrome. *Lancet,* 2004, 363:1699–1700.

[27] Lipsitch M et al. Transmission dynamics and control of severe acute respiratory syndrome. *Science,* 2003, 300:1966–1970.

[28] Hung IFN et al. Viral loads in clinical specimens and SARS manifestations. *Emerging Infectious Diseases,* 2004, 10:1550–1557.

[29] Wong RSM et al. Haematological manifestations in patients with severe acute respiratory syndrome: retrospective analysis. *British Medical Journal,* 2003, 326:1358–1362.

[30] Nicholls JM et al. Lung pathology of fatal severe acute respiratory syndrome. *Lancet,* 2003, 361:1773–1778.

[31] Franks TJ et al. Lung pathology of severe acute respiratory syndrome (SARS): a study of 8 autopsy cases from Singapore. *Human Pathology,* 2003, 34:743–748.

[32] Chow KC et al. Detection of severe acute respiratory syndrome-associated coronavirus in pneumocytes of the lung. *Americal Journal of Clinical Pathology,* 2004, 121:574–580.

[33] To KF et al. Tissue and cellular tropism of the coronavirus associated with severe acute respiratory syndrome: an in situ hybridization study of fatal cases. *Journal of Pathology,* 2004, 202:157–163.

[34] Nakajima N et al. SARS coronavirus-infected cells in lung detected by new in situ hybridization technique. *Japanese Journal of Infectious Diseases,* 2003, 56:139–141.

[35] Chong PY et al. Analysis of deaths during the severe acute respiratory syndrome (SARS) epidemic in Singapore: challenges in determining a SARS diagnosis. *Archives of Pathology and Laboratory Medicine,* 2004, 128:195–204.

[36] Leung WK et al. Enteric involvement of severe acute respiratory syndrome-associated coronavirus infection. *Gastroenterology*, 2003, 125:1011–1017.

[37] Wong CK et al. Plasma inflammatory cytokines and chemokines in severe acute respiratory syndrome. *Clinical and Experimental Immunology*, 2004, 136:95–103.

[38] Zhang Y et al. Analysis of serum cytokines in patients with severe acute respiratory syndrome. *Infection and Immunity*, 2004, 72:4410–4415.

[39] Ng PC et al. Inflammatory cytokine profile in children with severe acute respiratory syndrome. *Pediatrics*, 2004, 113(1): e7-e14 (http://www.pediatrics.org/cgi/content/full/113/1/e7, accessed 1 April 2005).

[40] Jones BM et al. Prolonged disturbance of in vitro cytokine production in patients with severe acute respiratory syndrome (SARS) treated with ribavirin and steroids. *Clinical and Experimental Immunology*, 2004, 135:467–473.

[41] Openshaw PJM. What does the peripheral blood tell you in SARS? *Clinical and Experimental Immunology*, 2004, 136:11–12.

[42] Yang ZY et al. pH-dependent entry of severe acute respiratory syndrome coronavirus is mediated by the spike glycoprotein and enhanced by dendritic cell transfer through DC-SIGN. *Journal of Virology*, 2004, 78:5642–5650.

[43] Simmons G et al. Characterization of severe acute respiratory syndrome-associated coronavirus (SARS CoV) spike glycoprotein-mediated viral entry. *Proceedings of the National Academy of Sciences USA*, 2004, 101:4240–4245,

[44] Hofmann H et al. Susceptibility to SARS coronavirus S protein-derived infection correlates with expression of angiotensin converting enzyme 2 and infection can be blocked by soluble receptor. *Biochemical and Biophysical Research Communications*, 2004, 319:1216–1221.

[45] Li W et al. Angiotensin-converting enzyme 2 is a functional receptor for the SARS coronavirus. *Nature*, 2003, 426:450–454.

[46] Wang P et al. Expression cloning of functional receptor used by SARS coronavirus. *Biochemical and Biophysical Research Communications*, 2004, 315:439–444.

[47] Hamming I et al. Tissue distribution of ACE-2 protein, the functional receptor for SARS coronavirus: a first step in understanding SARS pathogenesis. *Journal of Pathology*, 2004, 203:631–637.

[48] To KF, Lo AWI. Exploring the pathogenesis of severe acute respiratory syndrome (SARS): the tissue distribution of the coronavirus (SARS-CoV) and its putative receptor, angiotensin-converting-enzyme 2 (ACE-2). *Journal of Pathology*, 2004, 203:740–743.

[49] Jeffers SA et al. CD209L (L-SIGN) is a receptor for severe acute respiratory syndrome coronavirus. *Proceedings of the National Academy of Sciences USA*, 2004, 101:15748–15753.

[50] Yount B et al. Reverse genetics with a full length infectious cDNA of severe acute respiratory syndrome coronavirus. *Proceedings of the National Academy of Sciences USA,* 2003, 100:12995–13000.

[51] Lin M et al. Association of HLA class 1 with severe acute respiratory syndrome coronavirus infection. *BMC Medical Genetics,* 2003, 4:9.

[52] Ng MHL et al. Association of human-leukocyte-antigen class 1 (B*0703) and class II (DRB1*0301) genotypes with susceptibility and resistance to the development of severe acute respiratory syndrome. *Journal of Infectious Diseases,* 2004, 190:515–518.

[53] Heymann DL et al. Hot spots in a wired world: WHO surveillance of emerging and re-emerging diseases. *Lancet Infectious Diseases,* 2001, 1:345–353.

[54] Smolinski MS, Hamburg MA, Lederberg J (eds). *Microbial Threats to Health: Emergence, Detection and Response.* Institute of Medicine, The National Academies Press, Washington, DC, 2003.

[55] Heymann DL. The international response to the outbreak of SARS in 2003. Philosophical Transactions of Royal Society, London, B. *Biological Sciences,* 2004, 359:1127–1129.

[56] Mackenzie JS et al. The WHO response to SARS and preparations for the future. In: Knobler S, Mahmoud A, Lemon S, Mack A, Sivitz L, Oberholtzer K, eds. *Learning from SARS: Preparing for the Next Disease Outbreak.* Institute of Medicine, The National Academies Press, Washington DC, 2003; 42–50.

23 LABORATORY DIAGNOSTICS

This chapter reviews the capabilities and limitations of the main methods of laboratory diagnostics of SARS. Several potentially good diagnostic approaches are not mentioned because they have not been evaluated extensively on clinical samples.

ANTIBODY TESTING

Screening. It became clear early during the 2003 epidemic that virtually all patients with a clinical picture of SARS develop specific IgG antibodies against SARS-coronavirus (SARS-CoV).[1] In 92% of 417 probable SARS cases in Hong Kong (China), the IgG serum antibody titre rose four times or more between paired samples, using immunofluorescence assays (IFA).[2] The time course of seroconversion using IFA was first documented in a cohort of 70 SARS patients from Hong Kong.[3] IgG was detected within a mean of 20 (±5.1) days after the onset of symptoms. Another study of IFA found IgG in sera of six SARS patients starting from the ninth to the eighteenth day after the onset of illness.[4] In general, a negative IgG result using IFA cannot exclude SARS, unless it is taken at least 28 days from onset of symptoms.

IFA has become the "method of choice" for serological testing (testing for antibodies). This is not only because IFA tests were the first methods available, but also because of other obvious advantages of the method, including its high general sensitivity and low technical requirements for setting up the method. However, experienced laboratory personnel are needed to interpret results and to prepare slides with infectious virus.

Enzyme immunoassays (EIA) have been used in several studies to overcome these drawbacks. Such tests are easy to handle and do not require subjective interpretation of results. Recombinant test antigens can be used in EIA without risk of infection. Recombinant nucleocapsid protein of SARS-CoV or synthetic peptides homologous to the nucleocapsid or U274 proteins have proven to be appropriate test antigens in several studies [Table 23.1]. Sensitivities were largely concordant with IFA methods. One EIA study showed that IgM antibodies do not appear significantly earlier than IgG antibodies but disappear after about three months from the onset of symptoms.[5] Similarly, IgA antibodies were not detected earlier or more often than IgG.[6] Whether IgM testing may provide a differentiation between old and ongoing infections is questionable because detectable IgM antibodies do not develop in all patients with confirmed IgG seroconversion.[5,6]

Table 23.1. Synopsis of EIA methods for antibody detection

Study	Antigen	Days after onset	Sensitivity	Specificity	Gold standard
Timani KA et al[7]	Recombinant N	>20	16/16 (100%)	131/131 (100%)	Probable case definition
Guan M et al[8]	Recombinant (Gst-N and Gst-U274)	16–65	74/74 (100%)	209/210 (99.5%)	Probable case definition
Hsueh PR et al[9]	Peptides (S,M,N)	35–175	69/69 (100%)	1541/1541 (100%)	Probable case definition and whole virus ELISA
Chen W et al[10]	Whole virus	22–28	41/45 (91%)	NA	Probable case definition
Chen W et al[10]	Recombinant N	12–43	100/106 (94%)	142/149 (95.3%)	Whole virus IFA
Chen W et al[10]	Recombinant (Gst-N and Gst-U274)	21–30 >30	43/57 (75%) 18/19 (95%)	385/385 (99.5%)	Suspected case definition and IFA
Cumulative			(361/386) 94%	361/386 (99.6%)	

ELISA, enzyme linked immunosorbent assay; IFA, immunofluorescence assays; NA, not applicable

Confirmation. Although all published IFA and EIA methods have a specificity well above 90% [Table 23.1], the risk of obtaining false-positive results with any of these assays requires confirmatory testing by an alternative method. Western blot (WB) and virus neutralization tests (NT) are currently recommended methods used for serologic confirmation.

WB potentially provides greater specificity because the numbers and molecular weights of reactive test antigens can be used for interpreting results. The sensitivity of WB, as compared with that of IFA or EIA, has been determined to range between 85% and 100%.[11,12 13] WB can thus confirm IFA or EIA results in most patients.

NT provides enhanced specificity by examining not only the binding of antibodies to virus epitopes, but also their functional ability to interfere with virus entry, which is a very specific process. A significant rise in NT titre can reliably prove an infection. On the other hand, not all infected patients develop enough neutralizing antibodies to provide a positive NT.

Because NT is a cumbersome method, only few data exist on its clinical sensitivity. Among 623 patients with SARS in Beijing, 86% tested positive for neutralizing antibodies.[14] In a cohort of 469 patients in Taiwan, China, several of them sampled in the early phase of disease, NT was positive in 48% of patients, as opposed to 58% in EIA.[13] NT is an appropriate method for expert laboratories to provide definite confirmation of infection when virus cannot be detected.

VIRUS TESTING

Reverse transcriptase-polymerase chain reaction (RT-PCR). The first methods for detecting SARS-CoV in clinical samples were described along with the primary identification of the agent.[1,15,16] In each of these studies, RT-PCR detected SARS-CoV in most SARS patients, confirming the aetiology of the new disease. First-generation tests relied on conventional RT-PCR followed by agarose gel electrophoresis. A retrospective study compared two popular first-generation protocols.[1,15] These tests were distributed via a WHO Internet resource during the 2003 epidemic.[17] Nasopharyngeal aspirates, throat swabs, and urine and stool samples from serologically confirmed SARS patients in Hong Kong were tested. Sensitivities ranged between 50% and 72%, depending on the test and clinical material used [Table 23.2]. Crucially, the sensitivity of RT-PCR in respiratory samples reached reasonable levels only after one week of disease, leaving two thirds of patients who were later on confirmed with SARS undiagnosed on admission to hospital.[3] Stool samples give the highest rates of detection, 10 days after symptom onset, and are recommended.[3]

Table 23.2 Comparison of first-generation RT-PCR methods

Type of sample[a]	Sensitivity of first generation RT-PCR methods	
	Peiris JS et al[1]	Drosten C et al[15]
Nasopharyngeal aspriate	61%	68%
Throat swab	65%	72%
Urine	50%	54%
Stool	58%	63%

Clinical samples from 86 SARS patients, confirmed by seroconversion

Source: Yam WC et al. Evaluation of reverse transcription-PCR assays for rapid diagnosis of severe acute respiratory syndrome associated with a novel coronavirus. Journal of Clinical Microbiology, 2003, 41:4521–4524.

Different approaches have been explored to improve the sensitivity of RT-PCR. Testing two samples instead of one per patient increased detection rates slightly.[17] The same was achieved by testing one sample per patient two times, increasing the chance of detection of randomly distributed RNA in low-concentration samples.[18] Poon and colleagues increased the sample input volume in the RNA extraction, thereby improving the sensitivity of their first-generation RT-PCR from 22% to 44% in 50 nasopharyngeal aspirate samples.[19] However, this approach might not work with every assay, since RT-PCR has limited capacity to operate in the presence of background nucleic acids and other substances interfering with amplification. Inhibition control reactions, either by parallel testing of spiked patient samples or by internal inhibition control techniques, are mandatory for reliable diagnostic performance.

Real-time RT-PCR has been used early on, but only some laboratories could conduct clinical evaluation with sufficiently large cohorts of patients. SARS-CoV was detected in 80% of 50 nasopharyngeal aspirates on the first to the third day after admission with a probe-based assay, as opposed to 44% with a first-generation test.[20] However, in most other studies available, different highly optimized real-time RT-PCR assays provided sensitivities around or below 70% in respiratory swabs and aspirates [Table 23.3]. Similar figures were obtained for other types of clinical samples. Thus, real-time RT-PCR cannot be considered more sensitive than conventional assays.

The switching of the RT-PCR target gene within the SARS-CoV genome has been proposed as another means to achieve better sensitivity. During replication, coronaviruses generate an excess of subgenomic mRNA species, all of which contain the nucleocapsid (N) gene.[24] If virus-replicating cells were present in clinical samples, one would expect a higher sensitivity in N-gene-based RT-PCR. Though this hypothesis was supported by observations in experimental animals, it could not be confirmed in three independent studies on SARS patients.[18,19,25]

Table 23.3 summarizes the results of some of the larger clinical evaluation studies on SARS RT-PCR. Data from these studies indicate that samples from either the lower respiratory tract or nasopharyngeal aspirates should be tested. These samples should be complemented with stool specimens after 10 days of

Table 23.3 Cumulative sensitivity of RT-PCR in different clinical samples

Study	Nasopharyngeal aspirate specimens	Other upper respiratory tract	Lower respiratory tract	Stool	Urine	Blood/plasma
Cheng PK et al[1]	355/789 (45%)	116/489 (24%)	22/29 (76%)	150/540 (28%)	6/198 (3%)	20/89 (23%)
Chan KH et al[2]	29/98 (30%)	15/53 (28%)	5/9 (56%)	5/25 (20%)	0/15 (0%)	-
Tang P et al[2]		33/102 (32%)	10/17 (59%)	19/30 (63%)	-	2/81 (2%)
Drosten C et al[18]		11/19 (58%)	12/12 (100%)	20/23 (87%)	-	3/7 (43%)
Zhai J et al[3]	-	11/76 (15%)	113/180 (63%)	60/326 (18%)	-	96/426 (23%)
Poon LL et al[19]	43/98 (44%)	-	-	22/37 (59%)	-	-
Wu HS et al[13]	-	145/207 (52%)	-	-	-	-
Cumulative	**427/985 (43%)**	**287/825 (35%)**				
		758/1931 (39%)		162/247 (66%)	276/981 (28%)	6/213 (3%) 121/603 (20%)

[a]Clinical samples from 86 SARS patients, confirmed by seroconversion

Source: Yam WC et al. Evaluation of reverse transcription-PCR assays for rapid diagnosis of severe acute respiratory syndrome associated with a novel coronavirus. *Journal of Clinical Microbiology*, 2003, 41:4521–4524.

disease. An initially negative result should be confirmed by a second testing after two to three days. However, negative RT-PCR results will not rule out SARS in suspected patients because of the tests' general lack of clinical sensitivity.

Immunoassays. These 'bedside' methods are used to detect viruses; however, data on their effectiveness for detecting SARS are limited. The reportedly low amount of virus particles in early respiratory specimens will make a sensitive antigen test for these samples a difficult goal to achieve.[19] For serum, an antigen assay targeted at secreted nucleocapsid protein has been evaluated on 85 patients sampled from the first to the fifth day after the onset of symptoms. Sensitivity was high at 94%,[26] suggesting that this test could be a real alternative to RT-PCR in the early phase of disease. However, the same authors using the same test found in a different clinical cohort only 50% sensitivity on the third to the fifth day, and 71% on the sixth to the tenth day.[27] This is below the sensitivity of RT-PCR. Thus, the method must be evaluated further before it can be recommended as a standard procedure to complement RT-PCR.

SUMMARY

Several test methods are available that are fairly reliable in detecting antibodies to the virus or the virus itself. Each method has advantages and limitations. IFA is the method of choice for testing for antibody, but EIA has some advantages in terms of cost, requirements, and safety. RT-PCR is generally used for detecting virus. Unfortunately, there is no test that is reliably positive early in the course of SARS, when the result is needed for public-health actions to prevent spread.

REFERENCES

[1] Peiris JS et al. Coronavirus as a possible cause of severe acute respiratory syndrome. *Lancet*, 2003, 361:1319–1325.

[2] Chan KH et al. Detection of SARS coronavirus in patients with suspected SARS. *Emerging Infectious Diseases*, 2004, 10:294–299.

[3] Peiris, JS et al. Clinical progression and viral load in a community outbreak of coronavirus-associated SARS pneumonia: a prospective study. *Lancet*, 2003, 361:1767–1772.

[4] Hsueh PR et al. Microbiologic characteristics, serologic responses, and clinical manifestations in severe acute respiratory syndrome, Taiwan. *Emerging Infectious Diseases*, 2003, 9:1163–1167.

[5] Li G, Chen X, Xu A. Profile of specific antibodies to the SARS-associated coronavirus. *New England Journal of Medicine*, 2003, 349:508–509.

[6] Woo PC et al. Detection of specific antibodies to severe acute respiratory syndrome (SARS) coronavirus nucleocapsid protein for serodiagnosis of SARS coronavirus pneumonia. *Journal of Clinical Microbiology*, 2004, 42:2306–2309.

[7] Timani KA et al. Cloning, sequencing, expression, and purification of SARS-associated coronavirus nucleocapsid protein for serodiagnosis of SARS. *Journal of Clinical Virology*, 2004, 30:309–312.

[8] Guan M et al. Recombinant protein-based enzyme-linked immunosorbent assay and immunochromatographic tests for detection of immunoglobulin G antibodies to severe acute respiratory syndrome (SARS) coronavirus in SARS patients. Clinical and Diagnostic Laboratory Immunology, 2004, 11:287–91.

[9] Hsueh PR et al. SARS antibody test for serosurveillance. *Emerging Infectious Diseases*, 2004, 10:1558 562.

[10] Chen W et al. Antibody response and viraemia during the course of severe acute respiratory syndrome (SARS)-associated coronavirus infection. *Journal of Medical Microbiology*, 2004, 53:435–438.

[11] He Q et al. Development of a Western blot assay for detection of antibodies against coronavirus causing severe acute respiratory syndrome. *Clinical and Diagnostic Laboratory Immunology*, 2004, 11:417–422.

[12] Wang YD et al. Detection of antibodies against SARS-CoV in serum from SARS-infected donors with ELISA and Western blot. *Clinical Immunology*, 2004, 113:145–150.

[13] Wu HS et al. Serologic and molecular biologic methods for SARS-associated coronavirus infection, Taiwan. *Emerging Infectious Diseases*, 2004, 10:304–310.

[14] Nie Y et al. Neutralizing antibodies in patients with severe acute respiratory syndrome-associated coronavirus infection. *Journal of Infectious Diseases*, 2004, 190:1119–1126.

[15] Drosten C et al. Identification of a novel coronavirus in patients with severe acute respiratory syndrome. *New England Journal of Medicine*, 2003, 348:1967–1976.

[16] Ksiazek TG et al. A novel coronavirus associated with severe acute respiratory syndrome. *New England Journal of Medicine*, 2003, 348:1953–1966.

[17] Yam WC et al. Evaluation of reverse transcription-PCR assays for rapid diagnosis of severe acute respiratory syndrome associated with a novel coronavirus. *Journal of Clinical Microbiology*, 2003, 41:4521–4524.

[18] Drosten C et al. Evaluation of advanced reverse transcription-PCR assays and an alternative PCR target region for detection of severe acute respiratory syndrome-associated coronavirus. *Journal of Clinical Microbiology*, 2004, 42 (in press).

[19] Poon LL et al. Detection of SARS coronavirus in patients with severe acute respiratory syndrome by conventional and real-time quantitative reverse transcription-PCR assays. *Clinical Chemistry*, 2004, 50:67–72.

[20] Poon LL et al. Early diagnosis of SARS Coronavirus infection by real time RT-PCR. *Journal of Clinical Virology*, 2003, 28:233–238.

[21] Cheng PK et al. Viral shedding patterns of coronavirus in patients with probable severe acute respiratory syndrome. *Lancet*, 2004, 363:1699–1700.

[22] Tang P et al. Interpretation of diagnostic laboratory tests for severe acute respiratory syndrome: the Toronto experience. *Canadian Medical Association Journal*, 2004, 170:47–54.

[23] Zhai J et al. Real-time polymerase chain reaction for detecting SARS coronavirus, Beijing. *Emerging Infectious Diseases*, 2004, 10:300–303.

[24] Rota PA et al. Characterization of a novel coronavirus associated with severe acute respiratory syndrome. *Science*, 2003, 300:1394–1399.

[25] Ng EK et al. Quantitative analysis and prognostic implication of SARS coronavirus RNA in the plasma and serum of patients with severe acute respiratory syndrome. *Clinical Chemistry*, 2003, 49:1976–80.

[26] Che XY et al. Nucleocapsid protein as early diagnostic marker for SARS. *Emerging Infectious Diseases*, 2004, 10:1947–1949.

[27] Che XY et al. Sensitive and specific monoclonal antibody-based capture enzyme immunoassay for detection of nucleocapsid antigen in sera from patients with severe acute respiratory syndrome. *Journal of Clinical Microbiology*, 2004, 42:2629–2635.

24 THE ANIMAL CONNECTION

An important source of emerging diseases is the transfer of infectious agents from animals to humans through changes in ecology, human behaviour, technology or industry, international travel and commerce, or microbial characteristics, compounded perhaps by a breakdown in public-health measures.[1]

Since its discovery in 2003, the SARS coronavirus (SARS-CoV) has been thought to originate in animals. This chapter summarizes the published studies that support this hypothesis, and the issues that still have to be addressed to prevent the re-emergence of SARS.

EPIDEMIOLOGICAL LINKS

Evidence of an animal origin for SARS first came from epidemiological studies of early cases in Guangdong Province, China. The first cases or clusters occurred between November 2002 and February 2003 in several independent geographic areas in the southern part of the province.[2] This suggests multiple introductions of the virus from a common source, perhaps a wild animal used for food. Wild animals are commonly eaten in the Pearl River Delta region, sometimes to show social status or wealth. Several of the early patients

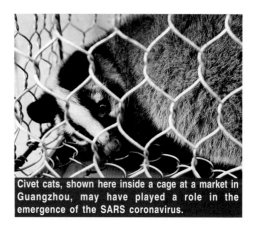

Civet cats, shown here inside a cage at a market in Guangzhou, may have played a role in the emergence of the SARS coronavirus.

were chefs or seafood merchants, or had contact in other ways with wildlife used for food.[3] Those who handled, killed, and sold wild animals or who prepared and served food made up 39% of those who fell ill before the end of January, but only 2%–10% of cases from February to April.[4] The early cases were also more likely to live within walking distance of a market where live animals were sold, killed, and butchered, than the later cases.[4]

SOURCE OF THE VIRUS

Researchers in China have tried to identify the natural reservoir of SARS-CoV by screening samples from wildlife and domestic species or from archived collections, but most of their findings are unpublished. Samples from six Himalayan palm civets, a raccoon dog, and a Chinese ferret badger from a live-animal market in Shenzhen showed infection with a SARS-like virus.[5] When researchers compared this virus with the human SARS-CoV, they found that the animal virus genome had a 29-nucleotide sequence not found in the human virus genome. But five isolates from patients in the early phase of the outbreak retained this 29-nucleotide sequence.[6] All of the patients had come into contact with some of the earliest independent cases in Guangzhou. These findings add compelling evidence to suggest that the virus originated in animals and then possibly mutated, becoming more readily transmissible between humans.

Four different studies have investigated SARS-CoV antibody levels among workers in live-animal markets.[5,7,8,9] Workers involved in the trade and slaughter of wild animals were consistently found to be at greater risk of having SARS-CoV antibodies; between 13% and 40% of them tested positive for the antibodies.[5,7,8] The proportion of antibody-positive workers was even higher among traders of palm civets, at between 59% and 72%.[7,8] Interestingly, in all of these studies antibody-positive individuals did not report having experienced symptoms of SARS.[5,7,8,9] These findings suggest either that infections can be asymptomatic or that these workers were exposed to a less severe SARS-like animal CoV, which might have cross-reacted with the SARS-CoV antibody test. The workers may also have acquired immunity from low-level exposure over time.

SARS CORONAVIRUS IN OTHER ANIMALS

Other groups have studied the effect of SARS-CoV in other species to develop animal models or to identify possible hosts for the virus. The first animal model developed was the cynomolgus macaque.[10] This study helped fulfil Koch's postulates and confirm SARS-CoV as the aetiologic agent of SARS. Ferrets develop SARS-like clinical signs and are therefore good alternative models, besides primates, for SARS research.[11] Domestic poultry and pigs were found to be unlikely reservoirs or amplifying hosts, following experimental infections to determine their susceptibility to the virus,[12,13] although it is not known if prior immunity of the pigs to another coronavirus had an effect. Civets,[14] golden hamsters,[15] and mice[16] have been shown in recent experiments to be susceptible to infection by SARS-CoV and may also be used as animal models for future studies.

After the first case of community-acquired SARS in China was identified in the winter of 2003–2004, findings from studies of animals from live-animal markets in the late fall of 2003 prompted the cull of about 10,000 palm civets and several other small mammals.[17,18] Dr Guan Yi reported that the viral genomic sequence obtained from a recently sampled palm civet was identical to that found in the patient.[17] In all, four community-acquired cases of SARS were identified between December 2003 and January 2004. According to a presentation on this cluster at the International Conference on Emerging Infectious Diseases in 2004, the only clear case of exposure to a palm civet was a waitress who worked in a restaurant that had the animals in a cage, with evidence of SARS-CoV, in front of the shop.[19]

ISSUES TO BE RESOLVED

While a growing body of evidence suggests that palm civets may have been involved in the spread of SARS-CoV, many questions persist regarding which other animals may have contributed to its spread, and which animals could serve as the reservoir host. For example, rats may have been a source or vector of the SARS virus in the outbreak in Amoy Gardens, Hong Kong (China) in 2003.[20] This theory has been largely discounted, but it remains a possibility. The studies of civet cats in markets may not be representative of

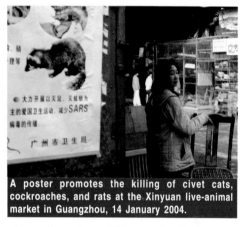

A poster promotes the killing of civet cats, cockroaches, and rats at the Xinyuan live-animal market in Guangzhou, 14 January 2004.

infection in other places, as seroprevalence has been found to differ markedly between civet cats in the market and those on the farm.[21]

A diagnostic test to screen animals for the virus or antibodies urgently needs to be developed and validated to help track the movements of the virus. The factors that influenced the emergence of the SARS-CoV in the winter of 2003 must also be investigated. As noted above, several studies into the origin of SARS have been done or are under way in China, but much of the data remains unpublished.

A research framework has been developed by WHO in collaboration with colleagues from the Government of China, but it needs to be fully implemented. The origin and ecology of the SARS virus must be understood before appropriate preventive measures can be developed.

Summary

Epidemiological, virological, and serological studies suggest that the palm civet in southern China may have played a role in the emergence of the SARS-CoV, but many questions remain unanswered. The close relationship between these animals and humans seems to have been a likely precondition. Appropriate preventive measures can be developed only with a clear understanding of the origin and ecology of the SARS-CoV. The scientific community must therefore continue to collaborate toward a better understanding of the chain of transmission to avoid future pandemics.

References

[1] Morse SS. Factors in the emergence of infectious diseases. *Emerging Infectious Diseases,* 1995, 1(1):7–15.

[2] Zhong NS et al. Epidemiology and cause of severe acute respiratory syndrome (SARS) in Guangdong, People's Republic of China, in February 2003. *Lancet,* 2003, 362:1353–1358.

[3] He JF *et al.* Severe acute respiratory syndrome in Guandong Province of China: epidemiology and control measures. *Zhonghua Yu Fang Yi Xue Za Zhi,* 2003, 37(4):227–232.

[4] Xu R-H et al. Epidemiologic clues to SARS origin in China. *Emerging Infectious Diseases,* 2004, 10(6):1030–1037.

[5] Guan Y et al. Isolation and characterization of viruses related to the SARS coronavirus from animals in Southern China. *Science,* 2003, 203:276–278.

[6] The Chinese SARS Molecular Epidemiology Consortium. Molecular evolution of the SARS coronavirus during the course of the SARS epidemic in China. *Science,* 2004, 303:1666–1669.

[7] Xu HF et al. An epidemiologic investigation on infection with severe acute respiratory syndrome coronavirus in wild animal traders in Guangzhou. *Zhonghua Yu Fang Yi Xue Za Zhi,* 2004, 38(2):81–83.

[8] Yu D et al. Prevalence of IgG antibody to SARS-associated coronavirus in animal traders, Guangdong Province, China, 2003. *Morbidity Mortality Weekly Report,* 2003, 52(41):986–987.

[9] Wang M et al. Analysis of the risk factors of severe acute respiratory symdrome coronavirus infection in workers from animal markets. *Zhonghua Liu Xing Bing Xue Za Zhi,* 2004, 25(6):503–505.

[10] Fouchier RAM et al. Koch's postulates fulfilled for SARS virus. *Nature,* 2003, 423:240.

[11] Martina BEE et al. SARS virus infection of cats and ferrets. *Nature,* 2003, 425:915.

[12] Swayne DE et al. Domestic poultry and SARS coronavirus, China. *Emerging Infectious Diseases,* 2004, 10(5):914–916.

[13] Weingartl HM et al. Susceptibility of pigs and chickens to SARS coronavirus. *Emerging Infectious Diseases*, 2004, 10(2):179–184.

[14] Wu D et al. Civets are equally susceptible to experimental infection by two different severe acute respiratory syndrome coronavirus isolates. *Journal of Virology*, 2005, 79:2620–2625.

[15] Roberts A et al. Severe acute respiratory syndrome coronavirus infection of golden Syrian hamsters. *Journal of Virology*, 2005, 79:505–511.

[16] Subbarao KJ et al. Prior infection and passive transfer of neutralizing antibody prevent replication of severe acute respiratory syndrome coronavirus in the respiratory tract of mice. *Journal of Virology*, 2004, 78:3572–3577.

[17] Normile D. Viral DNA match spurs China's civet roundup. *Science*, 2004, 303:292.

[18] Greenfeld KT. The inside story of one scientist's crusade to link SARS to civets. Will it avert an epidemic? *Time*, 19 January 2004, 26–28.

[19] Liang G, Xu RH. SARS in Guangdong: 2004. Late breaker presented on 1 March 2004 at the International Conference on Emerging Infectious Diseases 2004 in Atlanta, GA, USA.

[20] Ng SKC. Possible role of an animal vector in the SARS outbreak at Amoy Gardens. *Lancet*, 2003, 362:570–572.

[21] Tu C et al. Antibodies to SARS-Coronavirus in civets. *Emerging Infectious Diseases*, 2004, 10:2244–2248.

25 SARS VACCINE
___DEVELOPMENT___

As emphasized in a resolution of the World Health Assembly in May 2003,[1] a safe, highly effective and affordable SARS vaccine would be an invaluable complement to other containment or therapeutic measures to prevent a future epidemic.

Several countries have made the development of SARS vaccines a high priority, and will soon evaluate how safe and immunogenic the most advanced candidate vaccines are in humans. However, several key scientific questions still need to be answered. These relate notably to the need to generate data on: the genetic diversity and evolution of the SARS coronavirus (SARS-CoV); the nature of protective immune responses (including the potential for antibodies to worsen disease); and the natural history of the disease. In addition, current animal models need to be standardized to provide more reliable results on the efficacy of candidate vaccines, specific regulatory and licensing issues need to be dealt with, and strategies should be thought out for the deployment of future SARS vaccines.[2]

This chapter provides a brief overview of the challenges to the development of a SARS vaccine.

GENETIC DIVERSITY AND EVOLUTION

If it is like other coronaviruses, SARS-CoV is prone to genetic variations through frequent mutations and can diversify and continuously evolve through RNA recombination.[3] With some coronavirus infections, selected escape mutations appearing under immune pressure can result in major shifts in pathogenicity and tissue specificity. Most SARS-CoV isolates from the 2002–2003 outbreak are largely conserved, but some recent results suggest that more genetically diverse strains of SARS-CoV do exist and can cause a SARS-like illness. In addition, genetically diverse SARS-CoV could emerge as a result of cross-species transmission of SARS-like viruses from wild animals. Genetic and biological changes in the SARS-CoV might pose a problem for the development of broadly protective SARS vaccines. It is therefore important to continue monitoring variations in the virus to ensure that candidate vaccines will protect against all SARS-CoV strains.[4]

RELIABLE ANIMAL MODELS

Reliable animal models will be essential to the development and preclinical evaluation of candidate SARS vaccines. Extensive research being done in this area shows that various animal species, including mice, cats, ferrets, civet cats, pigs, hamsters, chickens, as well as nonhuman primates (*Macaca fascicularis, Macaca mulata*), can be infected with the SARS-CoV. Each of these animal models can vary significantly in levels of viral replication, demonstrated pathological events and clinical evidence of illness. However, none of the animal models tested to date has been able to reproduce the development of the severe disease observed in humans.

In addition, there is an urgent need to further standardize these animal models, to allow for a more robust evaluation of both the safety and the efficacy of SARS candidate vaccines. Likewise, well-characterized reagents should be developed and made widely available for challenge experiments to facilitate a comparison of results obtained by different groups.[5]

CORRELATES OF PROTECTION

To accelerate vaccine development, the correlates of immune protection should be known; this is not the case with SARS. The results of animal experiments suggest that a neutralizing humoral response can protect against infection by the SARS-CoV, but it is likely that both humoral and cellular immune responses would help protect against disease progression or virus transmission. There is some preliminary evidence that the viral S protein could be one of the targets for neutralizing antibodies, while cellular immune responses could be induced by the viral nucleoprotein. However, further research is needed to determine the role of different immune mechanisms of protection against SARS. The experience with cat coronavirus vaccines highlights the need to be aware of potential immune-mediated enhancement of susceptibility to infection or disease in vaccines (immunopathogenesis), which poses an additional challenge for safety monitoring with various candidate vaccines.[6]

In the absence of definitive information on correlates of immune protection, different vaccination strategies are being developed in parallel to stimulate different effectors of immunity at either the systemic or the mucosal level. Among the vaccines being explored are nonreplicating immunogens (whole-inactivated virus and subunit recombinant vaccines) and candidate vaccines that can induce cellular immunity (live attenuated, vectored, and DNA vaccines). Both types of vaccines could also be used in different "prime-boost" combinations to induce broadly reactive immune responses. The front-line SARS vaccine research has focused on the development of whole-inactivated candidate vaccines. Several of these have reached advanced stages of preclinical development and are being considered for testing in human clinical trials (by Sinovac, China; Aventis Pasteur,

France; Baxter Healthcare, Austria; Chiron, Italy; and several others). Other candidate vaccines based on novel technologies like recombinant candidate proteins, plasmid DNA, and viral-vectored vaccines are also being developed.[7,8,9,10]

REGULATORY ASPECTS

From a regulatory point of view, all these vaccine candidates must meet the required standards for good manufacturing practice (GMP) production, to ensure safe and high-quality products. The scientific and ethical review of protocols and the conduct of clinical trials in humans will need special consideration. Finally, a major hurdle on the pathway to a licensed SARS vaccine might be the difficulty or even impossibility of studying vaccine efficacy in humans. Indeed, with SARS cases currently absent, vaccine efficacy cannot be assessed. On the other hand, should the virus re-emerge on a scale to allow such assessment, this might have to be made under the pressure of an emergency epidemic situation, perhaps greatly complicating the conduct of efficacy trials. The national regulatory authorities of countries wishing to license a SARS vaccine will therefore need to establish the bases on which they will make decisions about surrogates of efficacy in humans for future products submitted for their approval.

SUMMARY

There are several important challenges to the development of a safe and effective SARS vaccine. All these challenges will need to be addressed through intensive and close international collaboration.

REFERENCES

1   Resolution WHA56.29. Severe acute respiratory syndrome. Geneva, World Health Organization, 2003.
2   Kieny M-P, Esparza J. SARS and the public good. *SCRIPS Magazine*, 2003, June:26–27.
3   Domingo et al. *Molecular Basis of Virus Evolution.* Cambridge, University Press, 1995, 181–191.
4   WHO Expert Group Consultation on "Needs and Opportunities for SARS Vaccine Research and Development", 31 October – 1 November 2003. Geneva, World Health Organization (http://www.who.int/vaccine_research/ , accessed 1 April 2005).
5   Report of the WHO Consultation on "SARS Animal Models", 5–6 February 2004, Rotterdam. *Vaccine*, 2004 (in press).
6   Corapi WV, Olsen CW, Scott FW. Monoclonal antibody analysis of neutralization and antibody-dependent enhancement of feline infectious

peritonitis virus. *Journal of Virology*, 1992, 66:6695–6705.

[7] Cavanagh D. Severe acute respiratory syndrome vaccine development: experiences of vaccination against avian infectious bronchitis coronavirus. *Avian Pathology*, 2003, 32:567–582.

[8] Marshall E, Enserink M. Caution Urged on SARS Vaccines. *Science*, 2004, 303:944–946.

[9] Yang ZY et al. A DNA vaccine induses SARS coronavirus neutralization and protective immunity in mice. *Nature*, 2004, 428:561–564.

[10] Choy WY et al. Synthetic peptide studies on the severe acute respiratory syndrome (SARS) coronavirus spike glycoprotein: Perspective for SARS vaccine development. *Clinical Chemistry*, 2004, 50 (in press).

26 BIOSAFETY AND BIOCONTAINMENT ISSUES

Following the identification of SARS coronavirus (SARS-CoV), a novel and previously unrecognized human pathogen causing significant mortality, concerns began to be raised about the safe handling of clinical specimens associated with SARS, as well as about safety issues related to culturing the virus, to avoid laboratory-acquired infections. In response to these concerns, the World Health Organization (WHO) developed biosafety guidelines for the handling of SARS specimens in April 2003.[1]

The guidelines recommended that any activities that required virus culture or manipulations involving the growth or concentration of the virus should be carried out in biosafety level 3 (BSL3) facilities, and routine diagnostic procedures (such as testing of serum and blood samples for serology, clinical chemistry, and haematology, or manipulations involving neutralised or inactivated virus) should be conducted under BSL2. Any procedure that could generate an aerosol should be performed in a class 2 biological safety cabinet within a BSL3 laboratory, and the operator should wear protective equipment, including disposable gloves, solid-front or wrap-around gowns with cuffed sleeves, eye protection, and a surgical mask. If a procedure was performed outside a biological safety cabinet, it should only be done in a BSL3 laboratory and a full-face shield should be used.

No case of laboratory-acquired infection was reported during the outbreak.

BIOSAFETY IN THE POST-OUTBREAK PERIOD

Once the SARS outbreak was over in early July 2003, and human transmission had ceased, biocontainment of SARS-CoV became increasingly important. The only known sources of SARS-CoV, other than wildlife, were diagnostic or research laboratories. It was suspected that many clinical specimens might have been stored in diagnostic pathology laboratories, especially in countries that had had SARS cases, and stored under inappropriate containment conditions. The risks were possibly greater for clinical specimens sent to nonmicrobiological laboratories, such as haematology, clinical chemistry, and pathology laboratories. In addition, strains of SARS-CoV had been distributed to many research laboratories around the world, and in many instances there was no record of which laboratories had received the virus, or whether they had in turn passed the virus on to other laboratories. Thus, there was a growing unease that accidental laboratory-acquired infections might give rise to renewed epidemic activity.

These concerns appeared to be realized in September 2003 when a laboratory-acquired case of SARS was confirmed in Singapore in a 27-year-old research worker. The patient had been working on West Nile virus in a laboratory that had also been doing research on SARS-CoV. Fortunately, the case was relatively mild and did not give rise to secondary infections.[2,3] An international investigation into the case concluded that cross-contamination of West Nile virus samples with the SARS-CoV in the laboratory was the source of the infection, and both viruses were detected in a research specimen. How this accidental laboratory contamination occurred is not known. The investigation identified several inappropriate laboratory practices, and made a series of recommendations for their correction.[3] There was also some concern about whether the BSL3 laboratory in which the infection occurred complied with internationally accepted standards, such as those published by WHO,[4] or from the United States of America.[5] This event showed the need to train all workers employed at the BSL3 level, and the importance of facilities meeting accepted international biocontainment/biosafety standards.

Laboratory biosafety was a major topic of discussion at an informal SARS Laboratory Workshop in Geneva in October 2003.[6] The participants discussed a number of biosafety issues, including the biocontainment level for culturing SARS-CoV; working with the live virus; storing SARS-CoV cultures and clinical specimens; and the need for national inventories of SARS-CoV and for national certification of laboratories working with the virus.

The participants endorsed the WHO biosafety guidelines with respect to biosafety levels for culturing the virus (BSL3) and for diagnostic activities (BSL2, using BSL3 work practices). They recommended that SARS-CoV cultures be stored at least at BSL3, and that clinical specimens known or suspected to contain SARS-CoV be stored preferably at BSL3, or at a minimum in a locked freezer in a BSL2 facility. It was also recommended that national governments keep an inventory of laboratories working with or storing SARS-CoV, including clinical specimens.

The workshop's deliberations and recommendations were used in developing the post-outbreak biosafety guidelines for handling SARS-CoV specimens and cultures.[7]

Laboratory-acquired infections in China

A second laboratory-acquired infection with SARS-CoV occurred in Taipei in December 2003. A senior research worker became infected while attempting to decontaminate a safety cabinet in a BSL4 facility at the Institute of Preventative Medicine, National Defence University.[8] An international investigation concluded that poor laboratory practice was at fault. There was no further transmission. Once again, the need for good training in laboratory practice, at the BSL3/BSL4 levels, was brought out.

A third and potentially more serious event occurred between February and May 2004. The index case in the outbreak was a 26-year-old postgraduate medical student from Anhui Medical University who was working at the National Institute of Virology of China's Centre for Disease Control Beijing. She became ill in late March and transmitted the infection to seven others, one of whom, her mother, later died. A second postgraduate student working in the same laboratory also became infected but did not transmit the virus to anyone else. Thus, between late March and late April, there were nine cases of SARS, one death, and three generations of transmission.[9,10,11,12,13,14,15,16]

Subsequent investigations of staff working at the National Institute of Virology revealed two other cases of infection in February resulting in SARS-like illnesses among workers in the same laboratory.[17] The main cause of the outbreak was the transfer of an incompletely inactivated culture of SARS-CoV from the BSL3 laboratory into the laboratory where the infections had occurred.[17] There was also an additional concern that instances of SARS-like disease had occurred in laboratory workers and in hospitalized patients with a history of working in a facility in which SARS-CoV was being cultured, yet none of these individuals were tested for SARS-CoV infection until mid April 2004, three weeks after symptoms first occurred. Furthermore there was no monitoring of the health of staff in the Institute of Virology.

The lessons learnt from this outbreak included the need to ensure training of laboratory workers at the requisite biosafety levels, the need for good and safe laboratory practices, the need for monitoring the health of all research workers using cultures of live SARS-CoV or in contact with those so doing, and the importance of taking a proper patient history at the time of admission to hospital.

Biosafety and biocontainment of sars coronavirus

A new epidemic of SARS would most likely emerge from an animal reservoir or a laboratory doing research with live cultures of SARS-CoV or handling stored clinical specimens containing SARS-CoV. The risk of re-emergence from a laboratory source is thought to be potentially greater.[18,19] For this reason, WHO provided guidelines for the handling, packing, and shipping of SARS-CoV or specimens containing SARS-CoV, and clearly indicated the laboratory practices that required BSL3 facilities and those that could be done under BSL2 conditions.[1,7] The laboratory-acquired infections in Singapore, Taipei, and Beijing indicate that these guidelines have not been strictly followed and reaffirm the importance of strong national monitoring of their implementation.[20] In addition, WHO has recently published an extensively revised and expanded third edition of its *Laboratory Biosafety Manual*,[4] which significantly extends and supports the guidelines.

However, concerns have been raised about the current levels of containment and the lack of consistency found in different national biocontainment/biosafety manuals. Varying requirements are evident between guidelines for BSL3 laboratories for human and animal pathogens in the United States of America, and between the guidelines set out by the United States, the United Kingdom, Australia, Europe, Canada, and WHO. Many of the guidelines do not provide sufficient protection, such as against possible aerosol transmission in the event of an accidental breakage outside a biosafety cabinet within BSL3 containment. To circumvent these possible scenarios, a "BSL3 plus" standard is urgently needed to provide greater operator protection through personal air pressure respirators, negative pressure environment, HEPA filtration of exhaust air, and showers. To maintain strict biocontainment, it may also be necessary to chemically treat waste. To ensure conformity and the guideline enforcement, the International Organization for Standardization should develop a set of international standards for laboratory design, maintenance, and operator training at the different biosafety levels.

There are a number of crucial lessons from the SARS outbreak and from the subsequent laboratory-acquired infections with respect to biosafety and biocontainment.

- Personnel working in BSL2, BSL3 and BSL4 laboratories should be properly trained. No research staff should be permitted to work with agents under these conditions unless they have been fully trained and understand the work practices essential to these levels of biosafety, including the use of personal protective equipment.

- National biosafety levels for laboratories must, at a minimum, meet the standards required in the WHO *Laboratory Biosafety Manual, 3rd ed.*[4] An international agreement should be sought to develop standards for the building and maintenance of biologically secure laboratories, based on the currently accepted biosafety levels with additional safeguards to protect against accidental spillages, preferably through an independent organization such as the International Organization for Standardization.

- The health of all those working with SARS-CoV and others who may be in contact with them must be monitored so that laboratory infections can be detected at an early stage.

- BSL2, BSL3, and BSL4 facilities must be regularly maintained so they continue to operate effectively.
- Laboratory workers must strictly adhere to the WHO guidelines when working with live cultures of SARS-CoV or with animals infected with live SARS-CoV.

In addition to these lessons, WHO strongly encourages countries to undertake an inventory of laboratories holding SARS-CoV or clinical samples or material potentially containing SARS-CoV. These clinical samples and other infective materials must be stored appropriately and all work with these materials must be done at the correct containment level. The intention is not to restrict laboratories from working with SARS-CoV; indeed, the more work that is done, the greater our knowledge about this novel virus. Rather, it is hoped that a detailed up-to-date inventory will make a laboratory accident or escape of virus less likely. Countries are also urged to set national guidelines and standards for biosafety and biocontainment based on those described by WHO.[4]

Finally, it is important to emphasize the basic components of laboratory biosafety that ensure a safe workplace: facility design; laboratory practices; safety equipment; and medical surveillance. Each aspect must be addressed, especially medical surveillance, which is often overlooked.[21]

SUMMARY

Laboratory-acquired SARS infections, which were a theoretical concern during the outbreak, have become an actual risk in the post-outbreak period. Biocontainment and biosafety issues need to be properly addressed to ensure that SARS does not re-emerge from a laboratory-acquired infection. All countries should develop their own national guidelines for biosafety and biocontainment, compliant with those described in the Laboratory Biosafety Manual, 3rd ed., so that SARS-CoV and other dangerous pathogens remain contained. The lack of consistency in the national biocontainment and biosafety guidelines for design, building, maintenance, and operator training of BSL 1-4 laboratories needs to be addressed, and more stringent guidelines should be developed through the International Organization for Standardization.

References

1. *Biosafety guidelines for handling of SARS specimens.* Geneva, World Health Organization, 25 April 2003 (http://www.who.int/csr/sars/biosafety2003_04_25/en/, accessed 1 April 2005).

2. *Severe acute respiratory syndrome (SARS) in Singapore: an update.* Geneva, World Health Organization, 16 September 2003 (http://www.who.int/csr/don/2003_09_16/en/, accessed 1 April 2005)

3. *Severe acute respiratory syndrome (SARS) in Singapore, update 2.* Geneva, World Health Organization, 24 September 2003 (http://www.who.int/csr/don/2003_09_24/en/, accessed 1 April 2005).

4. *Laboratory Biosafety Manual, 3rd ed.* Geneva, World Health Organization 2004.

5. Centers for Disease Control and Prevention (CDC) and National Institutes of Health (NIH). *Biosafety in Microbiological and Biomedical Laboratories*, 4th ed., Washington, DC, US Government Printing Office, 1999.

6. Summary of the discussion and recommendations of the SARS Laboratory Workshop. Geneva, World Health Organization, 22 October 2003 (http://www.who.int/csr/sars/guidelines/en/SARSLabmeeting.pdf, accessed 1 April 2005).

7. *WHO post-outbreak biosafety guidelines for handling of SARS-CoV specimens and cultures.* Geneva, World Health Organization, 18 December 2003 (http://www.who.int/csr/sars/biosafety2003_12_18/en/, accessed 1 April 2005).

8. *Severe acute respiratory syndrome (SARS) in Taiwan, China.* Geneva, World Health Organization, 17 December 2003 (http://www.who.int/csr/don/2003_12_17/en/, accessed 1 April 2005).

9. *SARS: one suspected case reported in China.* Geneva, World Health Organization, 22 April 2004 (http://www.who.int/csr/don/2004_04_22/en/, accessed 1 April 2005).

10. *China reports additional SARS cases, update.* Geneva, World Health Organization, 23 April 2004 (http://www.who.int/csr/don/2004_04_23/en/, accessed 1 April 2005).

11. *Additional patients in China under investigation for SARS: WHO team travels to Beijing, update 2.* Geneva, World Health Organization, 26 April 2004. (http://www.who.int/csr/don/2004_04_26/en/, accessed 1 April 2005).

12. *China reports additional SARS case, update 3.* Geneva, World Health Organization, 28 April 2004 (http://www.who.int/csr/don/2004_04_28/en/, accessed 1 April 2005).

13. *China confirms SARS infection in two previously reported cases, update 4.* Geneva, World Health Organization, 29 April 2004 (http://www.who.int/csr/don/2004_04_29/en/, accessed 1 April 2005).

[14] *China confirms SARS infection in another previously reported case: summary of cases to date, update 5.* Geneva, World Health Organization, 30 April 2004 (http://www.who.int/csr/don/2004_04_30/en/, accessed 1 April 2005).

[15] *SARS in China: investigation continues, update 6.* Geneva, World Health Organization, 5 May 2004 (http://www.who.int/csr/don/2004_05_05/en/, accessed 1 April 2005)

[16] *China's latest SARS outbreak has been contained, but biosafety concerns remain, update 7.* Geneva, World Health Organization, 18 May 2004 (http://www.who.int/csr/don/2004_05_18a/en/, accessed 1 April 2005).

[17] *Investigation into China's recent SARS outbreak yields important lessons for global public health.* Manila, World Health Organization, 2 July 2004 (http://www.wpro.who.int/sars/docs/update/update_07022004.asp, accessed 1 April 2005).

[18] Mackenzie JS et al. The WHO response to SARS and preparations for the future. In: Knobler S et al., eds. *Learning from SARS: preparing for the next disease outbreak*, Washington, DC, The Institute of Medicine National Academy Press, 2004:42–50.

[19] Olowokure B et al. The laboratory containment of dangerous pathogens: the lessons learnt from severe acute respiratory syndrome (SARS) [submitted for publication].

[20] Heymann, DL, Aylward RB, Wolff C. Dangerous pathogens in the laboratory: from smallpox to today's SARS setbacks and tomorrow's polio-free world. *Lancet*, 2004, 363:1566–1568.

[21] *Keeping the 'Genome' in the Bottle: Reinforcing Biosafety Level 3 Procedures.* Atlanta, GA, Centers for Disease Control and Prevention, Public Health Training Network Webcast, 17 June 2004 (http://www.phppo.cdc.gov/PHTN/bsl3/, accessed on 1 April 2005).

PART V: THE FUTURE

27 WHAT DID WE _LEARN FROM SARS?_

"History teaches us that men and nations behave wisely once they have exhausted all other alternatives."
- Abba Eban, Israeli Minister of Foreign Affairs, 1966–1974

With the SARS virus contained, we can now look back at the 2003 global epidemic through the rosy spectacles of hindsight and congratulate ourselves on a major public-health success. Self-congratulation, however, is unbecoming, and often based on selective memory. But the nations affected by SARS certainly deserve recognition for their efforts to control a frightening and obstinate new disease. Their international partners can, in general, be proud of the way they worked together with the affected countries. The efforts recalled here deserve to be remembered and recorded, either because they were effective and led to the end of the outbreaks or because they were ineffective or inefficient. We recall as well some of the administrative, organizational, and institutional factors that may have helped or hindered the success of the control operations.

LESSON 1: WE WERE LUCKY THIS TIME

The SARS virus could have become a constant threat to human health in the world we live in. It did not. Thanks to the intense and skilful efforts of the governments of all affected areas, together with their regional and international partners, the virus was contained.

Certain characteristics of the SARS virus made containment possible. Infected individuals usually did not transmit the virus until several days after symptoms began and were most infectious only by the tenth day or so of illness, when they develop severe symptoms. Therefore, effective isolation of patients was enough to control spread. If cases were infectious before symptoms appeared, or if asymptomatic cases transmitted the virus, the disease would have been much more difficult, perhaps even impossible, to control.

The chains of transmission could be broken at various points. The incubation period was relatively long (two to 10 days, with a median of five days), giving more time for contacts to be traced and isolated before they fell ill and became infectious themselves. The incubation period also dictated how long contacts had to be supervised. If the incubation period were longer, observation or quarantine would have been much more difficult to manage.

SARS being largely an urban disease, concentrated in relatively well-equipped hospitals, it was easier to detect cases and trace contacts, isolate patients, limit infection, and therefore control the spread of the disease. Reporting was also more reliable.

Still, many questions remain. Why did the outbreaks stop so abruptly in Viet Nam after such an explosive start? There is no doubt that the strict application of infection-control measures was critical, but they were far from perfect. In particular, several patients were transferred from the Hanoi-French Hospital to Bac Mai Hospital at a stage of their illness when transmission should have been very likely. But despite the potentially serious lapses, there were no new cases. Apparently many SARS cases were simply not very infectious.

Why did the Philippines not have a huge epidemic? Certainly, case investigation was done well, and contract tracing was exemplary, thanks to the energy of the Secretary of Health and to the expert work of the field epidemiologists. But, again, things were not perfect. Isolation of patients and contacts was less than ideal. And thousands of overseas workers returned to celebrate the Holy Week before Easter from Hong Kong (China) and other countries where the virus was still spreading. Only one from Canada brought the infection back with them.

Using the research data that have accumulated since the human epidemics stopped, the epidemiology of those situations and others like them should be re-examined. There are certainly better explanations than "good luck". There is certainly still much that we do not understand about this disease.

LESSON 2: TRANSPARENCY IS THE BEST POLICY

In this globalized age, the world community expects accurate, complete, and timely information about diseases that do not respect international borders. Within countries, as modern communications technology makes people better informed and more sophisticated, they expect their governments to provide transparent, up-to-date information about communicable diseases that may threaten their communities. Governments will be held accountable, both internationally and nationally, for failures in conveying straightforward, reliable information.

Some of the affected countries did not acknowledge openly and squarely the presence of SARS, downplayed its extent, and attempted to prove that it was something else. Delays in acknowledging the presence of the disease contributed to a general mistrust of public health information. In China, for example, the severe respiratory infection eventually known as SARS was allowed to spread unreported in the southern province of Guangdong for at least three months, from November 2002, before its existence was even acknowledged. When the disease broke out in Guangzhou City, hospitals were caught unprepared, as others were in subsequent outbreaks in Beijing, Inner Mongolia and Shanxi. Inadequate infection-control measures amplified the outbreak, which eventually spread to Hong Kong, where the international airport is one of the busiest in the world. Hong Kong's hospitals were infected, and the disease was carried by travellers to Toronto, Singapore, Hanoi, and eventually around the world.

As local medical and public-health staff battled heroically with the virus, they learnt important lessons about its epidemiology and infectivity, occupational risk factors, and infection control in hospitals. If shared earlier, these lessons would have been invaluable to other countries as the virus reached their shores.

LESSON 3: PUBLIC HEALTH IS A SERIOUS BUSINESS

In a globalized world, where people and products travel vast distances virtually in an instant, threats to health, whether real or imagined, can be economically disastrous. The economic devastation wreaked by SARS is well documented. Billions of dollars were lost by countries ill prepared for such losses, particularly in the tourism, hospitality, and transport industries. A clearly reasoned, well-planned, and effectively managed and publicized response to such threats is important in mitigating the damage to the economy, and to public confidence in government.

Here Singapore set a very positive example. When the epidemic emerged in this island state, the Government had to make difficult policy decisions. Would its officials be content with hoping that SARS would burn itself out quickly and not need stringent measures that would certainly result in accusations of human-rights violations, extreme expenditures of public money, and a weakened economy? Or would they take the strong measures needed to contain this threat to public health? The officials chose to act and stop the spread of the disease. The unprecedented public-health effort, which included a well-planned campaign to enlist the commitment of the public, was a 21st-century model for epidemic control.

SARS also showed the importance of committing enough resources right from the start. Massive resources went to controlling the outbreaks almost as soon as they appeared, although in the view of some people, the relatively few cases and deaths, compared with those from other public-health challenges such as tuberculosis, hardly justified the level of spending. In retrospect, spending to get rid of the new public-health threat was infinitely more cost-effective than having to apply resources continuously over time to control the disease. No further outbreaks occurred, neither in the winter of 2003–2004 nor in the next one. If SARS had become endemic, the resources required to root it out would have been enormous, especially in the winter months, and the impact on the health system would have been incalculable.

Speaking for many others in the Region, a senior Chinese expert privately referred to SARS as "the best thing that has ever happened to public health in China". The public-health bureaucracy, under one of the most able ministers in the Government, has gained a new standing. Relations between the provinces and the centre have greatly improved. Reporting systems have been updated and streamlined, and important information usually flows regularly and with dispatch. Epidemiological services have never been better. Public-health workers, proud to be part of this high-profile and now clearly successful effort, are seen as the heroes they often are.

LESSON 4: HUMAN-RIGHTS ISSUES MUST BE ATTENDED TO

In Hong Kong, Taipei, and Singapore, stopping the spread of SARS meant taking drastic measures. Privacy issues and human rights were hotly debated. If the governments involved had not acted decisively, however, the virus could have spread further and become endemic. The experience suggests that there should be international standards for the carefully considered use of countermeasures against dangerous communicable diseases, such as accessing police databases and imposing quarantine. Community surveillance, for example, may be effective, but could infringe on personal freedoms if used inappropriately.

LESSON 5: THE MEDIA PLAY A CRITICAL ROLE IN PUBLIC-HEALTH EMERGENCIES

Perhaps never before in history had the media been so involved in a public-health emergency. At the height of the epidemics, the world was deluged daily with more than 4,000 articles in English alone. Until then, only the war in Iraq had generated more headlines. Predictably, the reporting was uneven in quality. The media were sometimes accused of overstating the epidemics, causing panic and therefore serious economic damage to affected countries. While this accusation may be partly true, overall the media were in fact important allies of the health workers. They generally behaved responsibly and insisted on accurate statistics, precise scientific descriptions, and expert opinions.

As the epidemics progressed, government public-health programmes made current, complete, factual information available to dispel misunderstanding and panic. They received support from WHO, which took the importance of the media to heart, to an extent previously unheard of. The Headquarters in Geneva assigned skilful media officers. At the Regional Office in Manila, an experienced and highly able press officer, newly appointed, collaborated with the technical staff in fielding hundreds of telephone calls daily, appearing on radio and television, and releasing information regularly to the press. In Beijing and Hong Kong, the most badly affected cities, WHO press officers relieved the country office of media demands that threatened to overwhelm it. WHO Representatives in Viet Nam, China, and the Philippines dealt with the media most effectively. Much of the interest came from within Asia—from Hong Kong and other parts of the region where representatives of major international media organizations were based. The Regional Office had never been so challenged.

The efforts were fortunately well received by the media. Despite the general taste in the media for institution bashing, the Organization got surprisingly little bad press. A senior reporter for an international newspaper remarked that he had never seen an international organization—or group of countries—be so forthright with the press. For that reason, he said, unfair attacks were highly unlikely.

On the other hand, besides the regular briefings, more proactive, systematic, and thoughtful dealings with the press and the general public might have resulted in a better-informed public and less panic.

For the partnership between WHO and the media to be most productive, much more needs to be done, as the events of 2005—avian flu and the health effects of the Indian Ocean earthquakes and tsunamis—suggest. The Organization should give this matter continued serious attention.

LESSON 6: 21ST CENTURY SCIENCE PLAYED A RELATIVELY SMALL ROLE IN CONTROLLING SARS; 19TH-CENTURY TECHNIQUES CONTINUED TO PROVE THEIR VALUE

While modern science had its role, none of the most modern technical tools had an important role in controlling SARS. Sequencing the genetic code of the virus, for example, helped identify the origin and spread of the virus but did not really help to control it. Even identifying the virus itself added nothing substantial to control efforts, particularly since diagnostic tests were severely limited. But laboratory tests were helpful in confirming SARS infections, especially in clinically atypical cases.

Most important in controlling SARS were the 19th-century public-health strategies of contact tracing, quarantine, and isolation.

LESSON 7: PARTNERSHIPS WORKED, BUT THE PARTNERS NEED TO CLARIFY AND AGREE ON THEIR RELATIVE ROLES

Possibly the greatest triumph from the SARS experience was how fiercely and well national governments, international public health institutions, donor agencies, and other bodies (including the media) laboured together for six months to control the outbreaks.

Governments. Within countries the ministry of health usually took the lead. But the higher levels of government always stayed deeply involved to ensure a multisectoral response. The foreign affairs, agriculture, home affairs, transport, and other ministries all looked forward to a speedy end to the epidemics. The collaboration had perhaps the most dramatic effect in China when the Government finally decided to wage an all-out war against SARS. A highly effective monitoring and reporting system materialized almost at once, a community-based surveillance and disease-control system was installed, and, most amazingly, a 1,000-bed isolation hospital went up in little more than a week. In Singapore, Senior Minister Lee Kwan Yew, whose wife was quarantined after possibly being exposed to SARS in the outpatient unit of a hospital, gave an extraordinary talk to the nation. The galvanizing effect of this "fireside chat" by a greatly respected leader can hardly be overestimated. And airport authorities collaborated admirably in screening departing and arriving passengers, even if not many cases were detected or prevented that way.

Inter-governmental associations. ASEAN+3 arranged meetings on subjects ranging from case detection to airport measures among senior political figures and heads of national bureaucracies. Although hastily planned and organized, these meetings helped enlist high-level commitment, collaboration, and support. But given the difficulty and expense of organizing such meetings, perhaps more could have been accomplished. A general plan could be developed for meetings of this type, stressing the priorities and the need to recommend practicable forms of cooperation. Before a communicable disease emergency occurs, potential roles could be considered for the inter-country mechanisms of countries in the Region, based on their comparative strengths, and plans of action might be drawn up and tested in simulated conditions.

Government collaboration with international agencies. An impressive amount of goodwill surfaced during the SARS outbreaks. By and large, government agencies set rivalries aside; governments were forgiving of minor incidents of high-handedness by foreign consultants and agencies; and friendly, productive channels of information were maintained throughout. Clearly, in outbreaks within their sovereign territory national governments must be in the driver's seat. In all the affected countries in Asia the governments expected WHO, the most prominent international partner of the ministry of public health, to take the lead in coordinating external inputs. This seems to have worked well in most cases. The Director of the United States Centers for Disease Control and Prevention, for one, announced several times that her agency would work with governments through WHO. If WHO's Member States agree that this system was indeed effective and should be a model for future actions of this sort, they should draw up a resolution that clearly says so.

Conduct and protection of international staff. International staff and consultants contributed expertise and energy in all the affected countries. In general, they behaved with admirable professionalism and in genuine collegiality with their national hosts. But in a very few cases, complaints of "data smuggling" and withholding of information in hopes of early publication were heard. Some complaints may have been prompted by distrust of "neo-colonial" approaches; others may have had at least some basis in fact. It must be emphasized that consultants and other foreign experts work in foreign countries only at the invitation of the governments and with their support.

Soon after the outbreaks made the news, it became impossible to arrange transport home or to regional medical centres for individuals who may have been infected. Even the international medical "rescue" agencies refused to transfer these people to isolation and care facilities. The issue of insurance and liability for consultants on short-term contracts was never fully resolved. In anticipation of future outbreaks of communicable diseases, these issues should be discussed and approaches agreed upon, to protect the individuals involved as well as the agencies coordinating the investigation and management of epidemics.

Lesson 8: Modern modes of communication dramatically changed the way we work

The use of modern methods of electronic communication to control a major disease outbreak was perhaps without precedent in the history of public health. WHO Headquarters and the Regional Office in Manila communicated by telephone dozens of times a day from the very first days of the epidemics, often several times in a single hour. The result was constantly updated information and synchronized reporting.

A Singaporean physician who had treated his country's first cases of SARS and then attended a medical conference in the United States of America became feverish while flying from New York to Singapore, via Europe. On his way, he called a friend in Singapore to say that he was ill. The friend at once phoned the Health Ministry, and the senior epidemiologist at the ministry relayed the information by phone to the Communicable Diseases Director at the WHO Regional Office in Manila. A call from the Director to Geneva roused an officer of the Emergency Response office in the middle of the night. He alerted German public health authorities and officials at the Frankfurt airport. Barrier infection-control equipment was rushed to the airport, and the physician and his family, as soon as their plane landed, were whisked off to an isolation facility. As a result, although the Singaporean physician, his wife, his mother-in-law, and a flight attendant were confirmed to have SARS, they eventually recovered fully and returned to Singapore. (The German physician who supervised their successful treatment later helped treat Dr Carlo Urbani of WHO. Despite expert care, however, Dr Urbani died of the disease he had first characterized.)

The multiparty teleconference connected many participants at different sites through office telephones, mobile phones, and specially designed multi-microphone telephones in conference rooms. At the Regional Office, teleconferences constantly under way, it seemed, in the operations room, took up much of the working day. A nightly teleconference at 10 p.m., Manila time, and usually lasting well over an hour, involved the Director-General and her staff in Geneva; regional offices in Manila, New Delhi, Cairo, Harare, and Washington, DC; WHO country offices in Beijing, Hanoi, Bangkok, and Kuala Lumpur; and consultants in Singapore and Hong Kong. There were often up to 50 participants. As the outbreaks waned, these mega-conferences became less frequent, taking place on weekends only when needed, and eventually happening only twice or thrice weekly.

The conferences lacked focus. While some participants were being briefed on the global outbreak, others were dealing with minute details. Inevitably, some participants took the opportunity to promote themselves; others were daunted by the high level of participation. It was an inefficient way to synchronize figures—case and death totals, for example—and the variety of participants, which included journalists in some offices, made politically sensitive discussion (such as negative remarks about government actions) risky. As the focus and usefulness of the conference became less and less clear, participants in the Manila office, who had generally been working continuously for 16 hours before then, began to show the strain and to participate with much less enthusiasm. Such conferences must be expertly planned in the future.

Videoconferences were held intermittently during the outbreaks. The conferences, at which key government figures and WHO officials sat arrayed before flags or emblems and addressed speeches to one another, were time-consuming; had to be held in a specially fitted room, away from the scene of action; were prone to technical disruptions; and served little purpose other than the political benefits that might accrue from participants being able to see one another face to face.

The Internet proved its public-health worth during the outbreaks. Email reached such a huge volume (upwards of 400 messages a day for key staff) that it could not be relied on to transmit breaking news—the telephone was better suited for that. But email was ideal for sending figures, documents, reports, guidelines, training presentations, tables, graphs and photos instantly, and was used fully for that purpose. Ground rules should be established for the use of email in future outbreaks.

The Canada-based Global Public Health Intelligence Network (GPHIN) has shown how the Internet can be used more creatively, and much can be learned from their experience [see Chapter 2].

LESSON 9: CLEAR TRAVEL GUIDANCE IS NEEDED

In the handling of the SARS outbreaks, this aspect was possibly the most controversial. The effect of the travel advisories on the overall global epidemic cannot be ascertained. WHO was accused of overplaying the danger of the epidemics, and of thereby being partly to blame for their economic severity.

Others questioned whether WHO even had a mandate for such drastic action. It must be remembered that the world was confronted with a highly infectious, frequently fatal disease for which the cause was not known, the modes of transmission were not understood, and no effective treatment was available. Health-care workers were disproportionately affected, and the virus was seen to spread by international travel. Its emergence had been sudden and explosive, and for a while at least it seemed as if the world was coming to an end.

WHO, in fact, was reluctant to recommend travel restrictions. When it did take this step for the first time, many countries had already asked their citizens to avoid non-crucial travel to affected areas, or had recommended even broader restrictions. Some had criticized what they saw to be WHO's timid reluctance to act decisively. But the WHO advisories, once issued, were taken very seriously, perhaps even more so than those of the United States. The Organization's mandate to take a similar step in the future must be made absolutely clear. Hopefully, the revised International Health Regulations will define the circumstances where such action is warranted, and the steps that should be taken before a firm recommendation is made to avoid certain destinations.

LESSON 10: ANIMAL HUSBANDRY AND MARKETING PRACTICES SERIOUSLY AFFECT HUMAN HEALTH

The SARS outbreaks, particularly in southern China, exposed shocking but all too common practices in the exotic food trade. Although it is still unclear how wild animals destined for human consumption help spread SARS, the ways in which they are handled, marketed, and slaughtered pose obvious dangers to human health. Good veterinary habits are rare in markets where live animals are sold for the table. Aside from the question of cruelty in handling and slaughtering, animals that would never meet in the wild are kept close to one another, often in stacked cages, raising the risk of cross-infection and the emergence of new pathogens potentially dangerous to man.

If the practice is to continue—and it will certainly be difficult to eradicate, or even make less prevalent, given increasing affluence in the region and the taste for exotic dishes—measures should be implemented for the least dangerous methods of provision of these exotic species for human consumption.

For domestic animals and poultry, the very close proximity of animal pens and cages to human habitation in many crowded settlements would also appear to make zoonotic infections more likely. This issue is especially relevant to the current H5N1 situation.

LESSON 11: WHO SHOULD BE ON THE FRONT LINES?

WHO was effective as the prime partner of national ministries of health, worldwide, in the region, and in the individual affected countries. The Organization not only helped with policy development and coordination, but also reassigned its own staff, redefined their terms of reference, provided emergency supplies and equipment, and fielded expert consultants. However, the question remains: Is WHO the most appropriate organization to plan and implement such activities in the field? Could the Organization take on this role again, in an emergency perhaps more complex? Earlier in its history, WHO had provided Member States with a wide range of field workers: epidemiologists, laboratory technologists, sanitarians, clinicians, and nurses, among other specialists. WHO country teams were large, young, and mobile. However, demands on the Organization have changed over the years. Member States today seldom request WHO staff to directly implement or participate in disease control operations. Staff numbers in country offices have shrunk, and the functions of WHO country teams have leaned more towards health planning, standards setting, research, high-level consultation, and policy formulation.

It surprised many that WHO could change its methods. Now, all of a sudden, WHO had created a "war room" coordinating function at headquarters and regional offices, and was sending staff to the field to investigate the outbreaks and implement control measures. Others wondered how the Organization could enlist overnight the participation of hundreds of consultants and dozens of partner agencies. WHO identified effective field workers and appropriate agencies through personal contacts, and innovatively reprogrammed available funds. Donor governments responded quickly and generously.

This time the arrangement worked. Can it work in an outbreak that might be more complex and prolonged? If WHO is to take on this responsibility in the future, it must clarify the roles of partner agencies and identify potentially available experts of proven worth. To act quickly, it should be able to mobilize resources rapidly and access stockpiles of supplies and equipment. Networks like GOARN can provide high-quality laboratory support and short-term expertise at very short notice, but a longer-term situation will require months or more of continued support from large numbers of people.

LESSON 12: WITH NATIONAL DISEASE SURVEILLANCE SYSTEMS IN DISREPAIR, INFORMAL AVENUES OF REPORTING MUST BE TAKEN SERIOUSLY

The SARS outbreaks revealed how ineffective disease surveillance and outbreak alert systems are in most countries, apart from the wealthier ones. Even where surveillance systems are well developed, they seldom function adequately as "early warning systems" because of inherent bureaucratic delays and insufficient collaboration among response agencies. Specifically, in most countries, information exchange, joint analysis, and monitoring do not take place between health care facilities (especially private ones) and the public health authority. As a result, "informal" reports have become crucial in identifying and monitoring outbreaks.

Ubiquitous mobile telephones and text messaging, mushrooming Internet cafés, newspaper websites, email and "blogs" with their instant information and opinions—these informal channels are much more likely to report unusual disease events first, long before government releases do. Without official information and analysis, rumours can spiral out of control, spreading fear and panic. Governments must become better able to collect credible information and report it early. They must replan their disease surveillance systems, assign them to adequately trained people, and supervise their operation.

Lesson 13: Training and expertise in barrier nursing and hospital infection control are sadly deficient in the region

This important topic deserves separate mention. Unlike other expertise needed to deal with SARS, infection-control practices were poorly developed in many countries of the region. Support staff and administrative personnel, and even nursing and medical professionals, knew little about how to protect themselves from contagious diseases. Outside the capitals, isolation procedures were quite primitive. There was little understanding of personal protection measures and patient rooms set up to limit air- and fomite-borne spread. Most hospitals lacked even the most basic equipment. The "developed" countries of the region had the expertise, but could transfer it only with difficulty to hospitals where conditions were less than ideal. Now national authorities, with the help of WHO and other agencies, are well placed to establish or strengthen training in infection control for physicians and nurses.

Conclusion

The SARS epidemics of 2003 showed what countries with limited resources, in collaboration with international partners, are capable of doing to limit outbreaks of disease. In many ways, the odds were stacked on the side of success. The virus itself was amenable to control, and the potential economic impact of a serious disease spread by international travel was such that governmental commitment was guaranteed. One would hope that such commitment, both by national governments and the international community, could be enlisted in support of less dramatic events, with less immediate economic importance, posing less of a threat to privileged citizens of industrialized countries. Many examples of inadequate commitment can be cited: the African malaria situation, or the global tuberculosis problem, or even localized but devastating conditions such as Ebola or Marburg virus.

The SARS experience has not been examined critically enough, and the lessons learnt have not been thoroughly analysed. It is repugnant to think of the SARS outbreaks, which killed nearly 800 human beings, as a "dry run" for the next major, perhaps even more deadly, outbreak. But it would be tragic if we did not learn from the experience of 2003 and make the most of it. We would not be fulfilling our responsibilities to those, including our medical colleagues and friends, who died of SARS.

APPENDICES

APPENDIX 1:

WHO ISSUES A GLOBAL ALERT

ABOUT CASES OF ATYPICAL

PNEUMONIA

CASES OF SEVERE RESPIRATORY ILLNESS MAY SPREAD TO HOSPITAL STAFF

12 March 2003 | GENEVA – Since mid-February, WHO has been actively working to confirm reports of outbreaks of a severe form of pneumonia in Viet Nam, Hong Kong (China), and Guangdong Province in China.

In Viet Nam the outbreak began with a single initial case who was hospitalized for treatment of severe, acute respiratory syndrome of unknown origin. He felt unwell during his journey and fell ill shortly after arrival in Hanoi from Shanghai and Hong Kong. Following his admission to the hospital, approximately 20 hospital staff became sick with similar symptoms.

The signs and symptoms of the disease in Hanoi include initial flu-like illness (rapid onset of high fever followed by muscle aches, headache and sore throat). These are the most common symptoms. Early laboratory findings may include thrombocytopenia (low platelet count) and leucopenia (low white blood cell count). In some, but not all cases, this is followed by bilateral pneumonia, in some cases progressing to acute respiratory distress requiring assisted breathing on a respirator. Some patients are recovering but some patients remain critically ill.

Today, the Department of Health Hong Kong has reported on an outbreak of respiratory illness in one of its public hospitals. As of midnight 11 March, 50 health-care workers had been screened and 23 of them were found to have febrile illness. They were admitted to the hospital for observation as a precautionary measure. In this group, eight have developed early chest X-ray signs of pneumonia. Their conditions are stable. Three other health-care workers self-presented to hospitals with febrile illness and two of them have chest X-ray signs of pneumonia.

Investigation by Hong Kong public-health authorities is ongoing. The Hospital Authority has increased infection-control measures to prevent the spread of the disease in the hospital. So far, no link has been found between these cases and the outbreak in Hanoi.

In mid-February, the Government of China reported that 305 cases of atypical pneumonia, with five deaths, had occurred in Guangdong Province. In two cases that died, *Chlamydia* infection was found. Further investigations of the cause of the outbreak are ongoing. Overall the outbreaks in Hanoi and Hong Kong appear to be confined to the hospital environment. Those at highest risk appear to be staff caring for the patients.

No link has so far been made between these outbreaks of acute respiratory illness in Hanoi and Hong Kong and the outbreak of 'bird flu', A(H5N1) in Hong Kong reported on 19 February. Further investigations continue and laboratory tests on specimens from Viet Nam and Hong Kong are being studied by WHO collaborating centres in Japan and the United States of America.

Until more is known about the cause of these outbreaks, WHO recommends patients with atypical pneumonia who may be related to these outbreaks be isolated with barrier nursing techniques. At the same time, WHO recommends that any suspect cases be reported to national health authorities.

WHO is in close contact with relevant national authorities and has also offered epidemiological, laboratory and clinical support. WHO is working with national authorities to ensure appropriate investigation, reporting and containment of these outbreaks.

APPENDIX 2:

WHO ISSUES EMERGENCY TRAVEL ADVISORY

15 March 2003 | **GENEVA** – During the past week, WHO has received reports of more than 150 new suspected cases of severe acute respiratory syndrome (SARS), an atypical pneumonia for which cause has not yet been determined. Reports to date have been received from Canada, China, Hong Kong (China), Indonesia, the Philippines, Singapore, Thailand, and Viet Nam. Early today, an ill passenger and companions who travelled from New York, United States of America, and who landed in Frankfurt, Germany, were removed from their flight and taken to hospital isolation.

Due to the spread of SARS to several countries in a short period of time, the World Health Organization today has issued emergency guidance for travellers and airlines.

"This syndrome, SARS, is now a worldwide health threat," said Dr Gro Harlem Brundtland, Director-General of the World Health Organization. "The world needs to work together to find its cause, cure the sick, and stop its spread."

There is presently no recommendation for people to restrict travel to any destination. However, in response to enquiries from governments, airlines, physicians, and travellers, WHO is now offering guidance for travellers, airline crew, and airlines. The exact nature of the infection is still under investigation and this guidance is based on the early information available to WHO.

TRAVELLERS INCLUDING AIRLINE CREW: All travellers should be aware of main symptoms and signs of SARS, which include:

- high fever (>38 ºC)

    AND

- one or more respiratory symptom including cough, shortness of breath, difficulty breathing

AND one or more of the following:

- close contact* with a person who has been diagnosed with SARS
- recent history of travel to areas reporting cases of SARS.

In the unlikely event of a traveller experiencing this combination of symptoms they should seek medical attention and ensure that information about their recent travel is passed on to the health-care staff. Any traveller who develops these symptoms is advised not to undertake further travel until they have recovered.

AIRLINES: Should a passenger or crewmember who meets the criteria above travel on a flight, the aircraft should alert the destination airport. On arrival the sick passenger should be referred to airport health authorities for assessment and management. The aircraft passengers and crew should be informed of the person's status as a suspect case of SARS. The passengers and crew should provide all contact details for the subsequent 14 days to the airport health authorities. There are currently no indications to restrict the onward travel of healthy passengers, but all passengers and crew should be advised to seek medical attention if they develop the symptoms highlighted above. There is currently no indication to provide passengers and crew with any medication or investigation unless they become ill.

In the absence of specific information regarding the nature of the organism causing this illness, specific measures to be applied to the aircraft cannot be recommended. As a general precaution the aircraft may be disinfected in the manner described in the *WHO Guide to Hygiene and Sanitation in Aviation*.

* * *

As more information has become available, WHO-recommended SARS case definitions have been revised as follows:

SUSPECT CASE

A person presenting after 1 February 2003 with history of:

- high fever (>38 ºC)

AND

- one or more respiratory symptom including cough, shortness of breath, difficulty breathing
- close contact* with a person who has been diagnosed with SARS
- recent history of travel to areas reporting cases of SARS.

---

* Close contact means having cared for, having lived with, or having had direct contact with respiratory secretions and body fluids of a person with SARS.

PROBABLE CASE

A suspect case with chest X-ray findings of pneumonia or Respiratory Distress Syndrome

OR

A person with an unexplained respiratory illness resulting in death, with an autopsy examination demonstrating the pathology of Respiratory Distress Syndrome without an identifiable cause

COMMENTS

In addition to fever and respiratory symptoms, SARS may be associated with other symptoms including: headache, muscular stiffness, loss of appetite, malaise, confusion, rash, and diarrhoea.

* * *

Until more is known about the cause of these outbreaks, WHO recommends that patients with SARS be isolated with barrier nursing techniques and treated as clinically indicated. At the same time, WHO recommends that any suspect cases be reported to national health authorities.

WHO is in close communication with all national authorities and has also offered epidemiological, laboratory and clinical support. WHO is working with national authorities to ensure appropriate investigation, reporting, and containment of these outbreaks.

APPENDIX 3:

AFFECTED AREAS AND PATTERNS

OF LOCAL TRANSMISSION

From 16 March 2003, WHO reported on "affected areas" defined as a region at the first administrative level where the country is reporting local transmission of SARS.

From 12 April, some of the affected areas were identified as lower risk if they had "limited local transmission **and** no evidence of international spread from area since 15 March 2003 **and** no transmission other than close person-to-person contact reported."

From 28 April, the definion of "affected area" was changed to "a region at the first administrative level where the country is reporting local transmission of SARS, within the last 20 days, or two maximum incubation periods."

From 2 May, WHO replaced "affected areas" with "countries with recent local transmission" using this definition: "Recent local transmission has occurred when, in the last 20 days, one or more reported probable cases of SARS have most likely acquired their infection locally regardless of the setting in which this may have occurred." In addition, the extent of local transmission was categorized:

+ Low	++ Medium	+++ High	Uncertain
Imported probable SARS case(s) have produced only one generation of local probable cases, all of whom are direct personal contacts of the imported case(s).	More than one generation of local probable SARS cases, but only among persons that have been previously identified and followed-up as known contacts of probable SARS cases.	High Transmission pattern other than that described in + and ++.	Insufficient information available to specify areas or extent of local transmission.

From 8 May, the definition of +++ (High) transmission pattern was "local probable cases occurring among persons who have not been previously identified as known contacts of probable SARS cases."

From 10 May, a new definition was used: "Local transmission has occurred when one or more reported probable cases of SARS have most likely acquired their infection locally regardless of the setting in which this may have occurred. If no new locally acquired cases are identified 20 days after the last reported locally acquired probable case died or was appropriately isolated, the area will be removed from this list."

The names of the three patterns of spread were changed. Pattern A, B, and C replaced + Low, ++ Medium, and +++ High, but the definitions stayed the same (i.e. the definion for pattern A was the same as had been used for +, etc.)

Table 1. Areas that experienced local transmission of SARS [a,b,c]

Country	Area	From[d]	To[e]
Viet Nam	Hanoi	23 Feb 03	27 Apr 03
Mongolia	Ulaanbaatar	5 Apr 03	9 May 03
Philippines	Manila	6 Apr 03	19 May 03
China	Jiangsu	19 Apr 03	21 May 03
China	Hubei	17 Apr 03	26 May 03
China	Tianjin	16 Apr 03	28 May 03
China	Jilin	1 Apr 03	29 May 03
China	Shaanxi	12 Apr 03	29 May 03
Singapore	Singapore	25 Feb 03	31 May 03
China	Inner Mongolia	4 Mar 03	3 Jun 03
China	Guangdong	16 Nov 02[f]	7 Jun 03
China	Hebei	19 Apr 03	10 Jun 03
China	Shanxi	8 Mar 03	13 Jun 03
China	Beijing	2 Mar 03	18 Jun 03
China	Hong Kong	15 Feb 03	22 Jun 03
Canada	Greater Toronto Area	23 Feb 03	2 Jul 03
China	Taiwan	25 Feb 03	5 Jul 03

APPENDIX 4:

CASE DEFINITIONS FOR SURVEILLANCE OF SEVERE ACUTE RESPIRATORY SYNDROME (SARS) (REVISED 1 MAY 2003)

OBJECTIVE

To describe the epidemiology of SARS and to monitor the magnitude and the spread of this disease, in order to provide advice on prevention and control.

INTRODUCTION

The surveillance case definitions based on available clinical and epidemiological data are now being supplemented by a number of laboratory tests and will continue to be reviewed as tests currently used in research settings become more widely available as diagnostic tests. *Preliminary clinical description of severe acute respiratory syndrome* (www.who.int/csr/sars/clinical/en/) summarizes what is currently known about the clinical features of SARS. Countries may need to adapt case definitions depending on their own disease situation. Retrospective surveillance is not expected.

Clinicians are advised that patients should not have their case definition category downgraded while awaiting results of laboratory testing or on the bases of negative results. See *Use of laboratory methods for SARS diagnosis* (www.who.int/csr/sars/labmethods/).

Suspect case

1. A person presenting after 1 November 2002* with history of:

    ·   high fever (>38 °C)

    AND

    ·   cough or breathing difficulty

    AND one or more of the following exposures during the 10 days prior to onset of symptoms:

    ·   **close contact**** with a person who is a suspect or probable case of SARS
    ·   history of travel to an area with recent local transmission of SARS
    ·   residing in an area with recent local transmission of SARS.

2. A person with an unexplained acute respiratory illness resulting in death after 1 November 2002,* but on whom no autopsy has been performed

    AND one or more of the following exposures during to 10 days prior to onset of symptoms:

    ·   **close contact** with a person who is a suspect or probable case of SARS
    ·   history of travel to an area with recent local transmission of SARS
    ·   residing in an area with recent local transmission of SARS.

Probable case

1. A suspect case with radiographic evidence of infiltrates consistent with pneumonia or respiratory distress syndrome on chest X-ray.
2. A suspect case of SARS that is positive for SARS coronavirus by one or more assays. See *Use of laboratory methods for SARS diagnosis.*
3. A suspect case with autopsy findings consistent with the pathology of respiratory distress syndrome without an identifiable cause.

---

*   The surveillance begins on 1 November 2002 to capture cases of atypical pneumonia in China now recognized as SARS. International tranmission of SARS was first reported in March 2003 for cases with onset in February 2003.
** Close contact: having cared for, lived with, or had direct contact with respiratory secretions or body fluids of a suspect or probable case of SARS.

EXCLUSION CRITERIA

A case should be excluded if an alternative diagnosis can fully explain their illness.

RECLASSIFICATION OF CASES

As SARS is currently a diagnosis of exclusion, the status of a reported case may change over time. A patient should always be managed as clinically appropriate, regardless of their case status.

- A case initially classified as suspect or probable, for whom an alternative diagnosis can fully explain the illness, should be discarded after carefully considering the possibility of co-infection.
- A suspect case who, after investigation, fulfils the probable case definition should be reclassified as "probable".
- A suspect case with a normal chest X-ray should be treated, as deemed appropriate, and monitored for 7 days. Those cases in whom recovery is inadequate should be re-evaluated by chest X-ray.
- Those suspect cases in whom recovery is adequate but whose illness cannot be fully explained by an alternative diagnosis should remain as "suspect".
- A suspect case who dies, on whom no autopsy is conducted, should remain classified as "suspect". However, if this case is identified as being part of a chain transmission of SARS, the case should be reclassified as "probable".
- If an autopsy is conducted and no pathological evidence of respiratory distress syndrome is found, the case should be "discarded".

REPORTING PROCEDURES

All probable SARS cases should be managed in the same way for the purposes of infection control and outbreak containment. See Management of severe acute respiratory syndrome (www.who.int/csr/sars/management/).

At this time, WHO is maintaining surveillance for clinically apparent cases only ie probable and suspect cases of SARS. (Testing of clinically well contacts of probable or suspect SARS cases and community based serological surveys are being conducted as part of epidemiological studies which may ultimately change our understanding of SARS transmission. However, persons who test SARS-CoV positive in these studies will not be notified as SARS cases to WHO at this time).

Where laboratory tests are not available or not done, probable SARS cases as currently defined above should continue to be reported in the agreed format.

Suspect cases with positive laboratory results will be reclassified as probable cases for notification purposes only if the testing laboratories use appropriate quality control procedures.

No distinction will be made between probable cases with or without a positive laboratory result and suspect cases with a positive result for the purposes of global surveillance. WHO will negotiate sentinel surveillance of SARS with selected partners to collect detailed epidemiological, laboratory and clinical data.

Cases that meet the surveillance case definition for SARS should not be discarded on the basis of negative laboratory tests at this time.

RATIONALE FOR RETAINING THE CURRENT SURVEILLANCE CASE DEFINITIONS FOR SARS

The reason for retaining the clinical and epidemiological basis for the case definitions is that at present there is no validated, widely and consistently available test for infection with the SARS coronavirus. Antibody tests may not become positive for three or more weeks after the onset of symptoms. We do not yet know if all patients will mount an antibody response. Molecular assays must be performed using appropriate reagents and controls under strictly controlled conditions, and may not be positive in the early stages of illness using currently available reagents. We are not yet able to define the optimal specimen to be tested at any given stage of the illness. This information is accruing as more tests are being performed on patients with known exposures and/or accompanied by good clinical and epidemiological information. We hope that in the near future an accessible and validated diagnostic assay(s) will become available which can be employed with confidence at a defined, early stage of the illness.

APPENDIX 5: PEOPLE WHO WORKED ON SARS RESPONSE, FEBRUARY TO JULY 2003

The following tables list the technical staff and consultants who provided WHO with support during the SARS pandemic. Key staff from WHO country offices (CO), regional offices and Headquarters, who were involved in the response, are also listed. It should be noted that many more people, other than technical experts, also devoted their time and skills. Areas of expertise are categorized into: clinical (Clin); communications (Com); epidemiological and public health (Epi); infection control (Inf C); laboratory (Lab); logistics (Log); psychological (Psy); and animal health (Zoo).

CAMBODIA

Name	Organization, Country	Area of work	Start date	End date
Clayton, Penelope		Inf C	13 May	13 Jun
Daily, Dr Frances	Independent consultant, Cambodia	Inf C	19 Apr	13 Jun
Merklen, Bernard	Independent consultant, Lao People's Democratic Republic	Log	19 Jun	29 Jul
Morita, Dr Kouichi	Nagasaki University, Japan	Epi	14 Apr	21 May
Vong, Dr Sirenda	Centers for Disease Control and Prevention (CDC), United States of America (USA)	Epi	10 May	11 Jun
Witt, Dr Clara	Walter Reed Army Institute of Research, USA	Epi	20 May	16 Jun

CHINA

Name	Organization, Country	Area of work	Start date	End date
Aguilera, Dr Ximena	Ministry of Health, Chile	Epi	15 May	15 Jun
Anderson, Dr Roy	Imperial College London Medical School, United Kingdom of Great Britain and Northern Ireland	Epi	11 Jun	14 Jun
Balasegaram, Mangai	Freelance writer, Malaysia	Com	13 Apr	17 May

Barboza, Philippe	Institut de Veille Sanitaire, France	Epi	12 Apr	17 May
Bekedam, Dr Henk	WHO Representative in China	CO	10 Feb	
Brantsaeter, Dr Arne Broch	Norwegian Institute of Public Health, Norway	Inf C	10 May	8 Jun
Breiman, Dr Robert Fredric	The International Centre for Diarrhoeal Disease Research, Bangladesh (ICDDR, B)	Lab	22 Mar	5 Apr
Broadbent, Clive		Inf C	25 May	17 Jun
Chin, Daniel	WHO, China	CO	10 Feb	30 Jul
Chow, Dr Catherine	CDC, USA	Epi	12 May	08 Jun
Chu, Dr May Chin-May	CDC, USA	Lab	07 Jun	08 Jul
Cocksedge, Dr Sandy	WHO Headquarters, Switzerland	Inf C	27 Apr	05 May
Coulombier, Dr Denis	WHO, Lyon, France	Epi	11 Jun	15 Jun
De Main, Yvonne	Australia	Inf C	10 May	20 July
Dietz, Mr Robert Karl	Communications expert, USA	Com	15 May	11 Aug
Doran, Dr Rodger	WHO, Viet Nam	CO	11 Jun	17 Jul
Dowell, Dr Scott	International Emerging Infectons Programme (IEIP), CDC, Thaland	Epi	26 Apr	1 May
Dumont, Serge	Springford Investment Ltd	Com	30 Apr	15 Jun
Dwyer, Dr Dominic Edmund	Westmead Hospital, Australia	Lab	9 May	9 Jun
Dziekan, Dr Gerald	Ministry of Health, Germany	Inf C	21 Jun	28 Jul
Evans, Dr Meirion	University of Wales College of Medicine, United Kingdom	Epi	23 Mar 27 Apr	6 Apr 15 May
Feikin, Dr Daniel Ross	National Center for Infectious Diseases, CDC, USA	Epi	8 Jun	3 Jul
Field, Dr Hume	Animal Research Institute, Australia	Zoo	4 May	18 May
Fleerackers, Dr Yon	Independent consultant, Belgium	Epi	11 Jun	10 Sep
Fukuda, Dr Keiji	CDC, USA	Epi	22 Feb 20 April	10 Mar 16 May
Giesecke, Dr Johan	Swedish Institute for Infectious Disease Control, Sweden	Epi	15 Jun	28 Jun
Giesecke, Dr Kajsa	Sodertalje Hospital, Sweden	Epi	15 Jun	28 Jun
Grein, Dr Tom	WHO Headquarters, Switzerland	Epi	11 Jun	14 Jun
Hardiman, Dr Max	WHO Headquarters, Switzerland	Epi	29 May	5 Jun
Heymann, Dr David	WHO Headquarters, Switzerland	Epi	11 Jun	14 Jun
Hoffman, Peter Nicholas		Inf C	21 May	17 Jun

Killingsworth, James	WHO, China		May	Jul
Lee, Dr Chin-Kei	Australian National University, Australia	Epi	5 May	
Lee, Dr Lisa Ann	WHO, China	CO	May	Jul
Legros, Dr Dominique	Epicentre, France	Epi	7 Jun	15 Jun
Li, Dr Ailan	WHO, China	CO	10 Feb	
Li, Dr Jin		Lab	25 May	5 Jun
Lu, Dr Xiuhua		Lab	16 Mar	29 Mar
Mackenzie, Professor John S.	University of Queensland, Australia	Lab	22 Mar	29 Mar
Maguire, Dr James Harvey	CDC, USA	Clin	22 Mar	25 May
McFarland, Jeff	WHO, Western Pacific Regional Office, Philippines	Epi	5 Apr	31 May
McMahon, Dr Shawn Renee	CDC, USA	Epi	7 Jun	29 Jun
Meyer, Dr Elizabeth	University Hospital Freiburg, Germany	Inf C	21 Jul	7 Sep
Mishima, Dr Noboyuki	SOS Clinic, China	Inf C	15 Jun	26 Jun
Ni, Dr Daxin		Epi	29 May	30 Jun
Nygard, Dr Karin	Norwegian Institute of Public Health, Norway	Epi	14 Jun	30 Jun
Oishi, Dr Kazunori	Nagasaki University, Japan	Clin	12 May	11 Jul
Oshitani, Dr Hitoshi	WHO, Western Pacific Regional Office, Philippines	Epi	23 Feb	10 Mar
Palmer, James		Com	5 Apr	19 Apr
Pappas, Tony	WHO Headquarters, Switzerland	Com	26 May	4 Jun
Patel, Dr Mahomed Said	Australian National University, Australia	Epi	10 Jun	15 Jun
Pickles, Dr Hilary	Health Protection Agency, United Kingdom	Inf C	22 May	4 Jun
Powell, Chris	WHO Headquarters, Switzerland	Com	23 Mar	30 Mar
Preiser, Dr Wolfgang	Institute of Virology, J.W. Goethe University, Germany	Lab	23 Mar	27 Apr
Rademackers, James		Com	5 Apr	19 Apr
Rodier, Dr Guenael	WHO Headquarters, Switzerland	Epi	11 Jun	14 Jun
Schnur, Alan	WHO, China	CO	10 Feb	5 Jul
Schuchat, Dr Anne	CDC, USA	Epi	12 May	12 Jun
Shapiro, Dr Craig	CDC, USA	Epi	12 Jun	30 Jun
Smyth, Garrett	WHO Headquarters, Switzerland	Com	3 Jun	13 Jun
Stielow, Janice	Royal Victorian Eye & Ear Hospital, Australia	Inf C	1 May	13 Jun
Stöhr, Dr Klaus	WHO Headquarters, Switzerland	Lab	24 Jun	10 Jul

Tam, Dr John	Chinese University of Hong Kong, China		25 May	5 Jun
Tashiro, Dr Masato	National Institute of Infectious Diseases, Japan	Lab	24 Feb	8 Mar
Tull, Dr Peet	National Board of Health and Welfare, Sweden	Epi	9 May	14 Jun
Uggowitzer, Steve	WHO Headquarters, Switzerland	Com	26 May	4 Jun
Watanabe, Dr Hiroshi	Nagasaki University, Japan	Inf C	2 May	15 Jun
Xu, Dr Fujie	CDC, USA	Epi	10 Jun	11 Jul
Xu, Dr Ruiheng		Epi	21 Apr	24 Apr
Xu, Dr Xiyan	CDC, USA	Lab	15 Mar	29 Mar
Yang, Dr Chen-Fu	CDC, USA	Lab	25 May	20 Jul
Yap, Dr Desiree Swei Lein	Australia	Inf C	9 May	5 Jul
Zhang, Dr Wenqing	WHO Headquarters, Switzerland	Lab	24 Jun	10 Jul
Zhang, Pengfei	WHO, Western Pacific Regional Office, Philippines		May	Jul
Zhou, Dr Sheng		Epi	16 Jun	30 Jun
Zhou, Dr Weigong	CDC, USA	Epi	14 May	14 Jun

Hong Kong (China)

Name	Organization, Country	Area of work	Start date	End date
Bresee, Joseph	CDC, USA	Epi	20 Mar	30 Apr
Brewster, Halijah Mokak	Independed consultant, Australia	Epi	7 Apr 24 Apr	10 Apr 30 Jun
Buchholz, Dr Udo		Epi	9 Apr	3 May
Cocksedge, Dr Sandy	WHO Headquarters, Switzerland	Inf C	23 Apr	26 Apr
Feldman, Heinrich	Health Canada, Canada	Lab	26 Apr	16 May
Flick, Ramon	Health Canada, Canada	Lab	26 Apr	16 May
Fukuda, Dr Keiji	CDC, USA	Epi	10 Mar	26 Mar
Grolla, Allen	Health Canada, Canada	Lab	26 Apr	16 May
Lee, Dr Chin-Kei	Australian National University, Australia	Epi	17 Mar	5 May
Li, Siu Mee Janet	Department of Health and Ageing, Australia	Epi	24 Mar	24 Apr
McNiece, Kay	Department of Health and Ageing, Australia	Com	25 Apr	24 May
Mock, Philip	CDC, USA	Com	18 Mar	17 Apr
Moren, Alain	Institut de Veille Sanitaire, France	Epi	25 Apr	23 May
Murphy, Dr Cathryn	NSW Department of Health, Australia	Inf C	4 May	10 May
Nakashima, Dr Kazutoshi	Oita University, Japan	Epi	7 Apr	19 Apr
Pappas, Tony	WHO Headquarters, Switzerland	Com	19 May	26 May
Schnitzler, Johannes	Robert Koch Institute, Germany	Epi	28 Apr	30 May

Sleigh, Dr Adrian Charles	National Centre for Epidemiology and Population Health, Australian National University, Australia	Epi	11 Jun	12 Jul
Sunagawa, Dr Tomimasa	National Institute of Infectious Diseases, Japan	Epi	18 Mar	17 Apr
Tilgner, Immo	Health Canada, Canada	Epi	26 Apr	16 May
Treadwell, Tracee	CDC, USA	Epi	7 Apr	7 May
Uggowitzer, Steve	WHO Headquarters, Switzerland	Com	20 May	26 May
Wang, Dr Julie Yung		Epi	9 Apr	21 May

MACAO (CHINA)

Name	Organization, Country	Area of work	Start date	End date
Murphy, Dr Cathryn	NSW Department of Health, Australia	Inf C	1 May	4 May
Morita, Koichi	Nagasaki University, Japan	Epi		

TAIWAN, CHINA

Name	Organization, Country	Area of work	Start date	End date
Barwick, Rachel	CDC, USA			
Bell, Michael	CDC, USA			
Bloland, Dr Peter	CDC, USA	Epi	13 May	6 Jun
Burlack, Paul	CDC, USA			
Burr, Gregory	CDC, USA			
Chang, Soju	CDC, USA			
Collins, Amy	CDC, USA			
Dowell, Dr Scott	IEIP, CDC, Thailand	Epi	16 Mar	23 Mar
Esswein, Eric	CDC, USA		17 May	2 Jun
Factor, Stephanie	CDC, USA			
Fisk, Tamara	IEIP, CDC, Thailand	Inf C	25 Mar	15 Apr
Greim, Bill	CDC, USA			
Jernigan, Dan	CDC, USA			
Kamara, Kande-Bure O'Bai	WHO Headquarters, Switzerland	Epi	19 Jun	7 Jul
Kaydos-Daniels, Susan	CDC, USA	Inf C	25 May	26 Jun
Keifer, Max	CDC, USA			
Lando, Jim	CDC, USA			
Macedo de Oliveira, Alexandre	CDC, USA			
Maloney, Susan	CDC, USA	Epi	24 May	17 Jun

Name	Organization / Position	Area of work	Start date	End date
Marx, Melissa	CDC			
Olowokure, Babatunde	WHO Headquarters, Switzerland	Epi	25 May	22 Jun
Olsen, Sonja	IEIP, CDC, Thailand	Epi	16 Mar 20 Apr	4 Apr 24 Apr
Park, Ben	CDC, USA			
Park, Dr Sarah	CDC, USA	Epi	25 May	27 Jun
Richards, Chelsey	CDC, USA			
Roth, Dr Cathy	WHO Headquarters, Switzerland	Epi	2 May	31 May
Shay, David	CDC, USA			
Shieh, Wun-Ju	CDC, USA	Inf C	6 Jun	15 Jun
Simmerman, Dr Mark	CDC/Thailand-Ministry of Public Health	Inf C	25 Apr	9 May
Sobel, Howard	WHO Headquarters, Switzerland	Epi	23 May	21 Jun
Wallingford, Kenneth	CDC, USA		28 Apr	12 May
Wang, Susan	CDC, USA	Epi	3 Jun	2 Jul
Watson, John	CDC, USA			
Wong, Dr David	CDC, USA			
Wong, Dr William	CDC, USA			

THE LAO PEOPLE'S DEMOCRATIC REPUBLIC

Name	Position and/or organization	Area of work	Start date	End date
Chojnacki, Astrid Laydia	Independent consultant, Lao People's Democratic Republic	Inf C	3 Apr	4 Jul
Clayton, Penelope		Inf C	13 May	13 Jun
Dowell, Dr Scott	IEIP, CDC, Thailand	Epi	3 Apr	4 Apr
Neu, Ingo		Epi	18 May	
Senaratana, Wilawan	Thailand	Inf C	7 Apr	24 Apr
Simmerman, Dr Mark	IEIP, CDC, Thailand	Inf C	3 Apr	5 Apr
Van Frachen, Veronique		Inf C	8 Apr	30 May

MALAYSIA

Name	Organization, Country	Area of work	Start date	End date
Patel, Dr Mahomed Said	Australian National University, Australia	Epi	20 Jun	24 Jun

MONGOLIA

Name	Organization, Country	Area of work	Start date	End date
Gresser, Norbert		Inf C	23 Apr	18 May
Hagan, Dr Robert	WHO Representative in Mongolia	CO	12 Apr	
Rojanapithayakorn, Dr Wiwat	WHO, Mongolia	CO	12 Apr	

THE PHILIPPINES

Name	Organization, Country	Area of work	Start date	End date
Brown, Sally E.		Inf C	26 Apr	7 Jun
Burr, Jodie Michelle	Women's and Children's Hospital, Australia	Inf C	26 Apr	5 Jun
De Main, Yvonne		Inf C	10 May	20 Jul
Harrington, Glenys Ann	Infection Control and Hospital Epidemiology Unit, The Alfred, Australia	Inf C	26 Apr	17 Jun
Mansoor, Dr Osman David	WHO, Western Pacific Regional Office, Philippines	Epi	2 May	30 Jun
Marano, Nina	CDC, USA	Inf C	4 Jun	3 Jul
Murphy, Dr Cathryn	NSW Department of Health, Australia	Inf C	27 Apr 14 May	1 May 6 Jun
Newman, Robert	CDC, USA	Epi	30 Apr	21 May
Noury, Dr Dominique	France	Log	21 May	22-Aug
Olivé, Dr Jean Marc	WHO Representative in the Philippines	CO	12 Mar	
Panlilio, Adelisa	CDC, USA	Inf C	30 Apr	21 May
Raghunathan, Dr Pratima	CDC, USA	Epi	30 Apr	21 May
Takahashi, Dr Hiroshi	Japan International Cooperation Agency, Japan	Epi	18 Apr	9 May

PACIFIC ISLAND COUNTRIES AND AREAS

Name	Organization, Country	Area of work	Start date	End date
Ewald, Dr Daniel Peter	Australia	Epi	27 May	16 Jun
Kitz, Dr Christa	Germany	Inf C	18 May	17 Jun
Pitman, Dr Catherine	Westmead Hospital and SDS Pathology Sydney, Australia	Lab	10 Apr	28 May
Zimmerman, Peta-Anne	Ryde Hospital and Community Health Services, Northern Sydney Health, Australia	Inf C	23 Apr	18 Jun

Papua New Guinea

Name	Organization, Country	Area of work	Start date	End date
Ewald, Dr Daniel Peter		Epi	27 May	16 Jun
Kitz, Dr Christa		Inf C	18 May	17 Jun

Singapore

Name	Organization, Country	Area of work	Start date	End date
Erickson, Bobbie Rae	CDC, USA	Lab	27 Apr	20 May
Kamara, Dr Kande-Bure O'Bai	WHO Headquarters, Switzerland	Epi	26 May	19 Jun
Khan, Ali	CDC, USA	Epi	9 Apr	16 May
Lambert, Dr Stephen	Murdoch Children's Research Institute, Royal Children's Hospital and University of Melbourne, Australia	Epi	11 Apr	24 May
Mansoor, Dr Osman David	WHO, Western Pacific Regional Office, Philippines	Epi	21 Mar	12 Apr
Murphy, Dr Cathryn	NSW Department of Health, Australia	Inf C	17 Apr 10 May	27 Apr 14 May
Rosen, Daniel	CDC, USA	Epi	7 Apr	7 May
Rotz, Lisa	CDC, USA	Epi	2 Jun	17 Jun
Shindo, Nikki	WHO Headquarters, Switzerland	Epi	25 May	20 Jun

Viet Nam

Name	Organization, Country	Area of work	Start date	End date
Aagesen, Dr Jesper	Ryhov County Hospital, Jonkoping, Sweden	Inf C	14 Mar	25 Apr
Anh, Bach Huy	Ha Noi Medical University, Viet Nam	Epi	20 Mar	21 May
Bausch, Dr Dan	CDC, USA	Epi	27 Mar	18 Apr
Bloom, Dr Sharon	CDC, USA	Epi	7 Apr	30 May
Brudon, Pascale	WHO Representative in Viet Nam	CO	3 Mar	
Chiarello, Linda	CDC, USA	Inf C	15 Mar	25 Mar
Depoorte, Dr Evelyn	Médecins Sans Frontières	Epi	18 Mar	26 Mar
Doran, Dr Rodger	WHO, Viet Nam	CO	10 Feb	
Hien, Nguyen Quang		Epi	23 Mar	6 May
Horby, Peter	PHLS Communicable Disease Surveillance Centre, United Kingdom	Epi	5 Apr	2 May
Hummel, Justin	Médecins Sans Frontières		2 Apr	30 Apr
Josse, Dr Evelyne	Médecins Sans Frontières	Psyc	1 Apr	20 Apr
Leitmeyer, Dr Katrin	WHO Headquarters, Switzerland	Epi	12 Mar	17 May
Maloney, Dr Susan	CDC, USA	Epi	17 Mar	28 Mar

Name	Organization, Country		Start date	End date
Miller, Dr Megge	Department of Health and Ageing, Australia	Epi	4 Apr	19 May
Montgomery, Dr Joel	CDC, USA	Epi	26 Mar	18 Apr
Nicholson, Professor Karl	Leicester Medical School, United Kingdom	Inf C	14 Mar	24 Mar
Oshitani, Dr Hitoshi	WHO, Western Pacific Regional Office, Philippines	Epi	10 Mar	18 Mar
Paquet, Dr Christopher	Institut de Veille Sanitaire, France	Epi	14 Mar	27 Mar
Plant, Professor Aileen	Curtin University of Technology, Australia	Inf C	15 Mar	30 May
Reynolds, Dr Mary	CDC, USA	Epi	15 Mar	5 Apr
Ronnevig, Hege Helene	Médecins Sans Frontières	Inf C	31 Mar	29 Apr
Sermand, Dan	Médecins Sans Frontières		31 Mar	29 Apr
Shah, Dr Jhankhana Jina	CDC, USA	Epi	8 Apr	8 May
Shieh, Wun-Ju	CDC, USA	Inf C	13 Mar	23 Mar
Thomson, Peter	Médecins Sans Frontières	Inf C	22 Mar	?
Urbani, Dr Carlo	WHO, Viet Nam	CO	28 Feb	11 Mar
Uyeki, Dr Timothy	CDC, USA	Epi	9 Mar	8 Apr
Viatour, Marianne	Médecins Sans Frontières	Admin	2 Apr	1 May
Wildau, Dr Huberta Lindeiner	Médecins Sans Frontières	Epi	9 Apr	5 May

WHO REGIONAL OFFICE FOR THE WESTERN PACIFIC

Name	Organization, Country	Area of work	Start date	End date
Antkowiak, Wayne	WHO, Western Pacific Regional Office, Philippines	Log	12 Mar	15 Jun
Atkinson, James	Independent Consultant, United Kingdom	Log	24 May	2 Nov
Bell, Dr David	WHO, Western Pacific Regional Office, Philippines	Log	10 Mar	1 May
Christophel, Eva Maria	WHO, Western Pacific Regional Office, Philippines	Epi	23 Feb	18 Jun
Clayton, Penelope		Inf C	13 May	13 Jun
Condon, Dr Robert	WHO, Western Pacific Regional Office, Philippines	Epi	12 Mar	19 Jun
Cordingley, Peter	WHO, Western Pacific Regional Office, Philippines	Com	12 Mar	
Cullen, Michele		Inf C	1 Apr	7 Jun
Doberstyn, Dr Brian	WHO, Western Pacific Regional Office, Philippines		10 Feb	
Kaku, Dr Mitsuo	Tohoku University, Japan	Inf C	3 Apr	13 Apr

Kasai, Takeshi	WHO, Western Pacific Regional Office, Philippines	Lab	12 Mar	30 Jun
Kojima, Dr Kazunobu	Sapporo Medical University, Japan	Lab	9 Apr	29 Apr
Lambert, Dr Stephen	Murdoch Children's Research Institute, Royal Children's Hospital and University of Melbourne, Australia	Epi	24 Mar	10 Apr
Libraty, Dr Daniel	USA	Lab	16 May	23 Jun
Miranda, Dr Elizabeth	WHO, Western Pacific Regional Office, Philippines	Vet	10 Feb	
Muller, Dr Rosanne	National Centre for Epidemiology and Population Health, Australian National University, Australia Centre for Disease Control, Darwin, Australia	Epi	9 Apr	7 Jun
Oshitani, Dr Hitoshi	WHO, Western Pacific Regional Office, Philippines	Epi	10 Feb	
Pappas, Tony	WHO Headquarters, Switzerland	Com	4 Jun	11 Jun
Patel, Dr Mahomed Said	Australian National University, Australia	Epi	1 May	10 Jun
Roces, Dr Maria Concepcion	Oak Ridge Institute for Science and Education (ORISE), CDC, Philippines	Epi	27 Mar	15 Apr
Saito, Dr Reiko	Niigata University, Japan	Epi	29 Apr	27 May
Sato, Yoshikuni	WHO, Western Pacific Regional Office, Philippines	Funding	22 Feb	
Senaratana, Wilawan	Thailand	Inf C	7 Apr	24 Apr
Shimada, Dr Yasushi	Field Epidemiology Training Programme, National Institute of Infectious Diseases, Japan	Epi	7 May	7 Jun
Spencer, Dr Jenean	Department of Health and Ageing, Australia	Epi	13 Jun	13 Aug
Suzuki, Dr Akira	Sendai National Hospital, Japan	Epi	2 Jun	1 Aug
Suzuki, Dr Satowa		Epi	23 Mar	24 Apr
Tanaka, Hiroko	WHO, Western Pacific Regional Office, Philippines		12 Mar	31 May
Uggowitzer, Steve	WHO Headquarters, Switzerland	Com	4 Jun	11 Jun
Vanquaille, Peter	Independent consultant	Log	7 Apr	27 May
Witt, Dr Clara	Walter Reed Army Institute of Research, USA	Epi	3 May	20 May
Yoshida, Dr Hideki	National Institute of Infectious Diseases, Japan	Epi	16 Apr	11 May

WHO Headquarters

Consultants

Name	Organization, Country	Area of work	Start date	End date
Gay, Nigel	Technical Adviser, Health Protection Agency, United Kingdom		24 Apr	2 Aug
Martin, Steve	European Programme for Interventional Epidemiology Training		6 Apr	30 May

Communicable Diseases, Department of Communicable Disease Surveillance and Response (CDS/CSR)

Ait-Ikhlef, Kamel

Anderson, Ruth

Andraghetti, Roberta

Anker, Martha

Bauquerez, Rachel

Breugelmans, Gabriele

Buriot, Diego

Carnicer-Pont, Dolors

Chaieb, Amina

Cocksedge, William

Costa, Ntanis (Danis)

Creese, Peggy

Drury, Patrick

Emami, Reza

Fitzner, Julia

Formenty, Pierre

Grein, Thomas

Hardy, Derek

Jenkins, P.G.

Jesuthasan, Emmanuel

Leitmeyer, Katrin

Lièvre, Maja

Merianos, Angela

Lorenzin, Eglé

Luy, Marie

Mathiot, Christian

O'Bai Kamara, Kande-Bure

Olowokure, Babatunde

O'Rourke, Suzanne

Poncé, Corrine

Preaud, Claire

Rashford, Adrienne

Roth, Cathy

Rodier, Guénaël

Shindo, Nikki

Sobel, Howard

Stöhr, Klaus

Thomson, Gail

Wilson, Williamina

Umali, Khristeen

Vandemaele, Kaat

Valenciano, Marta

van Rossum, Koen

Werker, Denise

Youssef, Mohammad

Communicable Diseases, Executive Director's Office (EXD)

Block Tyrrell, Sue

Cheng, Maria

Guilloux, Anne

Karahasanovic, Edin

Kindhauser, Mary Kay

Thompson, Dick

Tissot, Patrick

COMMUNICABLE DISEASES, MANAGEMENT SUPPORT UNIT (MSU)

Meloni, Jill	Pievaroli, Liliana	Tantillo, Chris
Pappas, Tony	Swanson, Michael	

OTHER DEPARTMENTS

Name	Department
Keiny, M.P.	Health Technologies and Pharmaceuticals (HTP), UNAIDS/WHO Research on Viral Vaccines (VABI/IVR)
Esparza, Jose	HTP/VAB/IVR/VIR
Bartram, James	Sustainable Development and Healthy Environments (SDE), Protection of the Human Environment (PHE), Water, Sanitation and Health (WSH)
Carr, Richard	SDE/PHE/WSH
Bos, Robert	SDE/PHE/WSH

OTHER WHO REGIONAL AND COUNTRY OFFICES

Name	Office
Gudjon Magnusson	Regional Office for Europe
Desiree Kogevinas	Regional Office for Europe
B. Ganter	Regional Office for Europe
Arun Ratnam	Regional Office for South-East Asia
Shipra Sharma	Regional Office for South-East Asia
David Wheeler	Regional Office for South-East Asia
Parmod Kapur	Regional Office for South-East Asia
Kumara Rai	Regional Office for South-East Asia
Duangvadee Sungkhobol	Regional Office for South-East Asia
Harsaran Pandey	Regional Office for South-East Asia
Alex Andjaparidze	Representative Office, the Democratic Republic of Timor-Leste
Sampath K Krishnan	Representative Office, India
S. J. Habayeb	Representative Office, India
Leonard Ortega	Representative Office, Myanmar
Marla Win	Representative Office, Myanmar
Mi Mi That	Representative Office, Myanmar
Patrick Wunna Htoo	Representative Office, Myanmar
Somchai Peerapakorn	Representative Office, Thailand
Bjorn Melgaard	Representative Office, Thailand
Richard Kalina	Representative Office, Thailand
Martin Eichel	Representative Office, Thailand
Mary Pinder	Representative Office, Thailand

ACKNOWLEDGEMENTS

AUTHORS

The principal writers of this report were Carolyn Abraham, Mangai Balasegaram, Mary Ann Benitez, Pascale Brudon, Maria Cheng, Dr Robert Condon, Dr Brian Doberstyn, Dr Christian Drosten, Dr Andrea Ellis, Dr Yi Guan, Dr David Heymann, Dr Marie-Paule Kieny, Mary Kay Kindhauser, Dr Stephen Lambert, Dr Katrin Leitmeyer, Professor John S Mackenzie, Dr Susan Maloney, Dr Osman David Mansoor, Dr Angela Merianos, Dr Elizabeth Miranda, Dr Rosanne Muller, Dr Jean-Marc Olivé, Dr Babatunde Olowokure, Dr Saladin Osmanov, Dr Mahomed Patel, Dr Malik Peiris, Professor Aileen Plant, Dr Leo Poon, Dr Guénaël Rodier, Dr Wiwat Rojanapithayakorn, Dr Cathy Roth, Professor Linda Saif, Professor Joseph Jao-Yiu Sung, and Floyd Whaley.

CONTRIBUTORS

Contributions were gratefully received from James Atkinson, Dr David Bell, Dr Robert Breiman, Oliver Cattin, Serge Dumont, Dr Heinz Feldmann, Troy Gepte, Allen Grolla, Mei-Shang Ho, Josh Jones, Peter King, John Leung, Dr Li Ailan, Dr Jamsran Mendsaihan, Dr Megge Miller, Ingo Neu, Sonja Olsen, Dr Sarah Park, Professor Aileen Plant, Doris Radun, Alan Schnur, Vu Hoag Thu, Immo Tilgner, Dr Timothy Uyeki, Peter Vanquaille, Denise Werker, and Peta-Anne Zimmerman.

PEER REVIEWERS

Valuable input was received from the following experts who reviewed the science chapters: Dr Ralf Altmeyer, Pasteur Institute, Hong Kong; Dr Larry Anderson, CDC, USA; Richard Bellamy; Dounia Bitar, l'Institut de Veille Sanitare, France; Mike Catton, Victorian Infections Diseases Reference Laboratory, Australia; Dr Mary Chu, WHO, Switzerland, Paul Garner, Liverpool School of Tropical Medicine, The University of Liverpool, United Kingdom; Matthias Niedrig, Robert Koch Institut, Germany; Janusz Paweska, National Institute for Communicable Diseases, South Africa; Dr Susan Poutanen, Toronto Medical Laboratories & Mount Sinai Hospital, Canada; Professor Linda Saif, Ohio Agricultural Research and Development Center, The Ohio State University, USA;

Lauren Stockman, CDC, USA; Sylvie van der Werf, l'Institut Pasteur, France; Dr Linfa Wang, Australian Animal Health Laboratory, Australia; and Denise Werker, WHO, Switzerland.

EDITORIAL TEAM

Editorial support was provided by Mary Ann Asico, Peter Cordingley, Alastair Dingwall, Dr Brian Doberstyn, Dr Osman David Mansoor, Dr Hitoshi Oshitani and Rhonda Vandeworp. Design by Alan Esquillon. Layout by Bhoie Hernandez and Grace Yu. Index by Indexing Specialists (UK) Ltd.

PICTURE CREDITS

Cover page, pp. 62, 63, 64, 65, 66, Alan Esquillon; p. 19, Dr Aiee Ling, Virology Unit, Singapore General Hospital; pp. 23, 29, 76, 81, 87, 89, 92, 142, 155, 157, Christian Keenan, Getty Images; pp. 24, 170 (bottom), Hanne Strandgaardh, WHO; pp. 34, 42, 50 (bottom), 51, 53, 79, 159, Pierre Virot, WHO; pp. 40, 56, Jay Directo, AFP, Getty Images; p. 41, JP Moczulski, AFP, Getty Images; p. 44, Jimin Lai, AFP, Getty Images; pp. 45, 82, 136, STR, AFP, Getty Images; p. 46, Liu Jin, AFP, Getty Images; p. 50 (top), Sam Yeh, AFP, Getty Images; p. 59, Dr Jenean Spencer and Steve Uggowitzer; p. 74, Peter Parks, AFP, Getty Images; p. 77, Frederic J Brown, AFP, Getty Images; p. 78, provided by Dr Robert Breiman; p. 80, Dr Johan Giesecke; p. 84, AFP, Getty Images; p. 91, Jean-Pierre Clatot, AFP, Getty Images; p. 95, Dr Joel Montgomery; p. 96, provided by Dr Sharon Bloom; p. 98, Dr Dan Bausch; pp. 99, 100, 170 (top) Hoang Dinh Nam, AFP, Getty Images; pp. 102, 105, 164 (bottom), Luis Ascui, Getty Images; pp. 106, 164 (top), 165, Roslan Rahman, AFP, Getty Images; pp. 110, 113 (top left), Sam Yeh, AFP, Getty Images; pp. 111, 113 (top right), Patrick Lin, AFP, Getty Images; p. 113 (bottom), provided by Dr Sarah Park, CDC; p. 117, provided by Dr Jean-Marc Olivé; p. 120, Penelope Clayton; pp. 121, 225, Richard A Brooks, AFP, Getty Images; pp. 122, 123, 125, Norbert Gresser; p. 128, Fred Lum, *The Globe and Mail*; p. 131, Louie Palu, *The Globe and Mail*; p. 153, Paula Bronstein, Getty Images; p. 158, Robert Ng, *South China Morning Post*; p. 171, Dr Carlo Urbani, WHO; p. 227, Katharina Hesse, Getty Images.

ABOUT THE
AUTHORS

Carolyn Abraham is an award-winning author and medical reporter for *The Globe and Mail*, Canada's national daily newspaper. She has won numerous prizes for her coverage of medical issues and covered Toronto's SARS outbreak from its beginning. At its end, Ms Abraham actually delivered her baby in a Toronto hospital under quarantine.

Mangai Balasegaram is a freelance writer who, for the past four years, has worked on public information for WHO in the Western Pacific Region, including WHO China office during the SARS outbreak. She began her career as a journalist, specializing in HIV/AIDS, and has won several awards and fellowships.

Mary Ann Benitez is a medical reporter for the *South China Morning Post* in Hong Kong. She has been a Hong Kong-based journalist for many years and a member of the "4.30 Club"-the core group attending the daily press briefings on SARS presided by government and hospital authority officials in Hong Kong.

Pascale Brudon was the WHO Representative in Viet Nam during the SARS outbreak. She received Viet Nam's "Medal for People's Health" for her work and the work of the WHO country office. She is currently Task Manager, General Programme of Work, at WHO Headquarters in Geneva.

Maria Cheng was a journalist in Hong Kong. She joined WHO as a communications officer in Geneva during the SARS outbreak.

Rob Condon is a public health physician in Suva, Fiji. During the outbreak, he was seconded from WHO South Pacific office (where he was responsible for Communicable Disease Surveillance and Response) to lead the response group of the SARS team.

Brian Doberstyn was Director of the Division for Combating Communicable Disease in the WHO Western Pacific Regional Office during the SARS outbreak.

Christian Drosten is Head of the Molecular Diagnostics laboratory group, Bernhard Nocht Institute for Tropical Medicine, Hamburg, Germany. His laboratory identified SARS-CoV from a sample of a patient who imported SARS into Germany and developed the first real-time RT-PCR test, which was made available as a diagnostic kit during the epidemic.

Andrea Ellis has been a senior epidemiologist for the Government of Canada for just over 10 years. She is currently the head of the Outbreak Response Section of the Foodborne, Waterborne and Zoonotic Infections Division at the Public Health Agency of Canada. Dr Ellis spent two years on secondment to WHO's Department of Communicable Disease Surveillance and Response in Geneva. There she provided training in disease surveillance and outbreak response and was involved in the response to the SARS and avian influenza outbreaks.

Yi Guan is a virologist and an associate professor in the Department of Microbiology at the University of Hong Kong. As a principal investigator, he identified animal reservoirs of SARS in southern China and helped the Chinese Government to avert the second SARS outbreak in early 2004.

David L. Heymann was Executive Director of Communicable Diseases at WHO Headquarters in Geneva from 1998 to 2004.

Marie-Paule Kieny is Director of the Initiative for Vaccine Research at WHO Headquarters in Geneva. She has spent most of her career working on the development of various human or veterinary vaccines.

Mary Kay Kindhauser is a science writer in the Communicable Diseases cluster at WHO Headquarters. She prepared the daily web updates during the SARS outbreak.

Stephen Lambert is a public health physician and senior research fellow at the Vaccine & Immunisation Research Group, Murdoch Children's Research Institute and School of Population Health, University of Melbourne. During the SARS outbreak, he worked in the WHO Regional Office and then in Singapore as a team leader.

Katrin Leitmeyer is a scientist at Robert Koch Institute in Berlin, Germany. She is a former WHO Headquarters staff member who was assigned to Viet Nam during the SARS outbreak. She is a physician with public health training in infectious-disease epidemiology; specialized in clinical, laboratory, and epidemiological management of hemorrhagic fever virus infections.

John S Mackenzie is a Premier's fellow and Professor of Tropical Infectious Diseases, Australian Biosecurity CRC, Curtin University of Technology, Perth, Australia. He is a member of the Steering Committee of the Global Outbreak Alert and Response Network (GOARN) and the WHO/CSR Strategic Advisory Committee for Global Health Security. During the SARS outbreak, he led an early WHO mission to China and worked in WHO Headquarters to establish the SARS Research Advisory Group and the SARS verification laboratory network.

Susan Maloney is a medical epidemiologist with the Division of Global Migration and Quarantine, Centers for Disease Control and Prevention (CDC), United States of America. She is a physician board-certified in both paediatrics and infectious diseases, and has extensive public health experience in infectious disease epidemiology and hospital and community infection control. During the 2003 SARS outbreak, she was a member of the WHO team in Viet Nam and Team Leader of the Taiwan CDC team.

Osman David Mansoor is a public health physician working as a consultant in New Zealand. He is a former WHO staff member (immunization unit in Manila) posted to Singapore and then to the Philippines during the SARS outbreak.

Angela Merianos is a medical epidemiologist/public health physician, Alert and Response Operations/Department of Communicable Disease Surveillance and Response, WHO Headquarters. Chair of the WHO Ad Hoc Working Group on the Epidemiology of SARS; and WHO SARS Disease Focal Point during the outbreak and in the post outbreak period.

Elizabeth Miranda was a field epidemiologist and a veterinary public health specialist in the Department of Communicable Disease Surveillance and Response, Regional Office for the Western Pacific, WHO, Manila.

Rosanne Muller was an epidemiologist and public health medical officer, based at the Centre for Disease Control in Darwin, Australia. During the SARS outbreak, she worked on regional rumour surveillance at the WHO Western Pacific Regional Office.

Jean-Marc Olivé is the WHO Representative in the Philippines.

Babatunde Olowokure is a Regional Epidemiologist, Regional Surveillance Unit, Health Protection Agency (West Midlands), Birmingham, United Kingdom. Formerly a WHO staff member, he worked on SARS as part of the Global Alert and Response team in Geneva, and then was posted to Taiwan during the SARS outbreak.

Dr Saladin Osmanov is Coordinator ad interim, WHO-UNAIDS HIV Vaccine Initiative for Vaccine Research. He was responsible for organizing the WHO consultation on "Needs and Opportunities for SARS Vaccine Research and Development", 31 October-1 November 2003, in Geneva, Switzerland.

Mahomed Patel is an epidemiologist and public-health physician at the National Centre for Epidemiology and Population Health, Australian National University. During the SARS outbreak, he was the Team Leader for Preparedness at the Regional Office in Manila and a team member for evaluating responses in China and Malaysia.

Malik Peiris is a professor in the Department of Microbiology at the University of Hong Kong and Chief of Virology at Queen Mary Hospital. He was involved in the discovery of the aetiological agent of SARS.

Aileen Plant is a professor of international health at the Australian Biosecurity Cooperative Research Centre for Emerging Infectious Disease, Curtin University of Technology; Perth, Australia. She was a member of the Global Outbreak Alert and Response Network and was WHO Viet Nam team leader during SARS outbreak. She was the first person in the world with SARS on her business card and received Viet Nam's Medal for People's Health.

Leo Poon is a molecular virologist at the LM Department of Microbiology, University of Hong Kong.

Guénaël Rodier was Director, Department of Communicable Disease Surveillance and Response, WHO Headquarters.

Wiwat Rojanapithayakorn is a WHO senior adviser in WHO China office. He was working as a medical officer in WHO Mongolia office during the SARS outbreak.

Cathy Roth is head of the Dangerous and New Pathogens cluster of the Epidemic and Pandemic Response department at WHO Headquarters in Geneva. She led the first WHO team that assisted Taiwan, China during the SARS outbreak.

Linda Saif is a distinguished university professor and researcher with The Ohio State University's Food Animal Health Research Program of the Ohio Agricultural Research and Development Center (OARDC). Saif is known internationally for her work on enteric viruses, including rotaviruses, caliciviruses, and coronaviruses. During the SARS outbreak, Dr Saif acted as a scientific adviser to the SARS Scientific Advisory Group of WHO, and her laboratory became part of the SARS international laboratory network organized to fight the disease. She also was a member of an ad hoc SARS scientific advisory team for CDC.

Joseph Jao-Yiu Sung is Chair of the Department of Medicine and Therapeutics at The Chinese University of Hong Kong. He is also Associate Dean, Faculty of Medicine; and Chief, Division of Gastroenterology and Hepatology. He is the author of six books and numerous book chapters, peer-reviewed papers and abstracts. He has won numerous awards, including *Time* magazine's Asian Heroes 2003 award for his work on SARS.

Floyd Whaley is a journalist who has been based in Asia-in the Philippines and in Thailand-since 1994. A former Special Correspondent for *Reader's Digest* magazine, he has also contributed to *The Los Angeles Times*, *The New York Times*, *USA Today*, Reuters News Service and many other publications. Currently, he works in media relations for the Manila-based Asian Development Bank.

GLOSSARY

Aerosol

A collection of very small particles or liquid suspended in air. A virus in an aerosol can be transmitted trough the air without direct contact. This was rare for SARS.

Aerosolization

The process of creating an aerosol. A SARS aerosol may have been created in the Amoy Gardens outbreak. Aerosols can also be produced during medical procedures, such as nebulization, tracheal suctioning, and intubation; however, there is no direct evidence that this happened during the care of a SARS patient.

Aetiology

The cause of a disease. The aetiology of SARS was at first unknown.

Aetiological agent

The specific agent that causes disease. Koch's postulates are used to establish the aetiological agent. For SARS, it was the SARS coronavirus.

Affected area

An area in which local chain(s) of transmission of SARS is/are occurring as reported by the national public health authorities. WHO defined an area as affected for 20 days after the last local case was isolated, 20 days being two incubation periods, to ensure that there was no further transmission of cases that had not yet been reported. From 2 May, WHO replaced the term "affected area" with "area with recent local transmission".

Agent

A factor, such as a microorganism, chemical substance, or form of radiation, whose presence, excessive presence, or (in deficiency diseases) relative absence is essential for the occurrence of a disease.

Alanine transaminase (ALT)

An enzyme most commonly associated with the liver, although it is found in every cell. Elevated levels of ALT often suggest the existence of medical problems. Mild elevation of ALT was commonly found in SARS patients.

Alveoli (plural of alveolus)
Terminal air sacs in the lungs where gases are exchanged. (The airtubes—bronchi and bronchioles—connect the outside air to the alveoli.) SARS damage in the lung was mostly at alveolar surface.

Antigen
A substance, often a protein, which stimulates an antibody response specifically targeted against it.

Asymptomatic
"Without symptoms". An asymptomatic case is an infected person who has no symptoms of the infection. Such cases of SARS were unusual. Asymptomatic transmission does not appear to have occurred in SARS.

Biopsy
Medical procedure that removes a very small piece of tissue for diagnostic procedures (e.g. microscopic examination). The material from the procedure is also called a biopsy.

Biosafety level (BSL)
There are four biosafety levels (BSL1 to BSL4) that categorize the minimum requirements (of work practices, safety equipment, and facilities) for handling infectious agents of different risk. BSL1 is for agents with no or low individual and community risk, while BSL4 is for agents with the highest risk.

Case
An individual with a particular disease. A SARS case is a person with SARS infection. A case can be classified as suspect, probable, or confirmed depending on contact history, clinical findings, and laboratory tests and according to the case definition. Defining who is and who is not a case is fundamental for studying the epidemiology of a disease.

Case definition
A set of standard criteria for deciding whether a person has a particular disease or health-related condition, by specifying clinical criteria and limitations on time, place, and person.

Chain of transmission	Describes the spread of a virus (or other agent) as it passes from one person to the next (for a disease that spreads from person to person). Transmission of a disease is stopped when all the chains are interrupted.
Close contact	In the context of SARS, "close contact" means having cared for or lived with someone with SARS or having direct contact with respiratory secretions or body fluids of a patient with SARS. Examples of close contact include kissing or hugging, sharing eating or drinking utensils, talking to someone within about one metre, and touching someone directly. Close contact does not include activities like walking by a person or briefly sitting across a waiting room or office. In practically all cases, "close contact" with a case was a prerequisite to be infected with SARS.
Cluster	An aggregation of cases of a disease. For a communicable disease, like SARS, a cluster is usually a group of cases directly or indirectly infected through a common exposure (person, place, or time). A cluster describes a group of cases that share epidemiological features— usually a group of cases that are closely grouped in time and place. A cluster can also be described as an outbreak, but the link between cases in a cluster is usually closer than that in an outbreak.
Contagious	Can be used to describe a disease or a person. It describes a disease as spreading from one person to another. It describes the stage or duration of the disease in a person when they can infect another person. Technically, contagious has the same meaning as infectious, but may be more emotive.
Coronavirus	A group of viruses that have a halo or crown-like (corona) appearance when viewed under an electron microscope. These viruses are a common cause of mild to moderate upper-respiratory illness in humans and are associated

with respiratory, gastrointestinal, liver, and neurologic diseases in animals. The SARS coronavirus is a new member of the coronavirus family.

Corticosteroid

A drug that suppress inflammation by mimicking the effect of a hormone that the body produces. It remains uncertain if corticosteroids have a beneficial impact on SARS.

Cytokine

A substance, usually a protein, which is produced by cells and sends chemical messages to other cells. These messages are the mediators of the body's inflammatory and immune response.

Droplet spread

SARS spread from person to person predominantly by droplet (as opposed to aerosol) spread. A droplet is too large to remain suspended in air. Infected droplets that are spread by talking, coughing, or sneezing can travel only a short distance (usually less than one metre), which is why close contact was usually needed for SARS transmission. Droplets can also be spread by hand or through fomites (inanimate objects that have had contact with contaminated body secretions). A droplet can be aerosolized (suspended in air) by medical procedures such as tracheal suctioning, intubation, and nebulization.

Epidemic

The occurrence of more cases of disease than expected in a given area or among a specific group of people over a particular period of time. Technically, has the same meaning as an outbreak. For infectious diseases like SARS, it implies the introduction and spread of the pathogen in a way that had not previously happened.

Epidemic curve

A graphical representation of the spread of the epidemic. This is usually shown by preparing a bar or line graph of the number of cases by time of onset. The pattern of the epidemic curve is a basic epidemiological tool that is used to help define the cause and control of an epidemic

Epidemiology

The study of the distribution (time, place, person) and determinants of disease, i.e. who gets the disease and why, so that appropriate control measures can be developed.

Epithelium (epithelial cells)

The outer lining of body surfaces (e.g. skin, gut, lung), which is composed of epithelial cells. Each body surface has its own special type of epithelial cells.

Fibrosis

The formation of fibrous tissue, which is histologically different than the original tissue, resulting from a disease process.

Genome

The genetic information of an organism.

Human leucocyte antigen

A protein on the surface of white blood cells that provides a genetic fingerprint and can be a marker for disease susceptibility in some diseases.

Host

A person or other living organism that can be infected by an infectious agent under natural conditions.

IgG / IgA / IgM

Different type of antibodies (immunoglobulins) produced by the immune system. Each one has a slightly different function, and antibody tests are usually directed at one or more of that type.

In vitro

"In glass". A test undertaken in the laboratory as opposed to in living organisms (*in vivo*).

In vivo

"In life". A test undertaken in a living organism as opposed to in a laboratory (*in vitro*).

Incubation period

Time from infection (exposure to the infectious agent) to the first manifestation of the disease it causes.

Index case

For a disease with person-to-person transmission, the index case is the source of a cluster or outbreak. He or she is the first person in the cluster or outbreak to become infected.

Infection	Identifying the index case helps to identify the chains of transmission and how the disease is spread.
	What happens when an infectious agent gets past the body's defences and takes hold. There are many kinds of infection. SARS produced what is called an "acute infection", meaning that infection led to disease soon after exposure (with a relatively short incubation period). As with other infections, the symptoms of SARS infection result not only from the presence of the virus in the body, but also from the body's efforts to fight off the virus. Fever, for example, is a symptom caused by the body attempting to destroy the pathogen.
International Health Regulations	The International Health Regulations (IHRs), which are administered by the World Health Organization, are the only legally binding international instrument covering measures for preventing the transboundary spread of infectious diseases. They provide a single code of procedures and practices, including routine measures at airports and seaports, for preventing the importation of pathogens and vectors. They also set out roles and responsibilities, for WHO as well as for individual countries, for responding to a limited range of disease outbreaks. They contribute greatly to the use of uniform and effective protective measures both on a routine basis and in certain crisis situations.
Koch's postulates	These postulates specify that to establish an organism as the pathogen for that disease: (1) the organism is found in all cases but not in healthy people; and (2) the organism when inoculated into a healthy subject causes the same disease. (Koch was a 19th-century German physician.)
Lymphocyte	A type of white blood cell responsible for the body's immune system. The two main types of

	lymphocytes are B cells (produce antibodies) and T cells (provide humoral immunity).
Lymphopaenia	A reduction in the number of lymphocytes in the blood. (a common finding in SARS).
Neutralizing antibody	An antibody that can inhibit the growth of a virus (or other infectious agent) from causing infection.
Nosocomial infection	Hospital-acquired infection.
Oedema	Abnormal, excess fluid that collects in the space between the cells in one or more parts of the body as a result of a systemic or local disease process.
Outbreak	The technical definitions of outbreak and epidemic are the same, but the term outbreak emotes a more 'neutral' description of the event. A cluster can also be described as an outbreak.
Pandemic	An epidemic occurring over a very wide area (several countries or continents) and usually affecting a large proportion of the population.
Pathogen	A virus, bacterium, fungus, parasite, or other type of microorganism that is the cause of that disease. (The SARS coronavirus is the pathogen that causes SARS.)
Pathogenesis	Origin and development of disease.
Polymerase chain reaction	A laboratory method for detecting the genetic material. The PCR test is a useful way of detecting infectious disease agents in specimens from patients, including SARS patients. The test involves making multiple copies of a small DNA fragment using the polymerase enzyme. In the case of RNA viruses such as SARS, the first step involves making a DNA copy of the RNA using the reverse transcriptase enzyme. Hence the test is called reverse transcriptase-polymerase chain reaction (RT-PCR).
Period of communicability	The period of time when a person infected with an agent can transmit it to others.

Prodrome (prodromal)	A symptom of a disease before it becomes fully manifest.
Pulmonary	Of the lung.
Sensitivity	A test's sensitivity is how accurately it picks up all cases, or 1-false negative rate (see also specificity).
Seroconversion	Describes the situation where a person who did not previously have the antibodies being discussed develops them, i.e. "converts" from having no antibodies (seronegative) to having them (seropositve), which means that the person was recently infected.
Serology	The results of antibody tests. Following an infection, the body makes antibodies against the pathogen. Tests for the specific antibodies against that pathogen can then show if there has been that infection. Antibody tests are commonly used to diagnose infectious disease, including SARS.
Seroprevalence	Percentage of a population with the antibody in question. It is a way of describing how common an infection is or has been.
Serosurvey (serological survey)	A survey of the blood of a population to measure what proportion have the antibody in question. This is used to test how common an infection is in that community.
Serum	The noncellular part of the blood where antibodies are present. As testing of antibodies is done on the serum (as opposed to whole blood), antibody testing is also called serological testing.
Specificity	A test's specificity is how accurately it rejects up all non-cases, or 1-false positive rate (see also sensitivity).
Super spreader	A person who passes an infection to many more people than the average. For nearly all SARS cases, transmission was limited to less than three other individuals. Only occasionally were the

numbers higher. *Note*: There is no precise numerical or statistical definition of how many cases make up a super spreader.

Super-spreading event

An occurrence of many people being infected by an index case. A super-spreading event is not defined by a precise number of cases. However, in most events, about 20 or more people were infected.

Syndrome

A collection of clinical manifestations (signs, symptoms, laboratory results) that describe a specific clinical entity.

Thrombocytopaenia

A reduction in the number of platelets in the blood (a common finding in SARS).

Vaccine

A substance that when given to a person protects against a specific infection. Vaccines are made from inactivated or modified pathogen, or some parts of it. If the person comes in contact with that pathogen, the body then fights it off easily and can protect against this disease in the future. This protection is called immunity.

Viraemia

The presence of virus in the blood.

Virus

A disease-causing microorganism that depends on a host cell to survive and reproduce. Unlike bacteria, which are larger, a virus needs to get inside a living cell and take over its machinery to reproduce. Once the virus has invaded a cell, it produces and releases copies of the virus, which go on to infect other cells.

Zoonosis (pl zoonoses)

An infectious disease that is transmissible under natural conditions from animals to humans.

ACRONYMS

ACE	angiotensin converting enzyme
ALT	alanine transaminase
ARDS	adult respiratory distress syndrome
BCoV	bovine coronavirus
BOOP	bronchiolitis obliterans organizing pneumonia
BSL	biosafety level
CDC	Centers for Disease Control and Prevention, United States of America
China CDC	Chinese Center for Disease Control and Prevention
CT	computed tomography
EIA	enzyme immunoassays
ELISA	enzyme linked immunosorbent assay
FIPV	feline infectious peritonitis virus
GMP	good manufacturing practice
GOARN	Global Outbreak Alert and Response Network
GPHIN	Global Public Health Intelligence Network
HE	hemagglutinin-esterase
IBV	infectious bronchitis virus
ICU	intensive care unit
IFA	immunofluorescence assays
ILO	International Labour Organisation
IMP	index of myocardial performance
M	membrane
MR	magnetic resonance
N	nucleocapsid
NT	neutralization tests
ORF	open reading frame
PCR	polymerase chain reaction
PEDV	porcine epidemic diarrhoea virus
PRCV	porcine respiratory coronavirus
RT-PCR	reverse transcriptase-polymerase chain reaction
SARS	severe acute respiratory syndrome
SARS-CoV	severe acute respiratory syndrome coronavirus
S	spike

TGEV	transmissible gastroenteritis virus
WB	Western blot
WHO	World Health Organization

INDEX

Easter in the Philippines 115
Ebola outbreak in Congo 51
EIA *see* Enzyme immunoassays
Electronic communications 52
Electronic tracing 91
Elevator lobby fans 147
ELISA *see* Enzyme linked
    immunosorbent assay
EM, Ms 9, 101, 102, 104, 118, 119,
    145, 146
EMH, Ms 145
Eng-kiong, Dr Yeoh 90, 92, 155, 157
Enteric animal coronaviruses 199–200
Enterocytes 212
Environmental aspects 39, 147–8,
    158–61
Enzyme immunoassays (EIA) 218–20
Enzyme linked immunosorbent assay
    (ELISA) 27–8, 219
Epidemic curves 87, 97, 103, 112, 156,
    187, 291–2
Epidemiology 49, 74–5, 185–93, 225,
    292
Epidemiology Surveillance Units (ESUs)
    (NEC, Philippines) 117
Escherichia coli 104
ESUs *see* Epidemiology Surveillance
    Units
Evacuation 155, 158
Evans, Dr Merion 78
Events chronology 3–47
Evolution of SARS-CoV 230
Exit screening 23, 69, 153
Expert recruitment 62–3

Faeces 159, 211, 220–1
Families A/B/C (Mongolia) 123
Family doctors, Toronto 129
Fans 147, 159
Feldmann, Dr Heinz 159
Field Epidemiology Training Programme
    62, 117
Filipino overseas workers 120–1
Finkelstein, Dr Sandy 128–30
Flick, Dr Ramon 159
Flight attendants 152, 153
Flight passengers 23, 97–8, 151
Flights 50, 69, 97–8, 125
    AF171 98, 153, 154
    CA112 16, 22, 24, 88, 122, 149–54
    CA115 150
    CZ355 152
    SQ25 15–16, 59, 153
    TG614 27, 152, 154

Flushing of toilets 159–60
Food trade 34, 41, 225–6, 227, 251
Fukuda, Dr Keiji 57
Funding 64, 125
Future aspects 243–54

Genetic aspects 30, 211, 213, 230
Genome sequence 211
Geylang Serai market (Singapore) 165
Giesecke, Dr Kajsa 80
Global alerts 13, 53, 54, 58–9, 169,
    257–8
Global collaboration 49–54, 185–7,
    247–9
Global Outbreak Alert and Response
    Network (GOARN) 11, 52, 62, 113,
    187
Global Public Health Intelligence
    Network (GPHIN) 5, 51, 53, 250
Glycosylated S protein 212
GOARN *see* Global Outbreak Alert and
    Response Network
Good laboratory practice 236
Good manufacturing practice 232
Government activities 91, 106, 124–5,
    164, 165, 247–8
GPHIN *see* Global Public Health
    Intelligence Network
Grace division (Scarborough Hospital,
    Canada) 126–32
Grolla, Allen 159
Guangdong Province (China)
    animal markets 225
    avian influenza A(H5N1) 74, 75
    Chlamydia 210
    LJL, Prof 141
    LTC, Mr 155
    SARS outbreak 3–9
    WHO experts 77–9
Guangzhou (China) 75, 78, 81, 135–6,
    141
Guidelines 54, 69, 234, 235, 236–8

Haematological manifestations 180
Hanoi-French Hospital (Viet Nam) 94–6,
    167–9
Health-care workers *see* Hospital staff
Hepatic manifestations 179–80
Heroism 96, 98, 100, 129–30, 167–71
Heymann, Dr David L. 50, 92, 284
'High transmission' 262–4
Hindsight 243–54
HIV/AIDS 50, 132